*The ultimate guide to heart health*

# MAYO CLINIC

# HEART BOOK

## Second Edition

Bernard J. Gersh, M.D.
Editor in Chief

**William Morrow**
*An Imprint of* HarperCollins*Publishers*

Layout and production by Craig R. King/Rudolph King Studios

Stock photography for lifestyle photos from Corel Corporation, PhotoDisc, and Stockbyte

Library of Congress Cataloging-in-Publication Data

The Mayo Clinic heart book / Bernard J. Gersh, editor in chief.—2nd ed.
    p. cm.
  "Completely revised and updated."
  Includes bibliographical references and index.
  ISBN 0-688-17642-9
   1. Heart—Diseases—Popular works.  2. Cardiology—Popular works. I. Gersh, Bernard J.

RC672 .M4 2000
616.1'2—dc21

99-053785

Printed in the United States of America

Second Edition

1 2 3 4 5 6 7 8 9 10

www.williammorrow.com
www.mayohealth.org

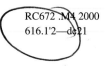

# Foreword

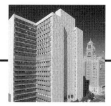
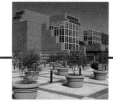
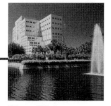

*Mayo Clinic*
*Rochester, Minnesota*

*Mayo Clinic*
*Scottsdale, Arizona*

*Mayo Clinic*
*Jacksonville, Florida*

Skilled and compassionate care of individual patients—that's what the Mayo Clinic story has been about for the past 100 years. And that's what continues to bring more than 400,000 people to Mayo Clinic annually for health care. Through the years we've served over 5,000,000 people in our primary facilities in Rochester, Minnesota; Scottsdale, Arizona; and Jacksonville, Florida. In addition, our Mayo Health System is a network of community-based health care providers who offer high-quality care close to home.

Mayo Clinic's success depends, in part, on its unique approach to medical practice. It is organized to enable physicians and other specialists to spend their time directly helping patients without worrying about scheduling appointments, locating records or X-rays, or handling an ever-expanding load of administrative details. It also promotes the concept of teamwork, so that many experts, in collaboration, can focus on the unique needs of individual patients. Our primary value is a simple statement: "The needs of the patient come first."

The quality of the Mayo style of health care hinges on the people we employ and the cooperation that characterizes their efforts. Extensive programs in medical education and medical research enrich the clinical care Mayo Clinic offers. Our physicians and scientists are continuously developing new and improved treatments and prevention strategies.

Health education is integrated with health care delivery at Mayo Clinic. In 1932, one of our founders, Dr. Charles H. Mayo, said, "The object of all health education is to change the conduct of individual men, women and children by teaching them to care for their bodies well." Dr. Mayo understood the importance of open, effective communication between patient and physician. He valued reliable, practical, easy-to-understand health information. He knew that people need authoritative information if they are to make well-informed health care choices.

The twenty-first century is heralding a new era in health care delivery. Choices are vast in today's managed care atmosphere. Individual responsibility is emphasized as never before.

Gone are the days of passive patients who knew only what their doctors told them. Knowledgeable health care consumers want, and need, facts upon which they can rely in building an effective partnership with their health care providers. That's why we prepared this expanded edition of our classic guide to heart health. Our first edition was published in 1993. This new edition has been extensively reviewed and updated by members of our Division of Cardiovascular Diseases and Internal Medicine and by other Mayo Clinic specialists.

On behalf of the 32,000 health professional, administrative and support personnel who make up our extended family of health care providers, thank you for selecting *Mayo Clinic Heart Book*. Between its covers you'll find everything you need to know about heart health.

**Michael B. Wood, M.D.**
President and Chief Executive Officer
Mayo Foundation

## Editorial staff

**Editor in chief**
Bernard J. Gersh, M.D.

**Editorial director**
Sara C. Gilliland

**Managing editor**
David E. Swanson

**Copyeditor**
Edith Schwager

**Contributing writers**
Linda Kephart Flynn
Michael J. Flynn

Lynn Madsen
Christina Verni

**Creative director**
Daniel W. Brevick

**Graphic design**
Garry J. Post
Kathryn K. Shepel
Karen E. Barrie
Craig R. King
Brian S. Fyffe

**Medical illustration**
John V. Hagen
Michael A. King
Stephen P. Graepel

**Photography**
Joseph M. Kane
Randy J. Ziegler

**Editorial assistant**
Penny Marshall

**Indexer**
Larry Harrison

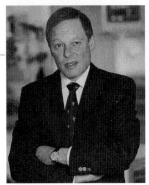

*Bernard J. Gersh, M.D.*

## Preface and acknowledgments

Why a book on heart disease? Consider these statistics from the American Heart Association:

- Since 1900, cardiovascular disease (CVD) has been the number one killer in the United States in every year but one (1918).

- Every day, more than 2,600 Americans die of cardiovascular disease. That's an average of 1 death every 33 seconds.

- Cardiovascular disease is the number one killer of women as well as men. Since 1984, CVD claimed the lives of more women than men, and the gap continues to widen.

- CVD kills more people each year than the next 7 leading causes of death combined.

- 58,000,000 Americans have one or more types of CVD. One in 3 men will deal with it personally before age 60.

Statistics, of course, offer an incomplete view of the impact of heart and blood vessel disease in our country. As a practicing cardiologist, I see it from a different perspective. I'm constantly reminded of the devastating effects of heart disease upon the lives of patients and their families.

Our purpose in preparing the first edition of this book 7 years ago was twofold:

**1.** To help people avoid CVD, and

**2.** To help those with the condition deal with it effectively, in partnership with their health care providers.

Our goals for this new edition are the same, but the medical world in which we live has changed. Advances are occurring more rapidly than ever before in all medical specialties, but especially in cardiology. We're beginning to understand the causes of CVD at the cellular, molecular and genetic levels, which no doubt will lead to a revolution in the prevention, diagnosis and treatment of CVD in the early part of the new millennium.

Moreover, we are living in the Information Age. Never before has so much health information been so readily available to so many people. The vast amount of information offered by an estimated 15,000 to 20,000 health-oriented Web sites is literally at your fingertips, instantly brought to your computer screen. Added to this are numerous health newsletters and the health sections of bookstores, which are filled with new titles. Some, but not all, of this information is reliable. Shop carefully. Consider the source as you travel the health information highway.

You can trust the information in the book you're holding. It provides a framework of the knowledge you need to enable you to make the most of the multiple resources available on cardiovascular health. Within these pages you'll find authoritative, easy-to-understand, basic information on the anatomy, physiology and pathology of cardiovascular disease and on its prevention, treatment and rehabilitation.

To bring you this latest information, the first-edition text underwent a complete review by Mayo Clinic cardiologists and others whose names are listed on this and the succeeding page. You'll find the most up-to-date information on causes, prevention, diagnosis and treatment. There's a completely new and expanded section on nutrition, because good nutrition and adequate exercise are essential to heart health.

You'll enjoy the new Healthy Heart Tip sidebars sprinkled throughout this edition. They're brief and easy to read. They offer practical self-help information—facts you can apply in daily living. Medical illustrations have been added and enhanced. We redesigned the book to make it more inviting to pick up and read.

Much of the information in this book is what Mayo Clinic doctors and other health care professionals use day in and day out in caring for their own patients.

If you put this information to work in your daily life, you'll live more comfortably and productively. You'll be able to communicate more effectively with your health care providers. You'll make better informed health care decisions.

Special thanks to the following for their special assistance:

- Dr. A. Jamil Tajik, chair of the Division of Cardiovascular Diseases and Internal Medicine at Mayo Clinic, Rochester, for his strong support and personal interest in this book.

- To my predecessor, Dr. Michael D. McGoon, for his enormous effort as editor in chief of the first edition, which provided a solid framework for this new book. And to Sara C. Gilliland, managing editor of the first edition.

- Drs. John W. Joyce and John A. Callahan for carefully reviewing each page of text.

- John V. Hagen, our lead medical illustrator, and assistant illustrators Michael A. King and Stephen P. Graepel, and photographers Joseph M. Kane and Randy J. Ziegler.

- Jennifer K. Nelson, Kristine A. Kuhnert and Dr. Donald D. Hensrud for their coordination of our expanded, new section on nutrition.

- Garry J. Post, Kathryn K. Shepel, Karen E. Barrie and Brian S. Fyffe for page design.

- Daniel W. Brevick for cover design and production.

- Craig R. King for page layout and production.

- Edith Schwager, for copyediting and proofreading.

- Penny Marshall for outstanding work as our editorial assistant.

- Toni Sciarra and her colleagues at William Morrow, our esteemed publisher, and the staff of Quebecor, our printer.

- Arthur M. Klebanoff, president, Scott Meredith Literary Agency, our literary agent.

In addition to these people, I would like to acknowledge the invaluable contributions of physicians and allied health professionals within the Division of Cardiovascular Diseases and Internal Medicine at Mayo Clinic, Rochester, and elsewhere in the Mayo Clinic Health System.

Here are their names:

| | | | |
|---|---|---|---|
| Tammy F. Adams, R.N. | William K. Freeman, M.D. | Verghese Mathew, M.D. | Charanjit S. Rihal, M.D. |
| Thomas Allison, M.D. | Paul A. Friedman, M.D. | Robert D. McBane, M.D. | Richard J. Rodeheffer, M.D. |
| Naser M. Ammash, M.D. | Robert L. Frye, M.D. | Robert B. McCully, M.D. | Veronique L. Roger, M.D. |
| William T. Bardsley, M.D. | Kirk N. Garratt, M.D. | Christopher G. A. McGregor, M.D. | Thom W. Rooke, M.D. |
| Gregory W. Barsness, M.D. | Gerald T. Gau, M.D. | Ann M. McLaughlin, R.N. | Maurice E. Sarano, M.D. |
| Thomas Behrenbeck, M.D. | Raymond J. Gibbons, M.D. | Michael A. Mikhail, M.D. | Hartzell V. Schaff, M.D. |
| Malcolm R. Bell, M.D. | Saima T. Goraya, M.D. | Fletcher A. Miller, M.D. | Alexander Schirger, M.D. |
| Marek Belohlavek, M.D. | Suellen K. Grice, R.N. | Todd D. Miller, M.D. | Kathy Schwab, R.N. |
| Peter B. Berger, M.D. | Martha Grogan, M.D. | Wayne L. Miller, M.D. | Gary L. Schwartz, M.D. |
| Johannes Bjornsson, M.D. | George M. Gura, M.D. | Michael B. Mock, M.D. | Robert S. Schwartz, M.D. |
| Daniel D. Borgeson, M.D. | Donald J. Hagler, M.D. | Nancy A. Moltaji | James B. Seward, M.D. |
| Jerome F. Breen, M.D. | Stephen C. Hammill, M.D. | Brian P. Mullan, M.D. | Win-Kuang Shen, M.D. |
| John F. Bresnahan, M.D. | David L. Hayes, M.D. | Charles J. Mullany, M.D. | Roger F. J. Shepherd, M.D. |
| John C. Burnett, Jr., M.D. | Sharonne N. Hayes, M.D. | Sharon L. Mulvagh, M.D. | Sheldon G. Sheps, M.D. |
| Mark J. Callahan, M.D. | John A. Heit, M.D. | Thomas M. Munger, M.D. | Clarence Shub, M.D. |
| Noel Caplice, M.D. | J. Richard Hickman, Jr., M.D. | Joseph G. Murphy, M.D. | Robert D. Simari, M.D. |
| Timothy F. Christian, M.D. | Stuart T. Higano, M.D. | Susan M. Nelson, L.P.N. | Lawrence J. Sinak, M.D. |
| Alfredo L. Clavell, M.D. | David R. Holmes, Jr., M.D. | Rick A. Nishimura, M.D. | Peter A. Smars, M.D. |
| Ian P. Clements, M.D. | Richard D. Hurt, M.D. | M. Kevin O'Connor, M.D. | Hugh C. Smith, M.D. |
| Roger L. Click, M.D., Ph.D. | Arshad Jahangir, M.D. | Jae K. Oh, M.D. | John A. Spittell, Jr., M.D. |
| Heidi M. Connolly, M.D. | Bruce D. Johnson, M.D., Ph.D. | Patrick W. O'Leary, M.D. | Peter C. Spittell, M.D. |
| Leslie T. Cooper, M.D. | Donald L. Johnston, M.D. | Byron A. Olney, M.D. | Ray W. Squires, Ph.D. |
| Mark G. Costopoulos, M.D. | Paul R. Julsrud, M.D. | Carol A. Olson | Randal J. Thomas, M.D. |
| Jack T. Cusma, Ph.D. | Barry L. Karon, M.D. | Lyle J. Olson, M.D. | R. Tom Tilbury, M.D. |
| Richard C. Daly, M.D. | Bijoy K. Khandheria, M.D. | Timothy M. Olson, M.D. | Teresa S. M. Tsang, M.D. |
| Ann E. Decker, J.D. | Kyle W. Klarich, M.D. | Steve R. Ommen, M.D. | Roger A. Warndahl, R.Ph. |
| David J. Driscoll, M.D. | Stephen L. Kopecky, M.D. | Thomas A. Orszulak, M.D. | Carole A. Warnes, M.D. |
| Brooks S. Edwards, M.D. | Thomas E. Kottke, M.D. | Michael J. Osborn, M.D. | Arnold M. Weissler, M.D. |
| William D. Edwards, M.D. | Iftikhar J. Kullo, M.D. | Douglas L. Packer, M.D. | Roger D. White, M.D. |
| Raul Espinosa, M.D. | Margo E. Kroshus, R.N. | Patricia A. Pellikka, M.D. | Douglas L. Wood, M.D. |
| Leo Evans, R.Ph. | Andre C. Lapeyre III, M.D. | Mary Jane Rasmussen, R.N. | Alan J. Wright, M.D. |
| Titus C. Evans, Jr., M.D. | Amir Lerman, M.D. | Robert F. Rea, M.D. | R. Scott Wright, M.D. |
| David A. Foley, M.D. | Margaret A. Lloyd, M.D. | Margaret M. Redfield, M.D. | Kathleen Zarling, R.N. |
| Robert P. Frantz, M.D. | Douglas D. Mair, M.D. | Guy S. Reeder, M.D. | Kenton J. Zehr, M.D. |

To one and all, as well as to those who contributed to the first edition of this book, my gratitude and sincere thanks for a task exceptionally well done.

**Bernard J. Gersh, M. D.**
Editor in Chief

# Contents

## Part 1  Your heart and blood vessels                                2

*The strength, rhythm and speed of your heart's pumping action to a large extent determine your health. This part describes how the normal heart and circulation perform night and day, year in and year out—with precision and efficiency.*

Chapter

## Part 2  What is heart disease?                                       24

*Heart disease takes many forms and varies widely in severity. Some people are born with it. More often it develops later in life. Most people detect warning signs or symptoms, but heart disease can strike without the slightest warning.*

## Part 3  Dealing with the risks of coronary artery disease     136

*You may not want to live forever, but you would certainly like to be healthy for as long as you can. Since your lifestyle affects your health, developing good habits and avoiding harmful ones can positively influence not only the length but also the quality of your life.*

## Part 4  Diagnosing heart disease                                220

*Fortunately, most tests—even those with high-tech names—aren't difficult to under-stand. A little detective work of your own about heart disease tests will boost your confidence and comfort levels.*

## Part 5  Treating heart disease                                   282

*Appropriate heart disease management entails selecting therapy that provides the best results for your particular medical problem while keeping risk, inconvenience and expense to a minimum.*

*The ultimate guide to heart health*

# MAYO CLINIC

---

# HEART BOOK

---

Second Edition

# Part 1

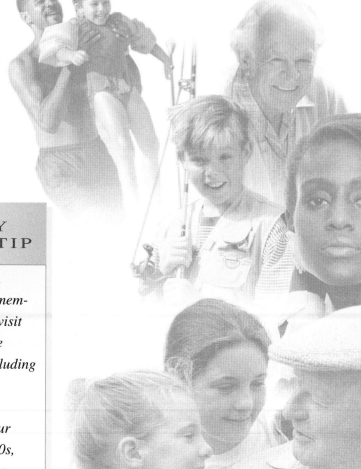

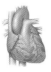

## HEALTHY HEART ♥ TIP

*As long as you're healthy, there's an easy way to remember how often a doctor's visit should include a complete physical examination, including heart screening: Plan on having a comprehensive medical exam twice in your 20s, three times in your 30s, four times in your 40s, five times in your 50s and every year if you're 60 or older.*

# Your heart and blood vessels

Although every tissue in your body depends on your heart, you may take for granted the faithful beating that literally keeps you alive from the moment of your birth until the day you die. How does this simple pump perform such an amazing task? As you gain a better understanding of your heart, you may also develop a sense of wonder at its elegant design.

The strength, rhythm, and speed of your heart's pumping action to a large extent determine your health. This part describes how the normal heart and circulation perform nonstop, night and day, year in and year out—with precision and efficiency.

## Chapter

# Chapter

# 1

# Heart muscle (myocardium)

Your heart, a muscular structure about the size of your fist, and a 60,000-mile network of blood vessels make up your cardiovascular system. Your heart is the focal point because it performs the main function of your cardiovascular system: pumping blood to all tissues of your body.

The muscle responsible for pumping the blood is called the myocardium (*myo* means "muscle," *cardia* means "heart"). Although the myocardium is the driving force of the circulation, it could not function as a pump without other components that combine with it to make up your cardiovascular system: the valves, the coronary vessels, the conduction (electrical) system, the arteries and veins throughout your body, and the pericardium (the sac around your heart).

Your heart is located slightly to the left of the center of your chest. It is protected by your breastbone (sternum) in front, your spinal column in back, and your lungs (see page A1).

The right side of your heart projects toward the front of your chest; the left side is toward your back. In the adult, the heart weighs about 3/4 pound.

Your heart has four chambers. Two atria on top are receiving chambers for blood returning from veins. Two ventricles underneath pump blood into your arteries.

The two sides of your heart are functionally linked in a figure-8 loop connected by arteries and veins of your lungs and the rest of your body (see page A2).

## What does it look like?

Your heart is shaped like a cone, with the point (apex) at the bottom and the broader part at the top. The apex of your heart is the tip of the ventricles. It points down to the left side of your chest. The wide upper part of your heart includes the right and left atria and the origins of the major blood vessels.

Your heart has three layers of tissue: the myocardium, the epicardium and the endocardium (see page A4). The myocardium is the thick main layer of heart muscle, made up predominantly of cells called myocytes. Its outside surface is covered by a thin, glossy membrane called the epicardium. Another smooth, glossy membrane, the endocardium, covers the inside surfaces of your heart's four chambers, the valves, and the muscles that attach to those valves.

## Role of muscle cells (myocytes)

Your heart muscle (myocardium) is made up of individual muscle cells called myocytes. These myocytes act together to contract and relax your heart's chambers in precisely the correct sequence to pump blood to your lungs and to the rest of your body.

Although these microscopic cells are individual units, they work together as a team to pump blood. This remarkable coordination is possible because of the way cells are arranged and because electrical messages pass easily between cells.

When muscle fibers within the cells relax, the cells lengthen and the heart muscle relaxes. The relaxation makes the pumping chambers expand. When the chambers expand, blood flows back into them. When the fibers contract, cells shorten. Shortening of the cells contracts your heart muscle. The pumping chambers become smaller and blood is pumped out.

## How your heart pumps

Your heart functions by squeezing blood out of its chambers (contraction) and then expanding to allow blood in (relaxation). The action is like squeezing water out of a soft plastic bottle while holding it under water, and then releasing your grasp so that water is sucked back into the bottle.

This cycle of contraction and relaxation causes blood flow to be "pulsatile." You can often feel your heart beat by touching your chest. The pulse of blood flow is also transmitted to your blood vessels, so you can feel your pulse at places where large arteries are close to the surface of your body, such as your wrist, neck and groin (see pages A2, A4).

*Apex*

*Your heart is cone-shaped, with the tip (apex) pointing down and to the left.*

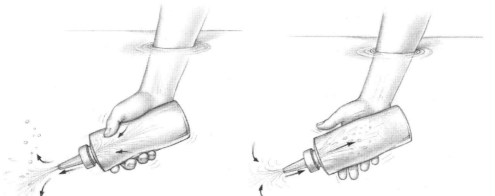

*Your heart's pumping action is similar to what happens when water is squirted out of a plastic bottle under water. Squeeze the bottle and water is forced out. Release your grip and the bottle refills.*

## Double pump

Your heart functions as two adjacent pumps, each with a receiving room (atria) and a pumping room (ventricles). The pumps beat simultaneously, and in a two-phase cycle. First, the atria contract and fill the relaxed ventricles with blood. Then the ventricles discharge their blood as the atria relax and refill.

The "right heart" pumps blood through your lungs, where it receives oxygen and rids itself of carbon dioxide. The "left heart" receives oxygenated blood from the lungs and pumps it through the body, where it gives oxygen to the cells and picks up carbon dioxide, a waste product. Blood that returns from the tissues of your body to the right heart chambers must circulate through your lungs before it can enter the left chambers.

Circulating blood performs many other transportation functions, such as distributing nutrients and hormones and carrying other waste products to elimination sites. Blood does not pass directly between the right and left sides if you have a healthy heart. The two atria are separated by a wall called the atrial septum. The two ventricles are separated by the ventricular septum.

The amount of blood that enters and leaves the left heart chambers is exactly the same amount as passes through the right heart. Thus, any increase or decrease in blood flow to the right heart will cause a similar change in the amount of blood pumped to your body by the left heart. Despite this similarity, the anatomy and functions of the right and left sides of your heart are different in many ways.

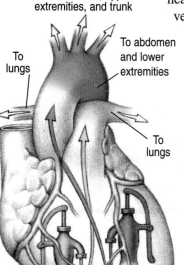

To head, neck, upper extremities, and trunk

To abdomen and lower extremities

To lungs

To lungs

*Your heart receives blood from your veins, pumps it to your lungs, receives blood from your lungs and distributes it through arteries to your body.*

## Right side of the heart

The right side of your heart is responsible for pumping blood to your lungs (the pulmonary circulation).

Used blood from your body returns to the right side of your heart through two large veins: the superior vena cava (from your head and arms) and the inferior vena cava (from your legs and abdomen). At this point your blood is a dark bluish-red because it has delivered oxygen to your body and its oxygen content is depleted (deoxygenated). The right side of your heart pumps this deoxygenated blood to your lungs, where it releases carbon dioxide and picks up oxygen. The carbon dioxide is expelled into the air as you breathe.

Lower pressure is required to push blood through the lungs. Therefore, the right side of your heart is less muscular and less powerful than the left side. Still, efficient performance of your right heart is important in ensuring optimal function of your whole cardiovascular system (see pages A2, A4).

## Left side of the heart

When the hemoglobin in your red blood cells picks up oxygen in your lungs, your blood becomes bright red. This oxygen-rich blood travels from your lungs to the left side of your heart. The left side of your heart is responsible for pumping oxygen-rich blood to the tissues and organs of your body.

While blood circulates throughout your body, substances other than oxygen and carbon dioxide are also transported from site to site. Your blood carries hormones from glands to their sites of activity. Waste products other than carbon dioxide go to your kidneys and liver, where they can be removed or broken down. Your blood picks up nutrients from your intestines and carries them to your liver and other locations in your body.

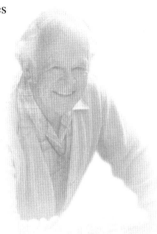

It requires more pressure to circulate blood throughout the entire body than to circulate blood through the lungs. The left heart is therefore more muscular and generates more pressure than the right heart. When you have your blood pressure checked, it is a measurement of the pressure in blood vessels throughout your body (see page 226). Your left heart must have enough strength to push blood forward under higher pressure. The left side of your heart is stronger than the right side.

## Atria

The atria are the small receiving chambers for blood returning from the body (right atrium) or from the lungs (left atrium) (see page A1). Although the atria contract, their contraction is rather weak and serves mainly to push blood into the ventricles.

Your heart could pump sufficient blood throughout your body even if the atria didn't contract at all. But the beating of the atria contributes to the overall efficiency of your heart and allows it to pump more blood with less effort. This added efficiency is particularly important if disease damages the ventricles.

Each atrium is about the size of a golf ball, or slightly larger. The walls of the right atrium are less than 1/8 inch thick. The walls of the left atrium are thicker and more powerful, but its volume is about the same.

## Ventricles

Your heart's ventricles are the main pumping chambers, propelling blood to your lungs and body. Your right ventricle sends blood to your lungs. Your left ventricle sends blood to your body.

Each ventricle holds about 1/8 cup of blood after your heart contracts and about 1/2 cup once your heart refills.

The walls of your right ventricle are 1/4 inch thick. The walls of the left ventricle are three times thicker. The left ventricle is by far the most powerful chamber in your heart. This chamber must generate enough pressure to drive blood to every region of your body.

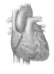

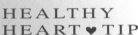
HEALTHY
HEART ♥ TIP

*Even though Americans have more low-fat food choices than ever, it's estimated that about half of the U.S. population has a total blood cholesterol count of more than 200 mg/dL. Of that group, 80 percent are classified as borderline-high risk, with readings between 200 and 240 mg/dL. About 20 percent have total blood cholesterol of more than 240 mg/dL, which is considered undesirable.*

## The cardiac cycle

The period from the beginning of one heartbeat to the beginning of the next is called the cardiac cycle. The cardiac cycle consists of a period of contraction (systole, SIS-toe-lee) followed by a period of relaxation (diastole, die-ASS-toe-lee) (see page A4).

Blood is pumped out of your heart during systole. During diastole, your heart relaxes and refills. During systole your heart pumps (squeezes). During diastole it relaxes (dilates).

Your heart must fully relax before it can pump again. This allows it to refill with blood. At 70 beats a minute, the cardiac cycle lasts about 8/10 second.

If you are a healthy, resting adult, your heart will beat about 60 times every minute, more than 86,000 times each day, and over 2 billion times in an average lifetime. Your heart will pump 3 ounces of blood with each beat. That amounts to 5.5 quarts every minute and over 2,000 gallons daily. An 18-foot-diameter swimming pool holds about 6,500 gallons—your heart could fill the pool in a little more than 3 days. And during strenuous exercise, your heart may have to pump four to seven times the amount of blood it pumps at rest.

## The heart's work

No matter how forceful the contraction, your heart does not pump all the blood out of both ventricles with each beat. Doctors call the portion of blood that is pumped out of a filled ventricle the "ejection fraction."

A normal ejection fraction is 50 percent or more. So at least half the blood in the ventricle is pumped out on each beat. The ejection fraction is a good indicator of the overall function of your heart. In a healthy person, the ejection fraction of the heart might increase by about 5 percent with exercise. It can diminish to 20 to 30 percent or lower if the ventricles are not functioning normally.

*During diastole (**left**), your heart relaxes and expands, allowing blood to flow into the pumping chambers (ventricles) from the upper holding chambers (atria). During systole (**right**), the powerful ventricles contract, pumping blood out of the chambers. The blood from the right ventricle is sent to your lungs. The blood from your left ventricle is sent to the rest of your body.*

Diastole

Systole

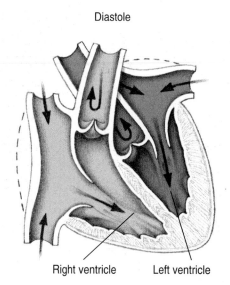
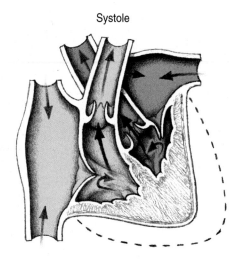

Right ventricle    Left ventricle

# The heart

Your heart is a muscular pump the size of your fist. Located to the left of the center of your chest between your lungs, its lower tip (apex) points toward the left.

Your heart pumps blood into your arteries (**bottom right**). The major arteries that emerge from the heart are the aorta and the pulmonary arteries. The coronary arteries, which supply the heart muscle itself with nourishing blood, branch off directly from the aorta.

Veins return blood to your heart. The large veins that enter the heart are the superior vena cava, the inferior vena cava, and the pulmonary veins.

Vessels carrying oxygen-rich blood are shown in red, while vessels containing blood with low oxygen levels are shown in blue.

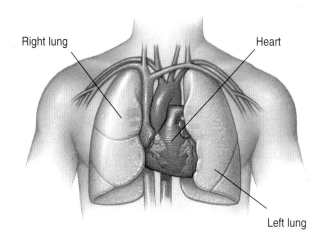

Right lung | Heart | Left lung

## Chambers and valves

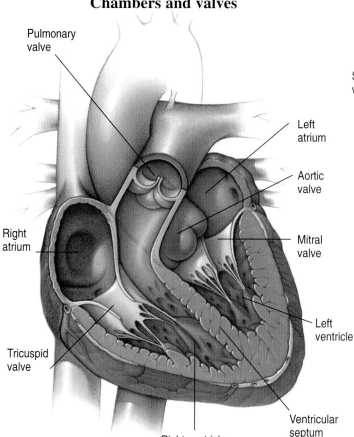

Pulmonary valve
Left atrium
Aortic valve
Right atrium
Mitral valve
Tricuspid valve
Left ventricle
Right ventricle
Ventricular septum

## Major arteries and veins

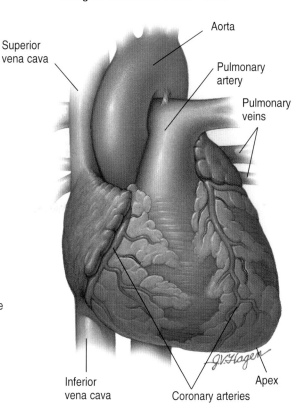

Aorta
Superior vena cava
Pulmonary artery
Pulmonary veins
Inferior vena cava
Apex
Coronary arteries

Your heart consists of four chambers (**left**). The two atria on top are receiving chambers for blood returning from veins. The two ventricles beneath pump blood into the arteries. Valves allow the blood to move in only one direction. The mitral valve on the left side, and the tricuspid valve on the right side, control the flow of blood from the atria to the ventricles. The aortic valve (between the left ventricle and the aorta) and the pulmonary valve (between the right ventricle and the pulmonary artery) control the flow of blood out of the ventricles.

# The circulation

## Figure-8 circulation

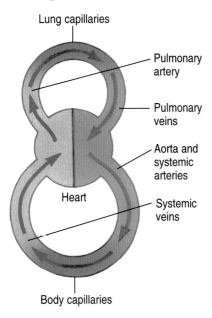

Lung capillaries

Pulmonary artery

Pulmonary veins

Aorta and systemic arteries

Heart

Systemic veins

Body capillaries

Circulating blood carries oxygen and nutrients to your body's organs and carries carbon dioxide and other waste products away from the organs to the sites of their elimination.

At its simplest, the circulation is like a figure-8 (**left**). One loop is the circulation to the lungs, in which blood is pumped through the pulmonary arteries, carbon dioxide is exchanged for oxygen in the capillaries, and the blood returns to your heart through the pulmonary veins. The other loop is the circulation to your body, in which blood is pumped through the arteries, oxygen and nutrients are exchanged for carbon dioxide and waste products in the capillaries, and the blood returns to your heart through your systemic veins.

## The circulatory system

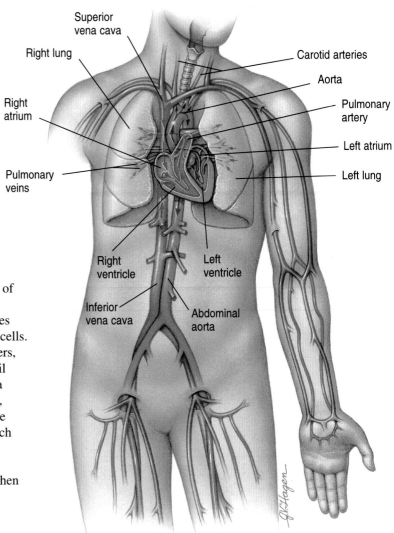

Superior vena cava

Right lung

Right atrium

Pulmonary veins

Right ventricle

Inferior vena cava

Carotid arteries

Aorta

Pulmonary artery

Left atrium

Left lung

Left ventricle

Abdominal aorta

Your circulatory system is quite complicated (**right**). Arteries branch repeatedly, transporting blood to all the cells of every organ. Veins join together, bringing blood back to your heart from every organ. The central focus is your heart: The right-sided chambers receive blood from your body and pump it into the pulmonary arteries. The left-sided chambers receive blood from your lungs and pump it into the aorta and systemic arteries.

Here is how a typical blood cell journeys through your circulatory system: It is pumped out of the left ventricle into the aorta, where it courses through smaller and smaller branches until it passes through a capillary in single file with other blood cells. Then it enters a tiny venule that joins up with others, like tributaries of a river, to form bigger veins until finally the blood cell passes through the vena cava (superior if it is returning from your head or arms, inferior if from your abdomen or legs) and into the right atrium. It passes into the right ventricle, which pumps it into the pulmonary artery. After going through a capillary in the lungs, it enters the pulmonary vein and is carried to the left atrium and then back to its starting point in the left ventricle.

# The capillaries

Arteries branch until they become capillaries, so tiny that only one blood cell can pass through at a time and so numerous that there is a capillary near each cell of your body. The capillary walls are thin enough that nutrients, wastes, and gases pass freely between the blood inside the capillaries and the nearby cells. In tissues of your body, such as your skin or muscles of a finger, oxygen passes from your blood to the cells, and carbon dioxide and other waste products pass into your blood.

In your lungs, carbon dioxide is released from blood in the capillaries into the nearby alveoli (air sacs), and oxygen passes from the air in the alveoli into the blood. This oxygenated blood flows from the capillaries into the pulmonary veins to the left-sided chambers of your heart. Then it is pumped into the arteries to the capillaries of your body. This cycle repeats itself throughout your lifetime.

## Capillaries in the lungs

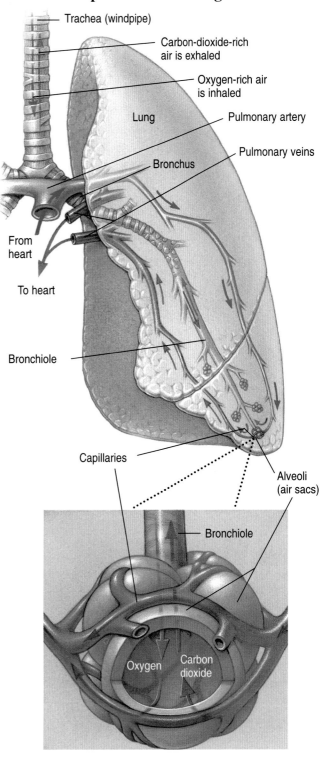

Trachea (windpipe)

Carbon-dioxide-rich air is exhaled

Oxygen-rich air is inhaled

Lung

Pulmonary artery

Pulmonary veins

Bronchus

From heart

To heart

Bronchiole

Capillaries

Alveoli (air sacs)

Bronchiole

Oxygen

Carbon dioxide

*Lung capillaries release carbon dioxide into alveoli in exchange for oxygen.*

## Capillaries in the body

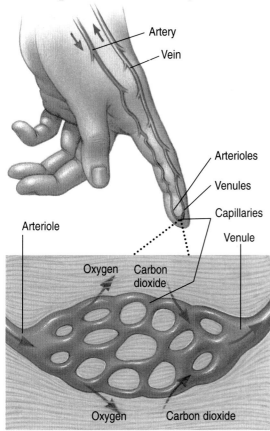

Artery

Vein

Arterioles

Venules

Capillaries

Venule

Arteriole

Oxygen

Carbon dioxide

Oxygen

Carbon dioxide

*In most tissues of your body, capillaries release oxygen and nutrients in exchange for carbon dioxide and waste products.*

# The heart muscle

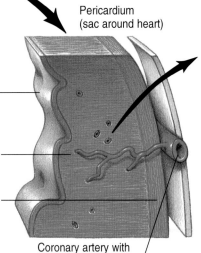

Your heart is a muscular pump that propels blood by squeezing it out of powerful ventricles into your arteries. The muscular wall of your heart has three layers: a thin inner lining (endocardium), the bulk of working muscle (myocardium), and the outer surface (epicardium).

The squeezing action of your heart is produced by coordinated shortening of the muscle fibers that make up the walls of your heart. When the muscles shorten (contract), the ventricular chambers become smaller, forcing blood out. Valves ensure that blood goes out in the right direction. This phase of the heart action is called systole. After contracting, your heart muscle relaxes, the muscle fibers lengthen, the ventricular chambers become more spacious, and blood flows into them from the atria. This phase is diastole.

Pericardium
(sac around heart)

Endocardium
(inner lining)

Heart muscle
(ventricular wall)

Myocardium
(heart muscle)

Epicardium
(outer surface)

Coronary artery with
branch into myocardium

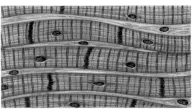
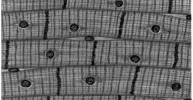

*When microscopic muscle fibers relax, they are long and thin (**top**). When they contract, they become short and thick (**bottom**).*

## MUGA scans

Diastole   Systole

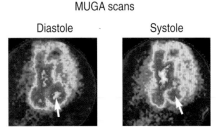

**Normal.** *These multigated acquisition (MUGA) scans show a normal heart. The ventricles (**arrows**) are large during diastole and contracted during systole.*

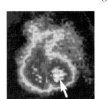

**Dilated.** *Abnormal scans show a weakened heart. It cannot squeeze as hard. Therefore, the size of the ventricles changes very little between diastole and systole (see page 248).*

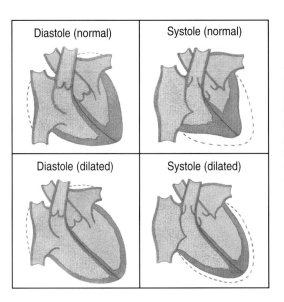

Diastole (normal)   Systole (normal)

Diastole (dilated)   Systole (dilated)

*If your heart muscle weakens, it cannot squeeze as hard. Your heart gradually enlarges (dilates) to compensate for its inability to expel the normal amount of blood.*

# Transplantation

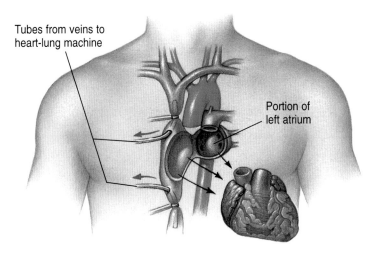

Tubes from veins to heart-lung machine

Portion of left atrium

Transplantation may be the best solution if other surgery or medications do not adequately improve symptoms or when life expectancy is short (see page 301). Your heart is replaced with a normally functioning heart donated by someone who died from a cause unrelated to heart disease.

The ventricles and part of the atria, together with the heart valves and coronary arteries, are transplanted during this operation. After the heart is removed from the donor, it is cooled and stored in special fluid. The time the heart is out of the body must be kept short, generally less than 4 hours.

*Before your weakened heart is removed, tubes must be positioned to take blood from your body and transport it to a cardiopulmonary bypass pump (heart-lung machine). This machine puts oxygen into the blood and then pumps the blood back into an artery (not shown). Because the machine functions as your heart and lungs, the weakened heart can be removed.*

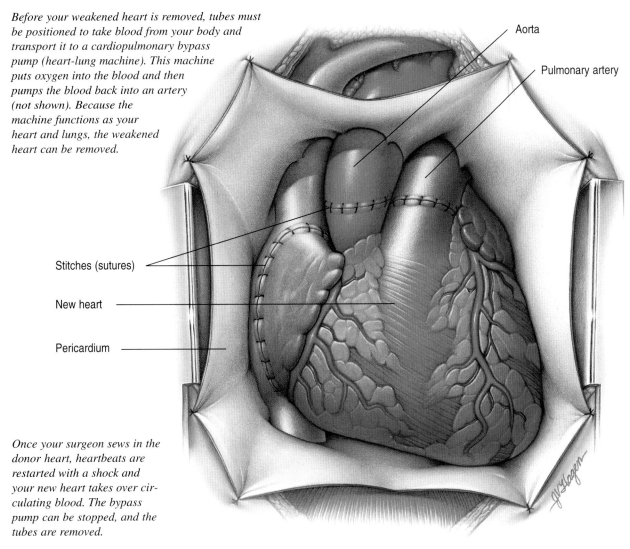

Aorta

Pulmonary artery

Stitches (sutures)

New heart

Pericardium

*Once your surgeon sews in the donor heart, heartbeats are restarted with a shock and your new heart takes over circulating blood. The bypass pump can be stopped, and the tubes are removed.*

# How the valves work

Valves keep blood flowing through your heart in one direction (see page 10). As the ventricles relax (diastole), the pressure within them decreases. The mitral and tricuspid valves are pushed open, allowing blood to flow from the atria to the ventricles. The aortic and pulmonary valves are closed, preventing the return of blood that was pumped out on the preceding beat. During contraction (systole), the pressure pushes the aortic and pulmonary valves open, and the mitral and tricuspid valves are pushed shut to prevent back flow of blood.

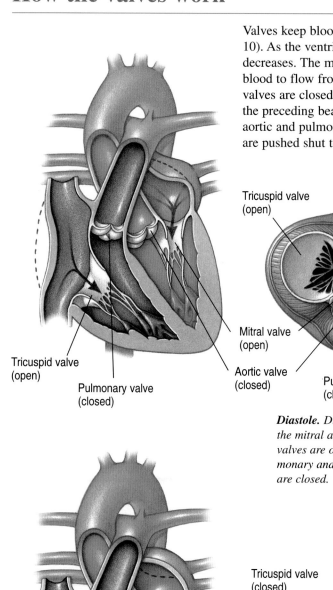

Tricuspid valve
(open)

Pulmonary valve
(closed)

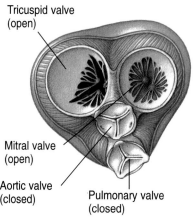

Tricuspid valve
(open)

Mitral valve
(open)

Aortic valve
(closed)

Pulmonary valve
(closed)

**Diastole.** *During diastole, the mitral and tricuspid valves are open; the pulmonary and aortic valves are closed.*

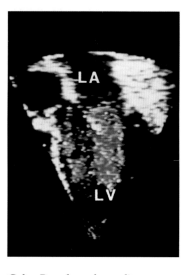

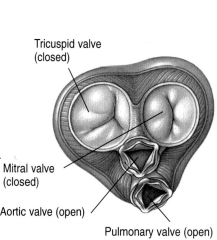

Tricuspid valve
(closed)

Mitral valve
(closed)

Aortic valve (open)

Pulmonary valve (open)

Tricuspid valve
(closed)

Pulmonary valve
(open)

**Systole.** *During systole, the mitral and tricuspid valves are closed; the pulmonary and aortic valves are open.*

*Color Doppler echocardiograms reveal blood flow through the chambers on the left side of the heart. In diastole (**above**) , blood flowing through the mitral valve from the left atrium (LA) to the left ventricle (LV) appears orange. In systole (**below**), blood is ejected through the aortic valve and appears blue (see page 254).*

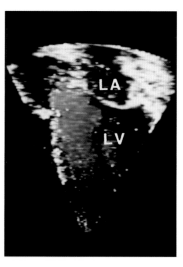

# Diseases of the valves

Diseases of heart valves may cause them to become too narrow, restricting blood flow (valve stenosis). Valves can also become "leaky," allowing blood to flow backward (valve regurgitation).

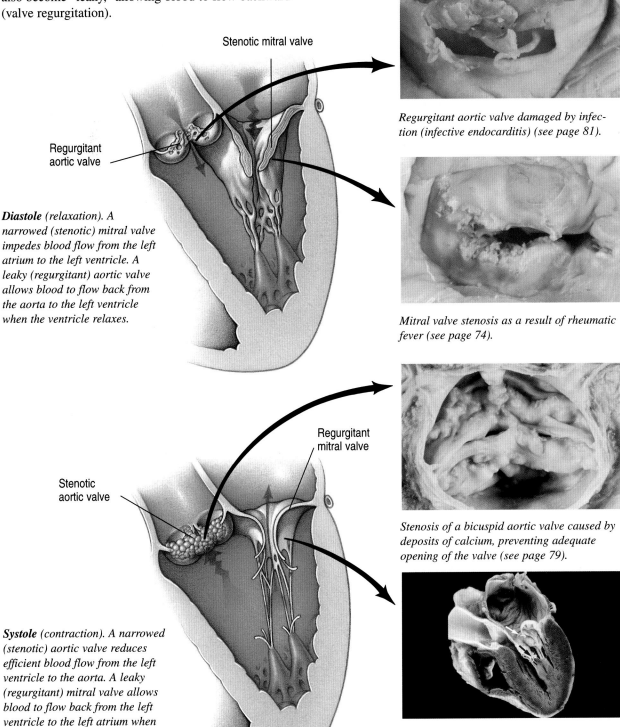

Stenotic mitral valve

Regurgitant aortic valve

*Diastole (relaxation). A narrowed (stenotic) mitral valve impedes blood flow from the left atrium to the left ventricle. A leaky (regurgitant) aortic valve allows blood to flow back from the aorta to the left ventricle when the ventricle relaxes.*

*Regurgitant aortic valve damaged by infection (infective endocarditis) (see page 81).*

*Mitral valve stenosis as a result of rheumatic fever (see page 74).*

Stenotic aortic valve

Regurgitant mitral valve

*Systole (contraction). A narrowed (stenotic) aortic valve reduces efficient blood flow from the left ventricle to the aorta. A leaky (regurgitant) mitral valve allows blood to flow back from the left ventricle to the left atrium when the ventricle contracts.*

*Stenosis of a bicuspid aortic valve caused by deposits of calcium, preventing adequate opening of the valve (see page 79).*

*Regurgitant mitral valve due to breakage (arrows) of the chordae tendineae that tether the valve leaflets (see page 76).*

# Artificial valves

One means of correcting a defective heart valve is for a surgeon to remove it and replace it with an artificial valve. Various artificial (prosthetic) valves are available, each with its own advantages (see page 310).

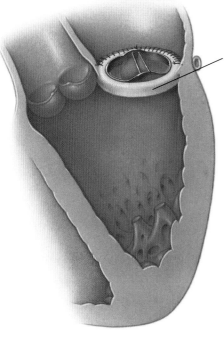

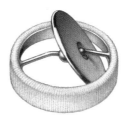

Bileaflet mechanical valve (open)

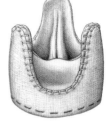

Tilting disc mechanical valve (open)

Stentless porcine tissue valve

*An artificial valve is sewn in by the surgeon after the diseased valve is removed. It is positioned to allow the blood to flow freely in the correct direction and not leak back.*

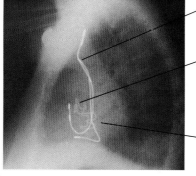

Pacemaker leads

Aortic stented tissue valve

Mitral stented tissue valve

X-ray of two artificial valves (side view)

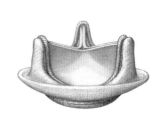

Stented pericardial tissue valve

# Balloon valvuloplasty

Mitral stenosis can often be effectively treated by threading a catheter with an inflatable balloon (**right**) through a vein and across the atrial septum (which is carefully punctured). It is positioned through the tight mitral opening. Then the balloon is inflated, pressing the valve leaflets apart, producing a wider opening (see page 308).

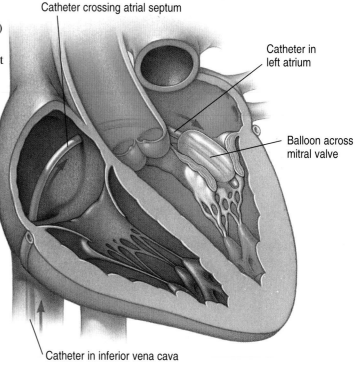

Catheter crossing atrial septum

Catheter in left atrium

Balloon across mitral valve

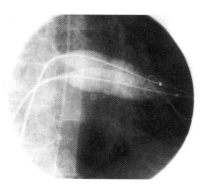

*In this X-ray, two inflated balloons extend across the mitral valve to produce a wider opening. The valve itself is not visible.*

Catheter in inferior vena cava

# Coronary arteries

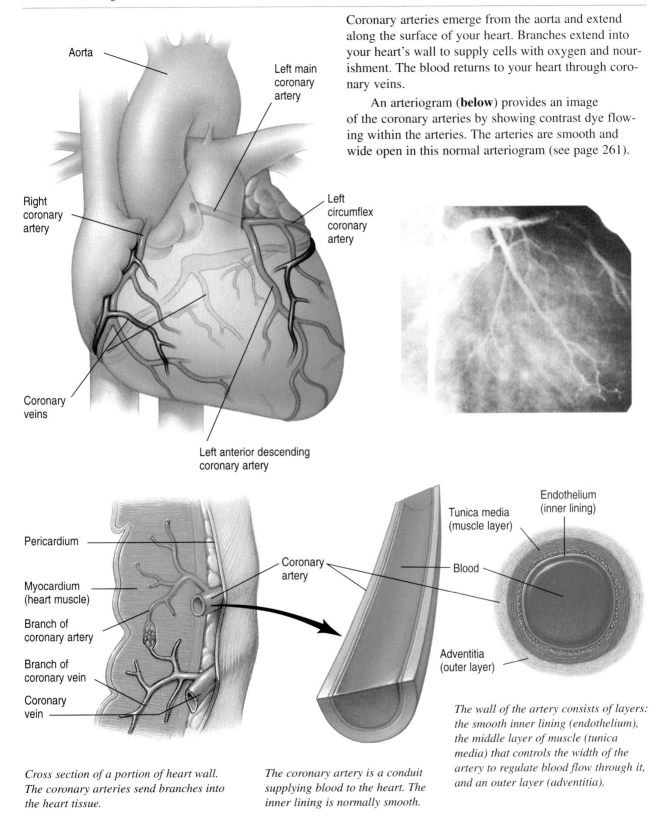

Coronary arteries emerge from the aorta and extend along the surface of your heart. Branches extend into your heart's wall to supply cells with oxygen and nourishment. The blood returns to your heart through coronary veins.

An arteriogram (**below**) provides an image of the coronary arteries by showing contrast dye flowing within the arteries. The arteries are smooth and wide open in this normal arteriogram (see page 261).

Aorta

Left main coronary artery

Right coronary artery

Left circumflex coronary artery

Coronary veins

Left anterior descending coronary artery

Pericardium

Myocardium (heart muscle)

Branch of coronary artery

Branch of coronary vein

Coronary vein

Coronary artery

Endothelium (inner lining)

Tunica media (muscle layer)

Blood

Adventitia (outer layer)

*Cross section of a portion of heart wall. The coronary arteries send branches into the heart tissue.*

*The coronary artery is a conduit supplying blood to the heart. The inner lining is normally smooth.*

*The wall of the artery consists of layers: the smooth inner lining (endothelium), the middle layer of muscle (tunica media) that controls the width of the artery to regulate blood flow through it, and an outer layer (adventitia).*

# Diseased coronary arteries

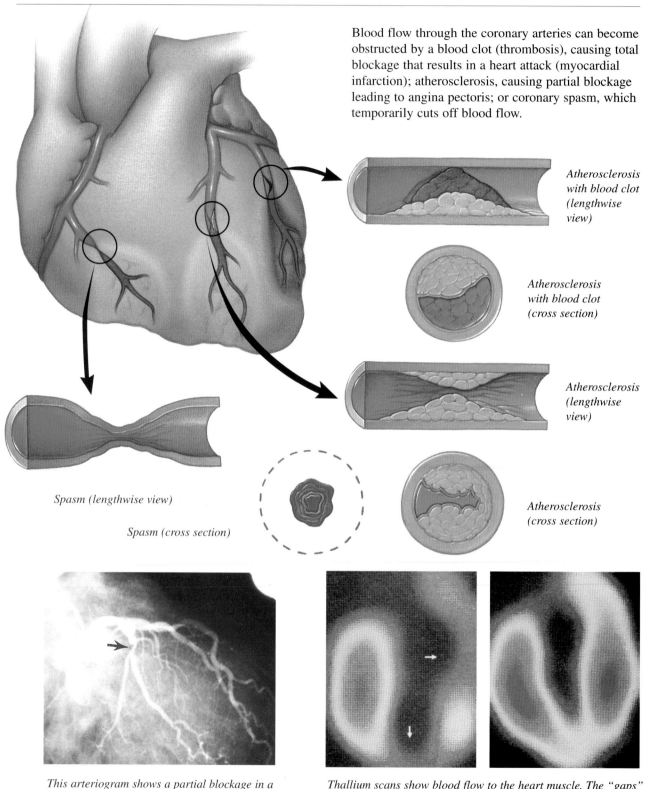

Blood flow through the coronary arteries can become obstructed by a blood clot (thrombosis), causing total blockage that results in a heart attack (myocardial infarction); atherosclerosis, causing partial blockage leading to angina pectoris; or coronary spasm, which temporarily cuts off blood flow.

*Atherosclerosis with blood clot (lengthwise view)*

*Atherosclerosis with blood clot (cross section)*

*Atherosclerosis (lengthwise view)*

*Spasm (lengthwise view)*

*Spasm (cross section)*

*Atherosclerosis (cross section)*

*This arteriogram shows a partial blockage in a coronary artery (**arrow**). Narrowing of the artery restricts the flow of blood to the heart muscle (see page 261).*

*Thallium scans show blood flow to the heart muscle. The "gaps" are areas that do not receive adequate blood flow during stress (**arrows**). During rest (**right**), blood flow is sufficient throughout (see page 249).*

# Restoring blood flow

In some circumstances, coronary blockages can be reduced with specially designed catheters. Various methods and techniques are available (see page 318).

*Coronary angioplasty. Your cardiologist inserts a long, hollow tube (catheter) into a large artery in your groin (**left, arrow**) or arm. The tube is guided to the narrowed coronary artery. Then a thinner, balloon-tipped tube is inserted into the first catheter and directed through the narrowing (**right, A**). The balloon is inflated (**B**), compressing deposits and widening the artery. Doctors also call this procedure balloon angioplasty, or percutaneous transluminal coronary angioplasty (PTCA).*

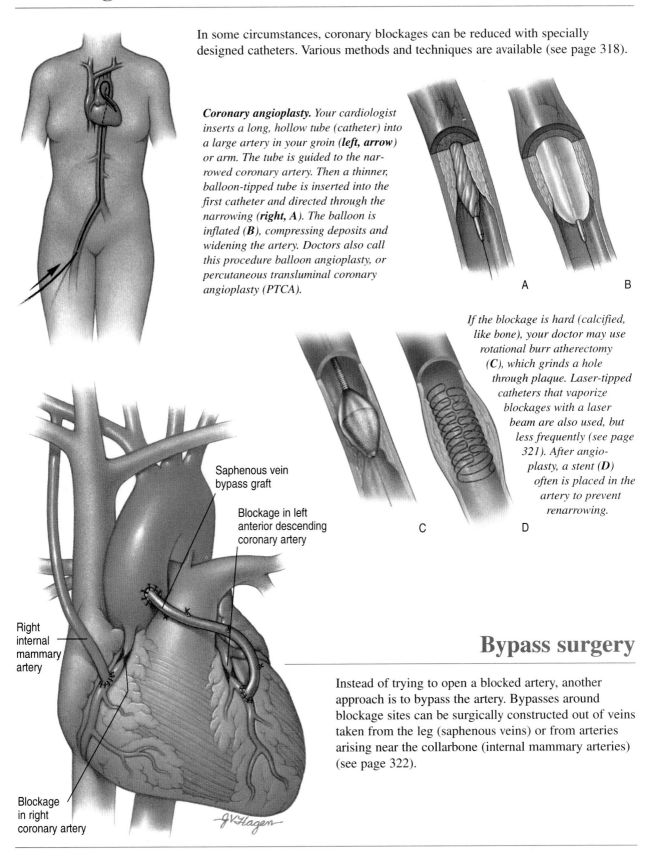

A          B

*If the blockage is hard (calcified, like bone), your doctor may use rotational burr atherectomy (**C**), which grinds a hole through plaque. Laser-tipped catheters that vaporize blockages with a laser beam are also used, but less frequently (see page 321). After angioplasty, a stent (**D**) often is placed in the artery to prevent renarrowing.*

Saphenous vein bypass graft

Blockage in left anterior descending coronary artery

C          D

Right internal mammary artery

Blockage in right coronary artery

# Bypass surgery

Instead of trying to open a blocked artery, another approach is to bypass the artery. Bypasses around blockage sites can be surgically constructed out of veins taken from the leg (saphenous veins) or from arteries arising near the collarbone (internal mammary arteries) (see page 322).

# The heart's conduction system

Sinus node

Atrioventricular
(AV) node

The conduction system is the "wiring" of your heart. It carries electrical impulses throughout your heart muscle. These electrical impulses cause your heart to beat. The wiring is not visible, but follows the paths shown in green.

The impulses begin in the sinus node, spread throughout the atria, pass through the atrioventricular node, and then are distributed throughout the ventricles. During each heartbeat (a duration of about 1 second during a resting state), these stages can be seen on an electrocardiogram (ECG).

The current flowing through the atria produces a small "blip" (**the P wave, bottom left**). As the impulse crosses the atrioventricular node, the ECG line becomes level (**the PR segment**). When the impulse spreads throughout the muscular ventricles, a larger "blip" (**the QRS complex**) is produced on the ECG.

Finally, the electrical system recovers in preparation for the next impulse. During this stage the **T wave** appears on the ECG (see page 16).

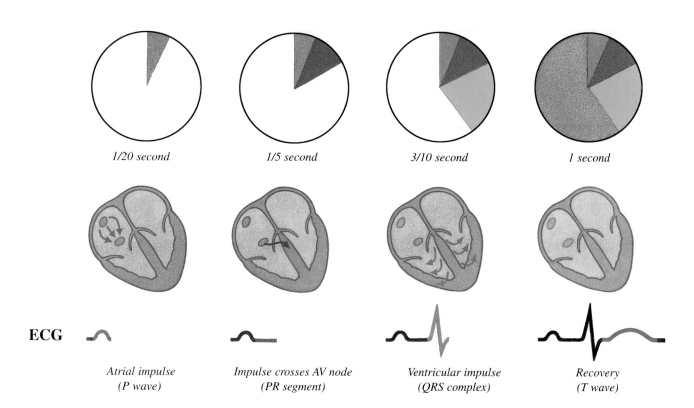

| 1/20 second | 1/5 second | 3/10 second | 1 second |

ECG

| Atrial impulse (P wave) | Impulse crosses AV node (PR segment) | Ventricular impulse (QRS complex) | Recovery (T wave) |

# Electrophysiology catheters

An electrophysiology test may be required for the evaluation of some heart rhythm problems (see page 268). This test consists of inserting electrode wire catheters through veins into the right-sided chambers of your heart. Several wires are often required so that different parts of the conduction system can be evaluated at the same time. In this way, your doctor can carefully assess the way in which electrical impulses travel through your heart and determine whether there are abnormalities that explain a rhythm problem or other symptoms. The wires can be used to detect and record impulses (like an "internal ECG"), or they can be used to pace your heart or stimulate it into abnormal rhythms that can be examined. Different catheters in various positions in the left and right sides of the heart can be used in a procedure called catheter ablation (see page 342).

*Cutaway view of heart shows placement of electrode catheters in an electrophysiology test. Not every procedure requires all of the catheters shown.*

Electrode threaded from the femoral vein to the right ventricle

Electrode threaded from the femoral vein to the region of the atrioventricular node

Electrode threaded from the femoral vein in the groin to the region of the sinus node

Electrode threaded from the neck vein into the coronary sinus (the main coronary vein). This catheter detects impulses on the left side of the heart

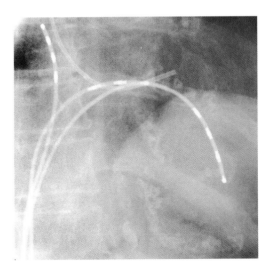

*An X-ray image of the electrophysiology catheters shown in the drawing above.*

# Pacemakers and implantable cardioverter defibrillators

**Pacemakers** produce small electrical impulses that stimulate the heart to beat. They are used when the natural heartbeat is too slow. Depending on the type of pacemaker, the impulses are carried by a lead (insulated wire) threaded through a vein into the right ventricle, the right atrium, or, as illustrated here, both chambers.

Occasionally, the leads can be placed surgically on the outer surface of the heart instead. Inserting a pacemaker and lead through a vein is a minor procedure that can be done with local anesthesia. The X-ray (**below right**) shows a pacemaker in place (see page 332).

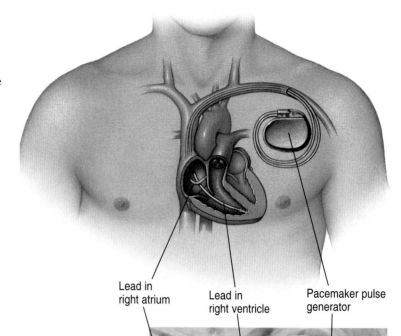

Lead in right atrium

Lead in right ventricle

Pacemaker pulse generator

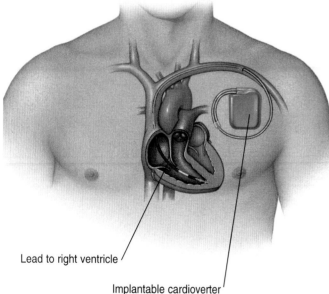

Lead to right ventricle

Implantable cardioverter defibrillator

**Implantable cardioverter defibrillators** (ICDs) can both pace and deliver shocks that can treat ventricular fibrillation or ventricular tachycardia (see page 337).

An ICD can monitor the heart rhythm at all times and will function as a pacemaker for slow heart rates. If a ventricular tachycardia or ventricular fibrillation rhythm occurs, the ICD treats the rhythm with the specific type of electrical therapy needed. There are three types of electrical therapy: rapid-pacing, low-energy shock and high-energy shock. Depending on the need, the electrical therapy will be delivered via pacing, a shock, or a combination of the two.

# Diseases of blood vessels

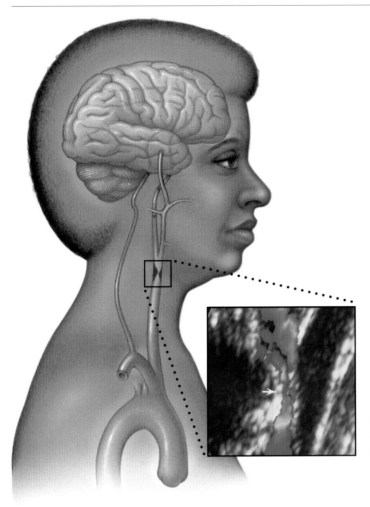

Several disorders of blood vessels are common. Atherosclerosis (deposits of cholesterol-containing plaques in the arteries) can cause partial or complete blockage of blood flow. Tissues downstream from the blockage receive insufficient oxygen-carrying blood.

Atherosclerotic plaque in a carotid artery (**left**) can impede blood flow to the brain. In addition, bits of blood clot or cholesterol can break off and plug smaller vessels in the brain, causing a stroke. One technique of detecting blockage in a vessel is color Doppler ultrasonography (**inset: arrow points to narrowing of the artery**). Turbulence in the bloodstream, caused by the blockage, is blue.

*Color Doppler ultrasound image of carotid artery shows blockage (see page 254).*

*An abdominal aortic aneurysm is an expanded region of the aorta (**arrow**) that runs the risk of rupturing or forming a blood clot at the site of expansion. Aneurysms can be viewed and measured with an ultrasound examination (see page 273).*

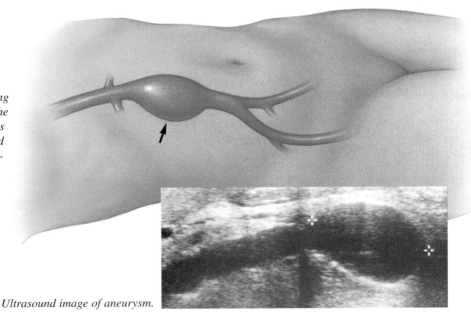

*Ultrasound image of aneurysm.*

# The pericardium

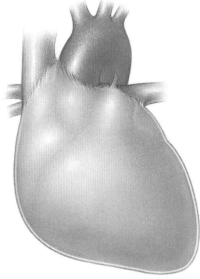

The pericardium is a thin sac surrounding your heart. It consists of an inner and an outer layer. Normally, a small amount of fluid fills the space between the heart and pericardium.

Some conditions cause excess fluid to develop in the pericardial sac (pericardial effusion). If a large amount of fluid accumulates, it can push in on the walls of your heart, decreasing the ability of your heart to expand and take in blood during diastole. This condition, called cardiac tamponade, can diminish the effective pumping function of your heart. The fluid may need to be drained by a needle carefully inserted through the chest wall (pericardiocentesis).

Inflammation of the pericardium is called pericarditis, a condition that can cause chest pain. Some types of pericarditis can lead to thickening and stiffening of the pericardium over time, encasing the heart in a rigid container. This constrictive pericarditis also leads to inefficient functioning of the heart, and it may require surgical removal of the pericardium.

*The normal pericardium forms a thin covering over the heart.*

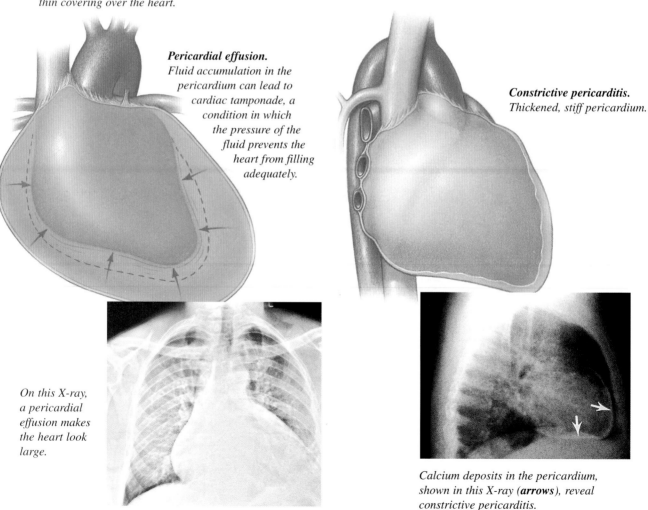

***Pericardial effusion.***
*Fluid accumulation in the pericardium can lead to cardiac tamponade, a condition in which the pressure of the fluid prevents the heart from filling adequately.*

***Constrictive pericarditis.***
*Thickened, stiff pericardium.*

*On this X-ray, a pericardial effusion makes the heart look large.*

*Calcium deposits in the pericardium, shown in this X-ray (**arrows**), reveal constrictive pericarditis.*

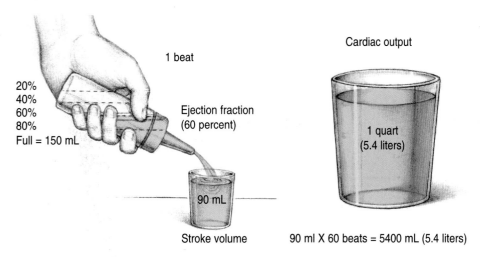

1 beat

Cardiac output

20%
40%
60%
80%
Full = 150 mL

Ejection fraction
(60 percent)

1 quart
(5.4 liters)

90 mL

Stroke volume

90 ml X 60 beats = 5400 mL (5.4 liters)

*Repeated squeezing of fluid from a bottle (**left**) illustrates the work of your heart's ventricles. The amount of fluid (blood) squirting into the cup (artery) is called the "stroke volume" (90 milliliters **above**). The portion of fluid squirted is called the "ejection fraction" (60 percent). If the bottle is squirted (or the heart beats) 60 times each minute, the total volume of fluid ejected in 1 minute is 5400 mL (5.4 liters, or about 1 quart). This amount is called "cardiac output."*

The actual amount of blood pumped by the left ventricle with one contraction is called the stroke volume. The stroke volume and the number of times the heart beats each minute (heart rate) determine your cardiac output. Your cardiac output is the amount of blood your heart pumps through your circulatory system each minute.

Your heart has an automatic mechanism to ensure that it pumps out the same amount of blood that it receives. When more blood enters than leaves your heart, your heart muscle can be stretched. The more the muscle is stretched, the more forceful will be the contraction and the more blood pumped with each beat. Imagine what would happen without this simple but vital adjustment mechanism. If your heart took in just a tiny bit more blood than it pumped out on each beat, it would gradually swell to the point of being unable to function.

Your heart can also increase the amount of blood it pumps by beating more times per minute, within limits. When the heart beats very fast, the strength of the heart muscle decreases and the period of diastole (when the heart relaxes and refills with blood) becomes too short for the chambers to fill adequately.

Although the pumping action of your heart seems simple, the mechanisms that make the pump perform are complex and elegant. Subsequent sections of this part describe how the valves, coronary vessels, conduction system, arteries and veins, and the pericardium are involved in your heart's work of pumping blood.

### How much blood does your heart pump?*

- Normal amount a minute = About 1 quart (5 to 6 liters)
- Without atria contracting = 4 to 6 liters
- Weakened heart, atria contracting = $3^{1}/2$ liters
- Weakened heart, atria not contracting = $2^{1}/2$ liters

*Measurements taken at rest.*

# 2

# Heart valves

Although the pumping action of your heart is certainly effective in ejecting blood from the chambers, it alone would not ensure effective blood flow through the figure-8 circulatory loop. Any pumping system requires a method to guarantee that the pumped fluid goes in the desired direction. This is the purpose of the valves.

Each valve in your heart opens and closes once with each heartbeat (or about once every second throughout your lifetime).

There are four valves in your heart: the tricuspid, mitral, pulmonary and aortic (see page A1). The valves are strong, thin leaflets of tissue attached to the myocardium. The leaflets consist of single sheets of fibrous tissue covered by endocardial cells. At the base of each valve leaflet, the fibrous layer merges with the myocardium to form a flexible hinge called the annulus.

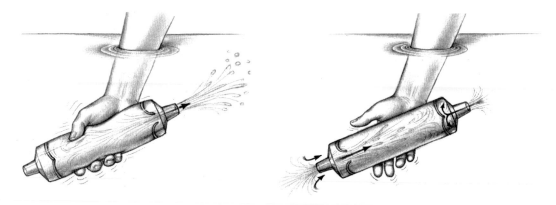

*During contraction of your heart (**left**), blood is ejected though a one-way valve at one end of the ventricle. Fluid cannot escape backward because another one-way valve prevents backward flow. During expansion of the ventricle (**right**), blood enters through the previously closed valve. The previously opened valve now closes to prevent leakage of the blood previously pumped out. Valves within your heart are designed to ensure one-way flow of blood.*

## The atrioventricular valves

The atrioventricular valves are the tricuspid (on the right side of the heart) and the mitral (on the left side). These valves regulate the flow of blood from the atria to the ventricles. Their leaflets are delicate flaps that open during ventricular diastole and close during systole. The leaflets are larger than needed to close the opening. Thus, some overlap and puckering of the leaflet tissue occur, ensuring a good seal when the valve is closed.

The leaflets are anchored and supported by chordae tendineae, strong cords that stretch from the valve edges to the myocardium and restrict how far the valve swings when it closes. They prevent the leaflets from flapping back into the atria from the pressure of ventricular contraction. These chordae are similar to the strings of a parachute in function and appearance (see pages A1, A6).

The chordae insert into mounds of myocardium, known as papillary muscles, inside the ventricle.

The tricuspid valve, separating the right atrium and the right ventricle, is named for its three tooth-shaped leaflets. Tricuspid leaflets tend to be thinner and more translucent than mitral leaflets, and tricuspid chordae tend to be thinner than mitral chordae.

The mitral valve (resembling the pointed shape of a bishop's miter) separates the left atrium and the left ventricle. In contrast to the three other heart valves, which each have three leaflets, the mitral valve has only two.

During diastole, when the ventricles relax and expand, the tricuspid and mitral valves open, allowing blood to flow into and refill the ventricles. When the ventricles contract again, blood pushes on the undersides of the leaflets and forces them to close. At the same time, the tiny tendons pull on the edges of the leaflets to keep them from bulging back into the atria and letting blood leak backward.

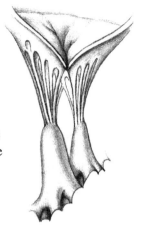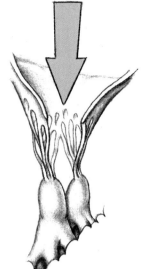

*The atrioventricular (mitral and tricuspid) valves as they appear when closed (**left**) and open (**right**). When open, they allow blood to flow from the atria to the ventricles.*

## The semilunar valves

The aortic and pulmonary valves are similar to one another in structure but are different from the atrioventricular valves. Their leaflets of delicate tissue are shaped like crescents, thus the name "semilunar" (half-moon) valves. The pulmonary valve is at the opening from the right ventricle to the pulmonary artery, and the aortic valve is at the opening from the left ventricle to the aorta.

In contrast to the atrioventricular valves, the semilunar valves have no chordae tendineae and are structurally simpler. The aortic valve leaflets are thicker and more opaque than the pulmonary valve leaflets.

HEALTHY
HEART ♥ TIP

*Fifty million Americans—one out of every three persons in the United States—have high blood pressure (hypertension), which means their hearts work harder to pump blood through their bodies. But one third of those people are unaware of their condition because they show no clear symptoms. That's why it's important to visit your doctor for regular blood pressure checks.*

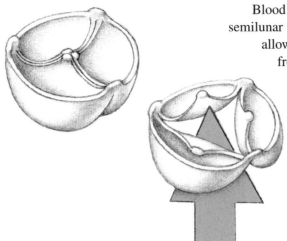

Blood flowing from the ventricles pushes the leaflets of the semilunar valves toward the artery walls during contraction, allowing blood to pass through freely. When the blood flow from the ventricles decreases, the pressure in the ventricles falls. The pressure in the artery soon becomes higher than that in the ventricles. When this happens, the blood under higher pressure in the arteries presses the leaflets downward, and the valves snap closed.

## One-way blood flow

The valves are designed to allow blood to pass in only one direction. The valves do not actively open and close; that is, they do not automatically open when blood is approaching. Instead, they function like a gate that opens only when it is pushed and only in one direction. The valves open and close in response to the naturally occurring pressure differences that build up within the heart's chambers during the systolic and diastolic portions of each cardiac cycle.

*The semilunar (aortic and pulmonary) valves as they appear when closed (**top**) and open (**bottom**). When open, they allow blood to flow from the ventricles to the aorta and pulmonary arteries.*

For example, the aortic valve opens to allow blood to eject from the left ventricle into the aorta, because during systole (contraction) the pressure in the left ventricle is higher than that in the aorta. This pressure difference forces open the leaflets and allows blood to flow through the aortic valve.

During diastole, when the left ventricle relaxes, the pressure in the left ventricle becomes low again, while the pressure in the aorta remains high. The valve is pushed closed by the pressure, and blood is prevented from leaking back.

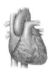

HEALTHY
HEART ♥ TIP

*For a heart-healthy diet, eat five or more servings of fruits and vegetables daily. Your best choices include fresh, frozen and dried fruits and vegetables. Go easy on canned fruits, because of their added sugar and decreased fiber, and canned vegetables, because of the added salt. Limit avocados, coconuts, and olives—they have a higher fat content. Limit or avoid breaded and deep-fried vegetables and fruits or vegetables in high-fat cream sauces, cheese, butter or dips.*

# Arteries and veins of your heart

Like any other organ or tissue in your body, your heart requires its own blood supply to get the oxygen and nutrition it needs for energy to contract again and again. Although the chambers of your heart are filled with blood, the heart muscle does not extract oxygen and nutrients from the blood in its chambers. Your heart receives its nourishing blood supply through the coronary arteries.

Because of its heavy work load, your heart requires a particularly rich blood supply. At rest, the blood flow through the coronary arteries averages about 225 milliliters (more than 7 ounces) a minute. This amount is 4 to 5 percent of the blood pumped by your heart, even though your heart makes up less than 1 percent of your body's weight.

The coronary arteries branch off from the base of the aorta just above the aortic valve. They run along the surface of the heart, encircling the top and branching toward the bottom like a crown (corona means "crown," hence their name).

The coronary arteries each have trunks and many branches, like trees. Each trunk is about the size of a soda straw. The smaller branches penetrate into the heart muscle, going from the outside toward the inner surface of the cardiac chambers to carry blood to the myocardial cells.

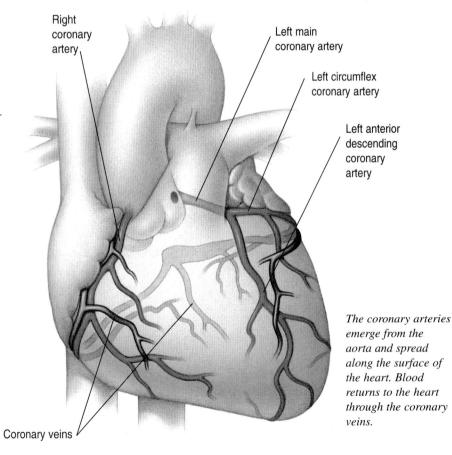

*The coronary arteries emerge from the aorta and spread along the surface of the heart. Blood returns to the heart through the coronary veins.*

*The coronary arteries, like all of the other larger arteries of the body, are tubes with walls that have three layers: the inner (intima), the middle (media), and the outer (adventitia). Blood flows through the opening called the lumen.*

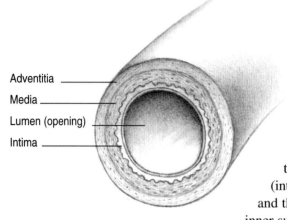

Adventitia

Media

Lumen (opening)

Intima

The smaller arteries branch into even smaller vessels and ultimately into capillaries. The capillaries are the places at which oxygen and nutrients are exchanged for waste products.

Like other arteries in your body, the coronary arteries have three layers: the inner layer (intima), the muscular layer (media), and the outer layer (adventitia). The inner surface of the blood vessel is lined with a layer of cells called the endothelium. The cavity (channel) within the vessel in which blood flows is called the lumen.

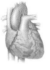

HEALTHY
HEART ♥ TIP

*Congenital cardiovascular defects may be the most frequent malformation in newborns, but heart problems at birth are relatively rare. Only 1 percent of babies are born with heart abnormalities.*

*Occasionally, viral infection is to blame. If a mother contracts German measles during pregnancy, for example, the infection can interfere with the baby's heart development. Heredity sometimes plays a role in congenital cardiovascular disease, and some prescription drugs, over-the-counter medicines, alcohol and illegal drugs may increase the risk of having a baby with a heart defect.*

## Coronary arteries

The left coronary artery carries blood to the front, top, and part of the back side of the left ventricle. The right coronary artery supplies most of the right ventricle and also a portion of the undersurface and back of the left ventricle (see page A9).

The left main coronary artery divides into the anterior descending artery, which carries blood down the front of the heart to both ventricles, and the circumflex artery, which winds around the back of the heart to nourish that portion of the left ventricle and left atrium.

The right coronary artery curves around the front of the heart between the right atrium and right ventricle, sending branches, the marginal arteries, along the front to bring blood to the right ventricle. Blood vessels extend through heart muscle to supply all layers of the muscle (see page A4).

Each person has a unique coronary artery tree. The coronary arteries can have various numbers of branches, and the placement and size of those branches vary greatly from person to person.

The left coronary, in all but rare circumstances, is the main source of blood supply to the left ventricle (the main pumping chamber of the heart). The right coronary artery may vary in size from small to large, and its contribution to the overall blood supply to the heart, while always important, is also variable. Usually, the left coronary artery supplies about 65 percent of the heart's blood flow (45 percent by the left anterior descending artery and

20 percent by the circumflex artery), and the right coronary artery supplies 35 percent. As the right coronary artery passes along the underside of the heart, it gives rise to the posterior descending artery, sending smaller arteries to both ventricles.

### Your heart may demand more oxygen if . . .

- You're excited, or you have a heart rhythm abnormality.
- You have strong heart contractions due to exercise.
- You have high blood pressure or heart valve problems.
- You have an enlarged heart chamber due to any condition that causes heart failure.
- Your heart muscle is thickened because of abnormalities, high blood pressure or valve problems.

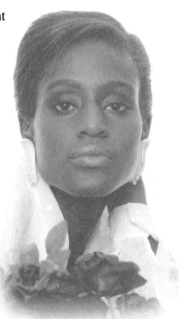

Blood flow through the coronary arteries is closely related to the amount of oxygen that the myocardial cells need at the moment. Therefore, in normal coronary arteries, blood flow increases as the demand for oxygen increases, such as during exercise.

During exertion, when the heart beats faster and more vigorously, more oxygen is needed. To get more blood to the myocardium, the muscular layer of the arteries relaxes and causes the arteries to expand, allowing a greater volume of blood to flow through them. More blood can flow through a wide vessel than through a small one in a given period, just as more water can flow through a wide pipe than a small one.

# Chapter

# 4

# Your heart's electrical (conduction) system

An intricate timing system underlies the rhythmic contractions of your heart. If the pumping is interrupted or erratic, your heart may not deliver enough blood to your tissues. To fulfill its task, your heart must beat at an appropriate rate, and the chambers of your heart must contract in a coordinated fashion.

The atria contract to help blood flow into the ventricles. Then the ventricles contract, propelling blood to the arteries of your body. The rate and sequence of these contractions are regulated by your heart's conduction system.

The conduction system is like microscopic wiring. It conducts electrical impulses throughout the muscle of your heart. These electrical impulses stimulate heart muscle to contract and squeeze blood out into your arteries.

## Parts of the system

The sinus node, a group of cells in the upper part of the right atrium, is the normal origin of the electrical impulse. It is your heart's natural pacemaker. The impulse is channeled into adjacent cells of the conduction system. This channeling, in effect, produces an electrical current that then passes from cell to cell.

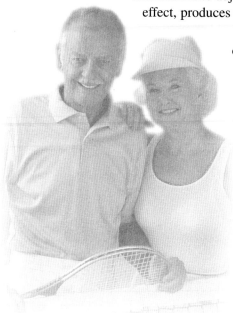

The second part of the conduction system is the electrical pathways in the atrium through which this electrical current travels on its journey toward the ventricles.

The third portion of the conduction system is the atrioventricular (AV) node, a cluster of cells at the center of your heart between the atria and the ventricles. The AV node is like a gate that slows down the electrical current before it is allowed to pass through to the ventricles. This conduction delay at the AV node ensures that the atria contract a short time before the ventricles contract, allowing more time for the ventricles to fill.

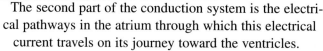

After the current leaves the AV node, it travels into specialized conduction tissue called the His-Purkinje system. This system of branching pathways of specialized electricity-conducting tissue rapidly distributes the current throughout the muscle cells of the left and right ventricles.

The interval from the beginning of the electrical impulse in the sinus node to completion of its delivery through the conduction system to the myocardial cells is brief, averaging about 1/4 second when the heart is beating 72 times a minute. More than half of this time is due to the built-in delay at the AV node (see page A12).

## How does it work?

In the conduction system, the flow of current in a cell is passed on to adjacent cells. In the heart muscle cells, the same thing happens, but in addition the electrical current activates the contractile apparatus of the muscle cell. When the contractile apparatus is activated, it starts the pumping action of the heart muscle. Thus, the conduction system, from the sinus node on down, is responsible for controlling the speed and rhythm of your heart's contraction.

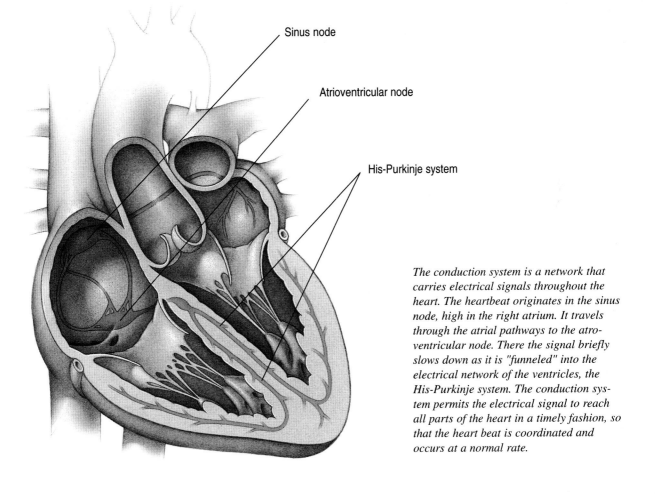

Sinus node

Atrioventricular node

His-Purkinje system

*The conduction system is a network that carries electrical signals throughout the heart. The heartbeat originates in the sinus node, high in the right atrium. It travels through the atrial pathways to the atroventricular node. There the signal briefly slows down as it is "funneled" into the electrical network of the ventricles, the His-Purkinje system. The conduction system permits the electrical signal to reach all parts of the heart in a timely fashion, so that the heart beat is coordinated and occurs at a normal rate.*

Unlike most other muscle cells in your body, cardiac cells can start their own electrical impulses and contractions. Although your nervous system can adjust the rate at which your heart beats, it is not the driving force that makes it beat. (Even a heart that has been removed from the body, such as with a heart transplant, or cardiac cells that have been separated from one another, can continue to contract for a while. In fact, even if the sinus node fails, other sites can take over the pacemaking function.)

The reason that the sinus node sets the pace is that its natural rate for formation of the electrical impulse is faster than the rates in other cells farther down in the conduction system, and the faster rate overrides the slower rates. As you go down the conduction system, the rate of spontaneous contraction gets slower and slower. In an adult, the usual sinus node rate at rest is 60 to 100 beats a minute. The spontaneous rate at the AV node is 40 to 60 beats a minute, and the rate in the ventricles is only 20 to 40 beats a minute.

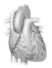

### HEALTHY HEART ♥ TIP

*You may be doing everything right, but still experience a narrowing of the coronary arteries. Perhaps 30 percent of Americans may have this so-called silent ischemia and not even know it.*

*This is one reason why people have heart attacks with no warning. In addition, people with chest pain also may have undiagnosed episodes of silent ischemia. Doctors can diagnose this condition with a variety of tests, such as an exercise test or a 24-hour portable electrocardiogram monitor. If you have other risk factors for heart disease, ask your doctor about undergoing these tests.*

Although the slower rate of impulse formation from an AV node site will keep you alive, your heart performs better under the direction of the sinus node. If neither the sinus node nor the AV node is working, another backup system (in the ventricles) takes over. However, it is even slower and is not designed to do the job alone.

## What's a normal heart rate?

The normal heart rate in a resting adult is 60 to 100 beats a minute. Remember, "normal" means most people have rates in this range most of the time. Small fluctuations outside the normal range do not necessarily indicate a problem. Some doctors might say the normal resting heart rate is 50 to 90 beats a minute.

As you run, climb stairs, or exercise, the sinus node responds and your heart rate speeds up. Your heart beats faster with increased activity to send more blood to nourish your muscles.

Along with exercise, several other things can increase your heart rate, including mental stress, tobacco, caffeine, alcohol, and some prescription and nonprescription drugs. Your heart rate normally slows during sleep and with some medications. Pulse rates in the range of 30 to 50 beats a minute are not unusual in healthy adults during sleep.

## Your autonomic nervous system

The message that prompts the sinus node to increase or decrease its rate is delivered by the autonomic nervous system. Your autonomic nervous system automatically controls many functions in your body, such as blood pressure, breathing, excretion and heart rate. You do not have to decide consciously to breathe or to change your heart rate, because your autonomic nervous system takes care of these vital decisions for you. It can make snap judgments. For instance, it can cause the sinus node to increase your heart rate to twice its normal rate within only 3 to 5 seconds.

## Heart rates for people of different ages*

| Normal rates at rest | |
| --- | --- |
| **Age group** | **Beats a minute** |
| Newborn | 140 |
| Young child | 100 to 120 |
| Adult | 60 to 100 |
| **Maximally attainable rates** | |
| **Age** | **Beats a minute** |
| 25 | 200 |
| 35 | 188 |
| 45 | 176 |
| 55 | 165 |
| 65 | 155 |

*Average rates.*

## How fast can your heart beat?

As you age, it may seem as if your body is slowing down. In fact, your heart rate actually does slow with age. The decrease is not noticeable during everyday activities, but your maximal heart rate during exercise decreases as you grow older. For example, your maximal heart rate at age 25 is about 200 beats a minute. By age 65, your maximal heart rate is only about 155 beats a minute. (Your maximal heart rate is approximately 220 minus your age.)

Your heart rate may also slow as a desirable result of being in good physical condition. An athlete's heart often beats slower than normal because training has allowed the heart to contract more strongly and pump more blood with each beat. As a result, the heart does not need to beat as fast to produce normal blood flow.

# Chapter

# 5

# Your body's arteries and veins

Your arteries and veins are essential for carrying blood pumped by your heart to and from all parts of your body. Your arteries carry blood away from your heart. Your veins bring it back (see page A2).

Think of your arteries as a tree in which the trunk branches into larger, then smaller branches, twigs (arterioles ), and finally microscopic twigs called capillaries. Capillaries are only slightly wider than a single blood cell. They accommodate only a single-file column of blood cells. It is through the thin walls of the capillaries that oxygen, carbon dioxide, nutrients and waste products are exchanged within each cell of the body (see page A3).

After the blood flows through the capillaries, it enters small veins (venules) that merge into larger and larger branches (veins) that go back to the atria.

## Aorta (the main artery) and pulmonary artery

The main artery in your body is the aorta. It carries bright red (oxygenated) blood to tissues throughout your body.

The ascending aorta emerges upward from your left ventricle. It makes a U-turn in the upper part of your chest and descends to become the abdominal aorta. Large branches lead from your aorta to your head, torso, arms and legs.

The main arteries supplying your head are the carotid arteries. Your arms receive their blood supply through the axillary arteries. Your legs receive their blood supply through the femoral arteries. These main branches divide into smaller ones as they extend out beyond your heart.

Your pulmonary artery carries blood from your heart to your lungs. It arises from your right ventricle and transports dark bluish-red (deoxygenated) blood to your lungs, where it is oxygenated.

## Venae cavae (the main veins)

The main veins in your body are the venae cavae. The superior vena cava receives blood from your head through jugular veins, and from your arms through axillary veins. The inferior vena cava receives blood from several veins in your abdomen and from your legs through the femoral veins. The superior and inferior venae cavae each empty into the right atrium.

As with arteries, your veins branch into increasingly smaller ones as they distance themselves from your heart. In this case, though, blood flows from the small vessels (capillaries) into bigger ones, and finally into your heart.

Your pulmonary vein carries newly oxygenated blood from your lungs to the left atrium.

At any given time, 9 percent of your blood is traveling to and from your lungs (through your pulmonary vessels), and about 7 percent is in your heart. By far the greatest volume of blood (84 percent) is in the vessels that travel to and from the rest of your body. These vessels are called systemic arteries and veins (your systemic circulation). Within the systemic circulation, 64 percent of your blood is in the veins, 13 percent is in the arteries and 7 percent is in the tiny branching arterioles and capillaries.

The structure of your systemic blood vessels is the same as that of the coronary arteries. The outside of the vessel is the adventitia. The middle muscular layer is called the media and the inner layer the intima. The opening (lumen) is lined with endothelium.

The blood vessels are more than just passive channels in which blood flows. They are a dynamic element of your circulatory system in their own right. The individual layers of these vessels interact in many ways.

The adventitia carries the vasa vasorum (small blood vessels supplying necessary nourishment to the other layers). It also contains nerves that can tell muscles in the media to contract.

The endothelial lining of the inner layer senses and produces messages that tell the muscle layer to contract or expand. Contraction and relaxation of muscles in the media help to control blood pressure and the amount of blood distributed to various organs. In these and other ways, your arteries and veins can have a great impact on your body's circulation.

Because your arteries transport blood under high pressure, they have strong elastic walls, and blood flows rapidly through them. The flow of blood in your arteries is said to be pulsatile. This means that the amount of blood flowing constantly increases and decreases as a result of the heart pumping a new volume of blood with each heartbeat, 70 times a minute. This effect is what causes the pulse that you feel over the arteries in your wrists and neck.

## The arterioles

Like other vessels, the arterioles also have strong muscular walls that can close off the vessel completely or dilate it greatly. This feature enables the arteriole to change the blood flow to the capillaries in response to the needs of your tissues.

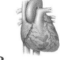

**HEALTHY HEART ♥ TIP**

*How fast is too fast? A normal heart usually beats in the range of 60 to 80 beats a minute, depending on your physical conditioning. Reasons for a heart that beats too fast can include fever, acute illness and anxiety. But an elevated heart rate may mean something more serious, such as anemia, an excess of thyroid hormone (hyperthyroidism), heart defects or disease, or abnormal connections between arteries and veins. If your heart rate is consistently high, you should have a medical evaluation to determine the cause.*

Muscles, for example, when active, may need as much as 20 to 30 times the blood flow that they need at rest. Because your heart can increase its output by only four to seven times, the tiny vessels continually monitor the needs in each tissue and control the blood flow in that portion of your body to the level required. When a large increase is needed in one area (for example, exercising muscles), the proportion of flow to other organs is temporarily decreased.

## Total cardiac output

*Your total cardiac output, the amount of blood your heart pumps in a minute, can vary considerably throughout the day. During strenuous exercise, your heart may pump as much as four to seven times more blood than it does when you're resting. Although the proportion of blood going to your heart and brain decreases during maximal exercise, the actual amount remains rather stable. Blood is distributed on the basis of need for oxygen and nutrients.*

### Cardiac output at rest

| | |
|---|---|
| 3.5 L ●●●◖ | Liver, kidney, intestine and other |
| 1 L ● | Muscle |
| 1 L ● | Skin and bones |
| 0.5 L ◖ | Brain |
| 0.5 L ◖ | Heart |

Approximately 6 liters (L) a minute

### Cardiac output during strenuous exercise

| | |
|---|---|
| 20 L ●●●●●●●●●●●●●●●●●●●●● | Muscle |
| 1 L ● | Liver, kidney, intestine and other |
| 1 L ● | Heart |
| 1 L ● | Brain |
| 0.5 L ◖ | Skin and bones |

Approximately 24 liters (L) a minute

## The capillaries

The capillary walls are microscopically thin, allowing only molecules to pass through. The role of the capillaries depends on the tissues in which they are located.

Pulmonary capillaries release carbon dioxide from your blood into air sacs (alveoli) in your lungs and at the same time absorb oxygen from those sacs into your blood.

The capillaries in your kidneys send waste products into tubules, where urine is formed. In the walls of your intestines, capillaries absorb nutrients from digested food. Capillaries in muscles exchange oxygen and nutrients for waste products and carbon dioxide.

## The veins

The pressure in your veins is very low, and their walls are thinner than the walls of your arteries. Your veins have valves that keep blood flowing only toward your heart. Veins are capable of contracting and expanding in response to the needs of your body. They can act as a reservoir because their walls are 6 to 10 times as expandable as those of your arteries. When you need blood drawn for most diagnostic tests, it is taken from a vein.

## The 'venous pump'

When you move your legs or even tense your leg muscles, blood in your legs is propelled toward your heart. This mechanism is called the "venous pump."

If you stand perfectly still for a long time, this pumping action is lost because of gravity, and as much as 15 to 20 percent of your blood volume pools in your legs. Because that amount of pooled blood is diverted from the overall circulation, other organs may not get their fair share.

The first organ to feel the consequences is the topmost—your brain. This effect may be the reason people sometimes feel dizzy or even pass out after standing rigidly for a long time, such as soldiers standing at attention or people stiffly standing in a wedding party.

## The pericardium

Your pericardium is a sac surrounding your heart (see page A16). The pericardial sac has two membranes, forming inner and outer layers, and with a fluid lubricant between them. This enables your heart to beat with minimal friction against adjacent structures, such as the lungs.

The inner lining of the pericardium is a thin, moist membrane. The tough outer layer adheres to several areas in your chest cavity to anchor your heart in place.

Although the pericardium provides some support and lubrication for the heart, it is somewhat expendable (like your appendix or gallbladder). You can get along without your pericardium should it ever have to be surgically removed.

**HEALTHY HEART ♥ TIP**

*Some people just can't find the right exercise program—especially when they don't have time for the recommended 20 to 40 minutes of aerobic activity three times a week.*

*Although the gain may not be as great, recent evidence indicates that you'll benefit even if you can manage only 10 minutes of activity at a time. Regular exercise, even for a brief period, leads to better cardiovascular health.*

# Part 2

*Can aspirin prevent a heart attack? If you've had heart trouble in the past, or you have narrowed arteries (atherosclerosis) now, a single, regular-strength aspirin daily might help prevent a heart attack. Even a baby aspirin daily or an asprin substitute such as Plavix (clopidogrel) may reduce your risk of heart attack or stroke by reducing the tendency for your blood to clot.*

*If you've had no heart trouble, the potential advantages of a daily aspirin are less clear. Some physicians believe aspirin can reduce your risk of an initial heart attack. Most doctors agree that aspirin's possible side effects (bleeding in your brain, intestines or urinary tract) don't justify its use by everyone. Ask your doctor if the benefits outweigh the risks for you.*

# What is heart disease?

Heart disease takes many forms and varies widely in severity. Some people are born with it. More often it develops later in life. Most people detect warning signs or symptoms, but heart disease can strike without the slightest clue. Managing your heart disease may require minor inconveniences or major lifestyle changes. Heart disease can also be fatal. It is the leading cause of death in the United States.

## Chapter

# Chapter

# 6

# Symptoms: signals of disease

Sometimes a specific symptom provides a warning. Or you may be unable to pinpoint the problem but you just do not feel right. Your doctor may be the first to discover a suspicious test result or physical sign or perceive the significance of a particular symptom. In other cases, a heart attack is the earliest warning.

The detective work of determining what problem is causing the symptoms is the cornerstone of diagnosis, and an accurate diagnosis is the best chance of finding an effective treatment.

## What is a symptom?

A symptom is a change in the way your body feels that may indicate illness or disease. A symptom is totally subjective. Doctors cannot detect a symptom; only you can do that. A symptom is not the disease itself.

Doctors are trained to listen to your description of symptoms and to ask questions to determine the significance of each. Doctors also look for "signs"—outward manifestations of the disease or problem.

Although neither the symptoms nor the signs are the disease, they are clues to a potential underlying problem. They are your body's way of telling you that something may be wrong.

Since symptoms are usually uncomfortable or distressful, one of the goals of medical treatment is to eliminate or reduce symptoms. Although some medications are capable of blunting symptoms, the very best treatment is to identify and reverse the problem that is provoking the symptom.

Because many symptoms are early warnings of underlying disease, it is important to respond to them in the right way. It would be futile to dwell on every minor ache, pain, and twinge in your body. These symptoms do not signal a serious illness. Over the years, you have learned to ignore certain symptoms because experience has shown that they have little impact on your overall health.

However, you may have symptoms of an actual problem, but because you have become familiar with the symptoms, you know what to do about them. For example, a runny nose, stuffy head, sore throat, and cough suggest that you have a cold. People with colds usually take it easy and may use a mild pain reliever and cough medicine as needed. A visit to the emergency room is unnecessary.

Questions may arise, though, when you experience a symptom for the first time or if it is worse than usual or accompanies other symptoms. When these situations occur, you might wonder whether an illness is present and whether you need medical attention.

The first step in answering these questions is to understand what the symptoms may mean. One purpose of this book is to help provide that working knowledge.

The second step is to decide whether the symptom is related to an underlying medical problem. Even if you are uncertain, it is advisable to consult a doctor.

The third step is to decide how urgently you need medical attention. On the one hand, it probably would be inappropriate, time-consuming, and expensive to call an ambulance or go to the emergency room for a momentary jab of pain on the right side of the chest. However, it might be appropriate to set up an appointment with a doctor for an examination.

On the other hand, it would be folly to ignore sustained chest pressure or breathing difficulty. You might hope it will go away, and you might not want to bother the doctor in the middle of the night, but you could be having a heart attack.

Neither this book nor any other book can cover all the possible symptoms you may experience, nor can it presume to make diagnoses. Unfortunately, no system or formula tells you in advance whether a symptom is significant. The same symptom or symptoms may indicate widely differing and unrelated types of conditions in different people; conversely, many different symptoms may be caused by one illness. No one can be expected to determine a diagnosis or its significance before seeing a doctor.

In general, however, you should consider seeing a doctor soon if a symptom meets any of the following general criteria:

- The symptom is new.
- The symptom is severe.
- The symptom is worsening.
- The symptom provokes anxiety.
- The symptom is unrelieved by a previously recommended medication.
- The symptom is a repetition of a symptom that was associated with a previous serious problem. This may be an indication that the problem has recurred.
- The symptom requires you to reduce or slow down a particular activity.

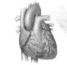

## HEALTHY HEART ♥ TIP

*Take a vitamin or eat an orange? In most cases, it's better to eat the orange. Whole foods have benefits you can't find in a pill. When you feast on whole foods such as fruits, vegetables, and grains, you also get phytochemicals and fiber. In addition, valuable vitamins and minerals are found in these foods as well as in lean meats and low-fat dairy products.*

*Nutritional supplements are recommended in certain situations, but remember: Even if you take a daily multivitamin, you still need to eat a balanced diet with whole foods as the focus.*

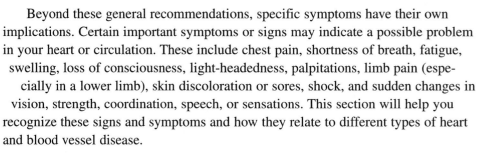

Beyond these general recommendations, specific symptoms have their own implications. Certain important symptoms or signs may indicate a possible problem in your heart or circulation. These include chest pain, shortness of breath, fatigue, swelling, loss of consciousness, light-headedness, palpitations, limb pain (especially in a lower limb), skin discoloration or sores, shock, and sudden changes in vision, strength, coordination, speech, or sensations. This section will help you recognize these signs and symptoms and how they relate to different types of heart and blood vessel disease.

This book does not take the place of a doctor's evaluation. If you have any questions, ask your doctor for advice.

## Talking to your doctor

Because symptoms are such important clues to underlying problems, and because no one but you can describe your symptoms, the better you can communicate your symptoms to your doctor, the more likely it is that your doctor can help you. Some doctors claim that 90 percent of the final diagnosis is revealed by what you tell them during your examination. Thus, you can save time, money, and effort, and increase the chances that your doctor will find an effective solution, by carefully describing your symptoms.

The more clearly you can describe your symptoms and other relevant factors (such as family history, medications and social habits), the more effective your evaluation will be. Admittedly, many symptoms are vague, but if you use precise terms, you will help your doctor find the problem.

## Symptoms: all the facts

Just as a beginning reporter learns to cover the "who, what, when, where, and how" of a story, doctors are taught in medical school to seek certain information to help them get the full story about your symptoms. You may be able to describe your symptoms more clearly if you specify these details. Write them down and bring the list along as a reminder when you visit your doctor. Here are things to consider:

How does it feel? (Quality)

Where does it bother you? (Location)

How bad is it? (Severity)

What brings on the symptoms? (Provocation)

Does it come on suddenly or gradually? (Onset)

What reduces or eliminates the symptoms? (Relieving factors)

How long have you had it? How long does it last? (Duration)

How often does it occur? (Frequency)

Do you have other problems along with it? (Associated symptoms)

Think ahead of time about what you want to tell the doctor. If you are vague, if you are quiet, or if you are unfocused, important information may be lost. Your doctor will ask questions to fill in the gaps, but usually the information you volunteer contains the key clues to a correct diagnosis.

Descriptions of major cardiovascular symptoms and signs may help you communicate more clearly with your doctor. At this point, the focus is on the symptoms, rather than what causes them. Some of the problems the symptoms suggest will be mentioned.

## Symptoms guide

### Chest pain

Chest pain is probably the symptom most commonly associated with heart disease. Cardiologists spend a large part of their time analyzing "chest pain." Ironically, the sensation associated with most types of heart disease is rarely described as pain. In fact, some people go out of their way to say that they are not experiencing pain, but rather a difficult-to-describe discomfort.

Chest pain usually falls into three categories: chest pain due to angina (pain caused by an insufficient oxygen supply to the heart muscle), chest pain from other cardiac causes such as an inflammation of the pericardium or the tearing pain from dissection of an artery, and chest pain from noncardiac problems such as chest wall, joint, nerve or gallbladder disease. This section focuses on angina and on chest pain from other cardiac causes.

### Angina pectoris

Angina pectoris is one of the most common symptoms of heart disease. Angina, like all other symptoms, is not a diagnosis. In most cases it is associated with any condition in which the heart muscle does not get an adequate supply of blood and oxygen.

#### *Qualities of angina pectoris*

Angina causes pain but not all chest pain is from the heart. The character of the pain may include burning, a discomfort, a dull ache or a full feeling. Occasionally the pain is sharp, although that's unusual.

Angina pectoris is often a constricting pressure or tightness of the chest. Not infrequently the symptoms are associated with sensations other than pain, for example: shortness of breath, nausea, sweating, light-headedness or a sense of impending doom. People experience angina pectoris in different ways, but in an individual the pattern is consistent.

## Symptoms and signs of heart disease

The symptoms and signs most commonly associated with heart and blood vessel disease include:

- Chest pain (angina pectoris)
- Shortness of breath (dyspnea)
- General fatigue
- Swelling (edema)
- Loss of consciousness (syncope)
- Light-headedness (presyncope)
- Palpitations
- Limb pain or tiredness (claudication)
- Abnormal skin color
- Sores on skin (ulceration)
- Shock (collapse)
- Sudden change in vision, strength, coordination, speech, or sensation

## Terms people use to describe angina

- Crushing
- Constricting
- Viselike
- Strangling
- Pressure
- Heaviness
- Fullness
- Feels like a weight
- Squeezing
- Burning
- Ache
- Feels like gas
- Tight
- Feels like indigestion
- Choking
- Coldness with perspiration or weakness

*Angina pectoris is usually experienced as discomfort, tightness, or pressure in your chest or in regions of your back, neck, jaw, shoulders, and arms (especially the left arm). Discomfort may be limited to a specific area, or it might radiate to various sites throughout your upper body, including the right side of your chest.*

Many people who experience angina have a difficult time explaining the nature of the discomfort to the doctor. Some people use images such as "like an elephant sitting on my chest" or "as if my chest is in a vise." They often describe the pain as dull rather than sharp.

### *Location*

When asked to show where the discomfort is located, many people put the whole hand or a clenched fist on the chest, because it is not possible to localize the sensation by pointing a finger. (This is a classic sign called "Levine's sign.")

The discomfort of angina pectoris is often described as spreading throughout the chest and occasionally radiating into the back, neck, shoulders, and arms, especially on the left side. Sometimes the discomfort is located only in the arm or the jaw, and not in the chest. Some people with angina have consulted with their dentists initially in the mistaken (but understandable) belief that the cause of their jaw pain was dental.

### *Provocation*

Angina pectoris is typically provoked by either mental or physical stress. Mental stress can be brought about by anxiety, fright, or other strong emotions. Physical stress can be brought about by walking (especially up a hill), stair climbing, running, housework, sexual intercourse, or other activities. The added stress requires more work from the heart, which produces a greater need for oxygen by the heart muscle. If this need is not met, angina results.

Angina is provoked more easily by performing physical activities in cold weather or after a meal. Cold temperatures and digestion require more work from the heart and may redistribute blood flow from the heart to other organs. In the cold, your body sends more blood to your arms and legs to keep warm. Digestion is a kind of "internal exercise" that requires that more blood be supplied to the digestive tract. As a result, your heart must work harder—perhaps hard enough to outstrip its supply of oxygen.

### *Duration*

Angina that is caused by a temporary insufficiency of the coronary blood supply typically lasts a matter of minutes, as opposed to momentary twinges. If you have angina that lasts more than 15 to 20 minutes, you could be having a heart attack. Seek medical attention immediately.

### Relief

If angina occurs during exercise, it will usually disappear within minutes of stopping the exercise or other stressful activity. People who have experienced the discomfort before or whose angina has been diagnosed may take nitroglycerin when they experience the symptoms. Relief usually comes within 10 minutes.

### Other Causes

Although some people have a classic constellation of symptoms suggesting angina pectoris, more often only some of the features point to angina, and others may be absent or atypical. Accordingly, you and your doctor must keep in mind possible diagnoses other than those associated with angina.

Not all chest pain is angina by any means. The less the symptoms sound like angina, the less likely the symptoms are caused by insufficient blood supply to the heart muscle.

Other types of chest pain may signal the presence of other heart problems. Sharp pain near the breast bone or front chest wall that becomes worse with breathing in or with lying down may point to inflammation of the pericardium (the sac that surrounds the heart).

### Chest pain due to problems other than angina

Chest pain can have many causes. Some causes are related to the heart and blood vessels. Others have nothing to do with the cardiovascular system but may be important nevertheless. The doctor considers a list of different possible causes, a process referred to as a differential diagnosis. Your careful description of the pain can often eliminate other possibilities.

Sometimes a person has alarming chest pain and yet has no identifiable problem with the heart. Conditions that often turn out to be present, although heart disease was suspected, include stomach disorders such as heartburn (esophageal reflux), stomach or duodenal ulcer, or gallstones with gallbladder irritation or inflammation. Other conditions that can mimic angina include costschondritis or chest wall pain (caused by soreness of the muscles between the ribs or the immovable joints between ribs and breastbone), a pinched nerve in the neck, inflammation of the membranes around the lung (pleuritis), blood clots in the pulmonary arteries, and shingles (herpes zoster).

## Shortness of breath (dyspnea)

Shortness of breath is another common symptom associated with some types of heart disease. Actually, it is a difficult symptom to describe. Usually it implies a sense of hunger for air that cannot be satisfied. Dyspnea (dys means "abnormal," pnea means "breathing" or "ventilation") is the medical term used to describe an abnormally uncomfortable awareness of breathing (which could mean labored, shallow, or rapid breathing).

Some people cannot distinguish dyspnea from chest discomfort, and dyspnea and angina sometimes occur together. Dyspnea may also be the consequence of lung disease.

### Shortness of breath with various levels of activity

Of course, everyone becomes short of breath after strenuous exertion. If you are not used to exercise, you may become short of breath with only moderate exertion. Therefore, this symptom is abnormal only when it occurs at rest or at a level of activity that is not expected to cause shortness of breath. It is important to distinguish when shortness of breath is due to actual health problems and when it is caused by being out of shape. You are the best judge of when your degree of breathlessness is abnormal for you.

For example, if you usually engage in an average amount of activity but find that you feel short of breath after climbing one flight of stairs, you may have an underlying disease process. Doctors refer to this as " dyspnea on exertion" ("DOE"). Many doctors evaluate the degree of dyspnea by asking how many blocks you can walk at a normal pace, how many flights of stairs you can climb, or how you cope with certain household chores. Shortness of breath at rest usually indicates a more advanced level of underlying disease.

Other factors may make you feel short of breath without an active underlying disease necessarily being present. For example, if you are overweight, you must carry that additional weight for any activity, which in itself may cause shortness of breath at an early stage of exercise.

Shortness of breath may occur in different patterns, which can help determine the underlying cause.

### Shortness of breath at night (paroxysmal nocturnal dyspnea)

"Paroxysmal" means a sudden onset, and "nocturnal" means occurring in the night. One classic pattern of shortness of breath occurs at night when you are asleep and lying down. You awake abruptly gasping for air and may sit up and fling open a window to try to catch your breath. Sometimes the episode is accompanied by coughing, wheezing, or a smothering sensation. To get any relief, you ultimately must sit straight up. Finally the symptoms subside, and you are able to return to bed and sleep for the rest of the night. If not, you may have to sleep sitting up in a chair.

This pattern of shortness of breath is a classic clue to the presence of extra fluid in the lungs due to one form of heart failure. Often, people who experience this find they can minimize the symptom by sleeping with the trunk and head in an upright position, either bolstered by pillows or sleeping in a chair or recliner. Difficulty breathing except in an upright position is called orthopnea (ortho means "straight" or "upright"). Other conditions not related to the heart can cause similar symptoms.

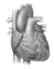

### HEALTHY HEART ♥ TIP

*Chest pains may not just get you a ride on a treadmill or an ECG. Your doctor may also order blood tests to check for increased levels of certain enzymes that are normally found in the heart muscle.*

*If you've experienced a heart attack, damage to your cells may allow these enzymes to leak into your blood over a period of hours. The blood test will detect these higher than normal levels and help the doctor decide on a further course of action.*

### Rapid breathing (tachypnea)

Any condition that makes a person short of breath tends to lead to more rapid breathing. Rapid breathing is called tachypnea (tachy means "fast"). Tachypnea occurs partly in an effort to get more oxygen and also because of anxiety.

### Hyperventilation

Labored, shallow, or rapid breathing as signs of underlying heart or lung disease must be distinguished from the sense of breathlessness and rapid breathing associated with hyperventilation. In hyperventilation, the problem (rather than the consequence) is anxiety. Hyperventilation due to anxiety is sometimes a repetitive sighing type of breathing and sometimes continued rapid breathing. You feel as though you cannot breathe deeply enough. Your arms and hands may tingle during hyperventilation.

The effect of hyperventilation is to reduce the carbon dioxide in the bloodstream to abnormally low levels. This can make you feel lightheaded or tingly (especially around the mouth), and muscle cramps may develop. An effective way of counteracting the low carbon dioxide level is to rebreathe the same air you breathed out, because it contains a lot of carbon dioxide. Do this by placing a small paper bag over your mouth and nose and breathing into it. Alternatively you may intentionally reduce your breathing rate and volume for several seconds, which can alleviate the symptoms. Ultimately, the psychological causes for your hyperventilation should be addressed to prevent its recurrence.

### Associated symptoms

Other signs and symptoms may occur with shortness of breath and provide clues as to the origin of the problem. Swelling of the feet and legs (edema), abdominal bloating, or shortness of breath while lying down suggests severe congestive heart failure. If you have these symptoms, you should promptly see your doctor.

If your shortness of breath is associated with angina, the dyspnea may be related to coronary artery disease. Sudden onset of shortness of breath may be a clue to various possible problems, including a blood clot in the lungs, fluid in the pericardium (the sac that surrounds the heart), heart attack, or anxiety-induced hyperventilation.

### Other causes

Of course, shortness of breath can be related to problems with the heart, lungs, or lung circulation, including emphysema, chronic bronchitis, and pulmonary hypertension. In contrast to cardiac dyspnea, the dyspnea of chronic obstructive lung disease or emphysema often occurs when you are in a position that prevents your lungs from expanding, such as when you bend over to tie your shoes.

### Fatigue

Many people complain of a generalized sense of fatigue that is not necessarily associated with shortness of breath or actual muscle weakness. Although fatigue certainly affects your life and may make you worry about heart disease, it is rarely associated with heart disease unless you also have other, more specific symptoms. If you are tired when you awaken and stay tired all day, the cause is most likely not your heart.

Nevertheless, if you complain of fatigue, especially if it has developed over a short time, your doctor will search for an underlying cause, among which heart failure is one possibility. Other possibilities include a low red blood cell count (anemia), low thyroid activity (hypothyroidism), various infections, and a disordered sleep pattern. Although in most people with isolated fatigue, a specific cause cannot be identified, noncardiac causes need to be excluded. Your doctor will know how far to go with testing.

### Swelling (edema)

Swelling (edema) is the leakage of fluid from the bloodstream into the surrounding tissue, like coffee through a coffee filter. Edema can occur for several reasons, including congestive heart failure, obstruction of the veins, and kidney failure. In all these cases, the fluid tends to collect at the lowest points because gravity forces fluid out of the lowest blood vessels.

You may first notice swelling in the feet and ankles, especially after a long day of standing or sitting, such as during a long plane trip. Crossing your legs, which partially obstructs the flow of blood from your feet, may make the condition even worse. A mild amount of this type of edema may not mean that anything is wrong.

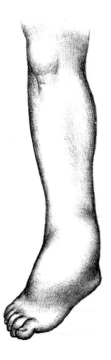

*Swollen feet and ankles indicate edema—leakage of fluid from the bloodstream into the surrounding tissues*

As the condition causing swelling worsens, the edema may ascend up to the thighs and even the torso. If you are confined to bed most of the time, the most significant edema may be in the lower back, again because gravity forces the fluid out at the lowest point.

In the early stages you may notice that your shoes and socks are leaving a more prominent impression than usual over your ankles and calves. As the edema becomes more severe, it is actually possible to indent the skin and leave an impression with your finger. (Doctors refer to this as "pitting edema.")

Edema may cause bloating of the stomach and poor digestion because of fluid in the walls of the intestinal tract. It can occur in the lungs (pulmonary edema), which is the basis for shortness of breath in congestive heart failure.

### Edema caused by heart disease

When edema is caused by a heart problem, it is because the heart cannot pump effectively. As the heart performs less and less efficiently as a pump, it becomes more and more of a dam. The fluid that was previously being pumped effectively through the bloodstream now collects behind the dam as though in a reservoir.

Tissues that are "sponge-like," such as the layers of tissue under the skin, the liver, and the lungs, are prone to "soak up" the excess fluid. Thus, people with decreased pumping function experience swelling of the legs, swelling and pain in the region of the liver under the right side of the rib cage, and shortness of breath from fluid in the lung air sacs.

Eventually, inadequate heart pumping decreases the amount of blood flow to your kidneys. Your kidneys respond as they would respond if you were losing blood through an injury—they "hold on to" fluid rather than excreting it as urine. Thus, you will gradually accumulate extra fluid in your body, which will show up as a weight gain. You can retain a lot of fluid—as much as 10 pounds in some people—before you can detect edema in the arms and legs from heart failure.

### Other causes

Another cause of edema is blockage of veins with a blood clot (thrombus). The most common site of vein blockage is in the legs (deep-vein thrombosis). Even after the blockage is resolved, damage to the veins from the blood clot and damage to the valves within the veins may cause an ongoing problem, causing edema in the legs and ankles.

Less common sites of vein blockage are the arms or under a collarbone. Blockage in these sites can cause swelling of the hand or arm. If the main vein that returns blood from the arms and head to the heart is blocked, both arms and the face may have swelling.

When your kidneys fail, your body cannot remove fluids, and the proteins that hold fluid in the bloodstream are reduced. Proteins can also be reduced in other diseases. When the proteins are low, fluid is more likely to leak from the bloodstream, as though through a sieve, into the surrounding tissues. Blockage of the lymphatics of the lower limbs and other conditions such as a lower level of thyroid hormone may also cause edema. An inherited trait for large calves and ankles (lipedema) is not related to a heart or circulatory problem, but may result in marked swelling of the lower extremities.

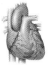

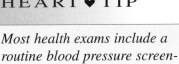

**HEALTHY HEART ♥ TIP**

*Most health exams include a routine blood pressure screening. But what really happens when your doctor performs this test?*

*After inflating a rubber cuff around your upper arm to compress a large artery, which momentarily stops the blood flow, your doctor releases the air and listens with a stethoscope. When the blood starts to pulse through the artery, it makes a sound, which continues until pressure in the artery exceeds pressure in the cuff.*

*Your doctor listens and watches the sphygmomanometer gauge, recording two measurements. The systolic pressure is the pressure of the blood flow when the heart beats (when the first sound is heard). The diastolic pressure is the pressure between heartbeats (when the last sound is heard).*

# Loss of consciousness (syncope)

One of the most alarming symptoms is sudden loss of consciousness (syncope). You lose consciousness when your brain does not get enough blood and oxygen. Heart disease can cause syncope if it reduces your heart's ability to pump enough blood to your brain. Heart problems that can cause syncope are related to rhythm disturbances, obstructed blood flow, a sudden fall in blood pressure, or severe heart muscle disease causing congestive heart failure.

### Pattern of syncope

Loss of consciousness can occur with or without warning. For example, it may be preceded by a sense of light-headedness (presyncope), sweating, nausea, palpitations, or a pale appearance, or it may occur suddenly with no warning whatsoever. It may occur during any activity, such as household chores or even while driving.

### Provocation and relief

In some cases, syncope is entirely unprovoked. In other situations, a factor or factors can be identified (such as fear, the sight of blood, stress, pain) that are related to the episode. Some unusual types of syncope occur during urination, defecation, or coughing.

What we typically think of as a simple faint (called vasovagal or vasodepressor syncope) can be resolved by lying down. After you lie flat, the blood flow to your brain is restored, and you regain consciousness. All people who faint should be placed in a lying-down position, preferably with their legs raised so their feet are 6 to 8 inches above the ground. This helps blood flow to the brain.

You may have occasionally felt light-headed from standing up quickly after lying down. In this case, the blood pressure control mechanism does not keep up with the need to pump blood "uphill" to the brain. Some people have particularly poor control mechanisms and may pass out or become very light-headed when they stand up—a condition called orthostatic hypotension.

### Duration

The duration of the loss of consciousness can be so short that you hardly know whether you lost consciousness. You just find yourself on the floor for no apparent reason. Little or no damage occurs to your brain from lack of oxygen if you quickly regain consciousness. Actually, the most serious risk is bodily injury from the fall itself.

Other episodes can be more sustained. The more prolonged the unconsciousness, the more likely that it will become permanent and that death (sudden cardiac death) will occur unless cardiopulmonary resuscitation (CPR) is initiated. Anyone who remains unconscious for more than several seconds requires on-the-spot evaluation to determine whether CPR is required. This involves answering the following questions: Is a pulse present? Is the person breathing?

*Frequency*

Syncope can happen once in a lifetime, or it can occur repeatedly. Your doctor will want to determine the likelihood of its happening again. If chances are high, a more aggressive approach to prevention is required.

*Associated symptoms*

Sweating, nausea, and pallor often precede fainting.

Palpitations leading up to a syncopal attack suggests an irregular, rapid, or unusually slow heartbeat as the cause of this spell. Sudden, unexpected loss of consciousness is usually related to a heartbeat abnormality that is so severe that the brain suddenly is deprived of its circulation and oxygen.

*Other causes*

Convulsions associated with loss of consciousness suggest a primary problem with the brain such as epilepsy, stroke, bleeding into the brain (cerebral hemorrhage), or tumor. However, convulsions can sometimes occur as a result of oxygen deprivation due to a heartbeat irregularity. Therefore, the presence of a seizure or convulsions does not rule out a heart-related basis for the episode.

Other noncardiac causes of syncope include a low blood sugar level (hypoglycemia), hyperventilation, and migraine headache.

## Light-headedness (presyncope)

Some people experience a sense that they will pass out but actually do not. The symptom is usually described as light-headedness and is referred to by doctors as presyncope or near-syncope.

## Light-headedness versus dizziness

Many people use the word "dizziness" to refer to light-headedness. However, a careful distinction must be drawn between light-headedness, which is the sensation that you are about to pass out, and true dizziness (vertigo), which is a sense that you or your surroundings are spinning or whirling around as if you just got off a merry-go-round.

Light-headedness may have many different causes, including heart rhythm abnormalities. The heart rhythm abnormalities responsible for the symptom of light-headedness usually are less severe and of shorter duration than those that lead to syncope.

*Other causes*

The symptom of vertigo suggests either an abnormality of the inner ear's balance mechanism or a brain-related problem. Occasionally, no specific cause for vertigo can be found. Sometimes obstructed arteries to the brain can cause a "drop attack" in which the individual may fall to the ground without losing consciousness. The heart is not the cause. A neurologic evaluation is required.

### Palpitations

Palpitations are an uncomfortable sensation of your heartbeat or a thumping sensation in your chest. The symptom may or may not be associated with heart disease, and it is the most common symptom in people who have an abnormal heartbeat (arrhythmia). However, as people age, extra beats (extrasystoles) tend to increase. These may be felt in people with otherwise apparently normal hearts.

Pertinent features of the thumping are the rate at which it is occurring, whether it is regular or irregular, whether there are individual thumps and how frequent and fast they are, or whether there are strings of rapid thumps. If the palpitations occur in series or strings, they may develop gradually and accelerate, or they may suddenly take off rapidly.

These characteristics are important in distinguishing the different types of heart rhythms that may be causing the palpitations, so you should describe them to the doctor with some care. A good descriptive technique is simply to tap out with your hand the pattern of palpitations as you recall it. Often, palpitations do not occur when you are in the doctor's office or being monitored, so an accurate description becomes all the more important.

### Provocation and relief

You should note whether anything provokes or stops the episodes. Some people find that certain types of rapid, regular palpitations can be interrupted by holding their breath or bearing down as though they were straining at a bowel movement (Valsalva maneuver). Sometimes a change in position will bring on or stop the palpitations.

Your doctor will want to know whether things such as exercise, eating, emotion, alcohol use, caffeine or medication have any effect on your palpitations.

### Associated symptoms

Key features helpful in diagnosing the cause of the palpitations and any underlying heart problems include the association of chest pain or pressure, light-headedness or syncope, or shortness of breath.

### Other causes

Although the apparent cause for thumping in the chest would seem to be the heartbeat, this is not always the case. Some people have a normal heart rate during their palpitations. Presumably, they are either anxious or experiencing chest wall twitching that is mistaken for the heartbeat.

## Palpitations: what to look for

- Fluttering in the chest
- Thumping in the chest
- Sensation of flip-flops
- Pounding in the chest
- Feeling the heartbeat in the neck
- Missing a heartbeat
- Skipping a heartbeat
- An extra heartbeat
- Racing in the chest
- Fast heartbeat

Some people describe "skipped heartbeats" or a sense of "vacancy" in the chest that quickly passes. The usual cause is early extra heartbeats (premature contractions or extrasystoles). After a beat comes a little too soon (premature), your heart waits a little longer before it beats again (this is called a compensatory pause). You may be sensing the beat after the pause because it tends to be a bit stronger than the average heartbeat.

## Limb pain or tiredness (claudication)

Leg pain can develop in the calves and feet with certain kinds of circulatory problems. Depending on the underlying cause, the pain may be crampy, sudden, and severe, or you may experience numbness. The location of the pain also depends on the location of the circulatory problem.

People with partially or totally blocked circulation to the legs have an insufficient oxygen supply to their muscles for the work that is required for walking. They typically complain of a sense of muscle fatigue, aching, or cramping when they use these muscles for walking, climbing stairs, or other activities.

### Provocation and relief

Depending on the degree of obstruction, the symptoms occur at various levels of exercise. The discomfort can usually be relieved by resting.

When the arteries become sufficiently blocked, the discomfort may persist and continue even if you rest. Simply elevating the legs may provoke pain if the circulation is blocked to a sufficient degree.

### Location

The site of the tiredness or cramping depends on where the artery is blocked. If the blockage is at the knee level or below, the discomfort may be confined to the foot, especially the instep. If the blockage is at the thigh level, the calf muscles are mainly affected. Blockage at the level of the groin or above results in cramping and fatigue in the muscles of the thigh and below, and the discomfort may also be felt in the buttocks.

### Other causes

Conditions other than arterial blockage can cause similar symptoms, and it is important for your doctor to make this distinction. For example, aching or pain in your legs that does not go away when you stop walking but actually requires you to sit or lie down may be caused by abnormalities that pinch your spinal cord. Venous insufficiency or varicose veins also may cause discomfort in your legs.

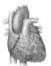

**HEALTHY HEART ♥ TIP**

*Hardened arteries is not just a problem of middle age. Atherosclerosis begins in childhood—decades before most people even think about heart-healthy lifestyles.*

*If your family has a history of heart disease, it's important to help your children reduce their future risks. Kids older than 2 should eat a low-fat diet of grains, vegetables and fruits. No more than 30 percent of total calories should be from fat.*

*Make sure your child gets enough exercise. Limit TV viewing to 2 hours daily. Routine blood pressure readings should begin around 3 or 4 years old. Doctors may prescribe special diets and physical activity for overweight children with high blood pressure.*

## Abnormal skin color

Skin color abnormalities can provide clues to underlying cardiovascular problems. Technically, skin color is a sign rather than a symptom. But if you notice a change in skin color, you may want to see your doctor.

Skin color in white people can vary from normal in several ways. It may be unusually white or pale (pallor), bluish (cyanosis), reddish (erythema), or black (necrosis, or tissue death).

### *Location*

Diffuse pallor may be caused by general depression of the circulation such as in shock or a fainting episode. Localized pallor is commonly caused by obstructed blood flow to a region that prevents adequate red (oxygenated) blood from reaching the skin. However, your skin may look red in areas where blood flow is abnormally abundant, as occurs in areas of an inflamed arthritic joint.

The location of skin color changes will lead your doctor to a conclusion about where the blood flow abnormality is and what blood vessels are involved. One classic constellation of symptoms is the occurrence of sequential white, blue, and red discoloration of one or more fingers, especially when exposed to cold. This is caused by spasm of the small vessels in the fingers and is referred to as "Raynaud's phenomenon." It may occur as an isolated "disease" in itself, or it may be associated with other illnesses.

### *Duration*

If the obstruction to blood flow is temporary, the pallor will disappear and the pinkish hue of the skin will return. However, if the blockage is prolonged, the skin may turn bluish (cyanotic) from lack of oxygen. If blood flow resumes after this stage, the skin may turn abnormally pinkish (erythematous). If the blockage is permanent and uncorrected, the tissue of the muscle and skin will eventually die and turn black (necrotic).

## Sores on the skin

Nonhealing sores on the skin (ulceration) of your lower limbs can also be a consequence of inadequate blood flow to the skin because an artery or vein is blocked or damaged. If tissue does not receive enough blood, it is vulnerable to even minor injury and infection. If the tissue does not receive enough oxygen and nutrients from the blood, it cannot heal.

Gangrene is the actual death of tissue. It usually appears as an area of black, shrunken skin in the region affected by the blockage.

*Associated symptoms*

Pain, paleness or other skin discolorations, and coldness may also accompany non-healing sores on the skin. Insufficient blood supply may cause inflammation and damage to the nerves (neuritis), resulting in burning, pain, and numbness. (These problems may occur in people with diabetes.)

## Shock

Shock is a constellation of severe symptoms and signs that imply a very serious circulatory abnormality. A person in shock has many problems:

- Very low blood pressure
- Confusion and altered consciousness (including possible unconsciousness)
- Generalized pallor and cold, clammy skin
- Evidence of malfunction of other organs because they are not getting enough blood
- Poor breathing function
- Low urine formation and inability to remove waste products

Shock can have various causes, including heart attack, trauma, hemorrhage, and overwhelming infection. If your heart's ability to meet your body's needs is limited, blood flow is directed to certain vital organs (the heart and the brain) at the expense of other organs such as skin, muscle, kidneys, and liver.

The constellation of symptoms from shock requires an emergency response by a medical team, including intravenous medication and fluids, help with breathing, blood transfusions if necessary, and urgent searching for the underlying cause so that it can be corrected if possible.

## Sudden change in vision, strength, coordination, speech, or sensation

A particular combination of symptoms indicates inadequate supply of blood to the brain. Depending on the duration of the symptoms, they may indicate a stroke or a transient ischemic attack (TIA). Specifically, the symptoms can include:

- Weakness, tingling, numbness, or paralysis typically involving one side of the body (or one limb or side of the face). Both sides of the body may be affected
- Vision loss or double vision
- Speech difficulty, slurred speech
- Incoordination, dizziness, severe headache

Two key factors that distinguish these symptoms from others are their rapid onset and their duration. Vision, speech, or sensation deteriorates over minutes to hours. If the episode lasts only a few minutes, it is classified as a TIA. The symptoms come on rapidly and last briefly, and then you return to normal. TIAs indicate a temporary deficiency of blood supply to the brain. TIAs are regarded as a warning

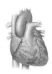

that a stroke may occur in the not-too-distant future. They warrant immediate evaluation by a doctor so that appropriate treatment can be started as soon as possible.

Another warning sign of stroke is amaurosis fugax. This is a temporary visual defect caused by inadequate blood flow to the eye. It seems as if a curtain is descending or rising over your field of vision, usually in one eye. Again, such a symptom requires immediate medical evaluation.

The symptoms of a stroke can be extremely varied because they correspond to the area of the brain that has been injured because of inadequate blood supply. In some cases, blood can be supplied to the injured area by way of another artery. This may explain, in part, the partial recovery after some strokes.

# Chapter
# 7

# Types of heart disease

Heart disease can affect any and all parts of your cardiovascular system—the myocardium, the valves, the coronary arteries, the conduction system, arteries and veins, and the pericardium. Disease in any of these areas may be called heart (or cardiovascular) disease.

The process of diagnosing heart disease is complicated. To begin with, more than one type of cardiovascular disease or problem can occur at the same time in the same person. In fact, this is often the case. However, one problem may overshadow the other. This problem may be the most direct cause of symptoms, or it may have the greatest effect on your overall health and life span.

When more than one problem occurs, the conditions can sometimes be related to a single underlying cause. For example, "hardening of the arteries" due to cholesterol plaque deposits (atherosclerosis) can occur in your coronary arteries (arteries to the heart muscle itself), carotid arteries (arteries carrying blood to the brain), aorta (the main artery leading from the heart), and leg arteries. Thus, you could have stroke (brain injury), and claudication (limb pain or tiredness), all of which are caused by insufficient blood flow due to atherosclerosis.

Knowing that certain problems occur, doctors must sometimes piece together evidence of associated disease even if you have only one symptom or evidence of only one problem. Suppose, for example, that your doctor has detected an abdominal aortic aneurysm and recommends an operation to repair it. Experience has shown that coronary artery disease is present in more than 50 percent of people with aortic aneurysms, even if it is not causing symptoms of angina. Because coronary artery disease might make the aneurysm operation risky, your doctor may recommend tests to see whether serious coronary artery disease is present. Looking for and treating the coronary artery disease first make the preparation for the aneurysm less risky and may also be important for long-term life expectancy once the aneurysm has been repaired.

Another complexity of diagnosis is that one type of heart disease can actually cause another, which in turn may become the main problem. For example, coronary artery disease can cause a heart attack, which may damage enough heart muscle that the heart becomes too weak to pump efficiently. After that, you may have no further symptoms directly from the coronary arteries (such as angina), but you may experience symptoms from the weak pumping of the ventricles (such as congestive heart failure).

As another example of one kind of heart disease causing another, a baby can be born with a hole in the heart wall separating the right and left ventricles (a ventricular septal defect). High blood pressure in the arteries to the lung (pulmonary hypertension) may develop if the defect is large enough and is not closed soon enough by an operation. Pulmonary hypertension may cause shortness of breath (dyspnea) and blue discoloration of the skin (cyanosis). Thus, dyspnea and cyanosis caused by lack of oxygen in the bloodstream become the prominent symptoms. In some cases, they may be the first signs of the original defect.

This section describes the gamut of things that can go wrong in each part of the cardiovascular system. Keep in mind that the problems can be—and often are—interrelated.

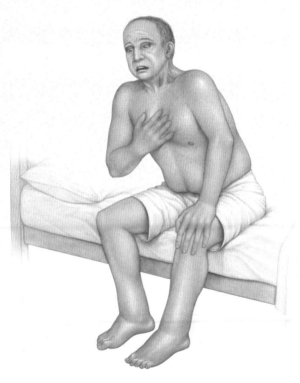

*See your doctor if you notice any of the following signs and symptoms of congestive heart failure:*

- *Fatigue, weakness and inability to exert yourself*
- *Shortness of breath soon after exertion begins*
- *Shortness of breath that awakens you from sleep*
- *Swelling in your legs, ankles or feet*
- *Rapid weight gain (such as a pound a day for three consecutive days)*
- *Swollen (distended) neck veins*

## Heart failure

The term "heart failure" is frightening, and heart failure is a serious problem, but it does not mean that the heart is not working at all. Heart failure is not a specific disease. It is a convenient way of describing a group of symptoms caused by diseases in which the heart is unable to circulate enough blood to meet the body's requirements. Heart failure has various degrees of severity, depending on what the problem is and how long the problem has existed.

Unfortunately, heart failure is common and on the increase, affecting 2 or 3 of every 100 people in the United States, or more than 4 million people. The impact of such widespread illness is enormous. Aside from suffering due to the symptoms, each year 35 percent of all people with heart failure require hospitalization.

Heart failure is the most common reason for hospitalization in people older than 65 years. Obviously, the expense to the nation is considerable. In 1999, heart failure cost the health care system $183 billion. Despite advanced medical care, 15 percent of all people with heart failure die within 1 year, and up to 50 percent of those with advanced symptoms die within 1 year.

## Causes of heart failure

Heart failure can be caused by anything that impairs the heart's ability to pump effectively, including congenital heart disease, valvular disease, and heart muscle disease (such as from a heart attack). These diseases are not the same as heart failure but are the result. You can have congenital heart disease, problems with the valves, or a heart attack and not have heart failure. But if one of these problems prevents your heart from pumping enough blood to your body, you are said to have heart failure.

Heart failure refers to the symptoms that occur when the heart muscle is weakened or when the workload is too great for the heart muscle to perform its task of pumping enough blood to meet the demands of the body. In either case, two things happen:

1. Your heart cannot pump enough blood to provide tissues with the nutrition, oxygen and waste removal functions they need.

2. Back pressure builds in your veins because your heart does not efficiently pump blood through the arteries. In other words, as your heart becomes less and less a pump, it becomes more and more a dam.

## Symptoms of heart failure

These two consequences of inadequate pumping function lead to all of the symptoms associated with heart failure: shortness of breath (dyspnea) and fatigue with exertion; shortness of breath at rest and especially when lying down (orthopnea) because of fluid accumulation in the lungs; swelling or accumulation of fluid in the feet, legs, and trunk; and general fatigue. Because many of the symptoms of heart failure are caused by congestion of the tissues and lungs with fluid, it is often called congestive heart failure.

With mild heart failure, you may not have any symptoms while sitting and resting. You may not be short of breath until you engage in physical activity. With severe heart failure, you may experience distress even at rest, including shortness of breath, pale skin color, coolness in the arms and legs, and blue color of the lips, fingers, and toes (cyanosis). These symptoms may become worse when you lie down.

With severe heart failure, you are also prone to various irregular heart rhythms and may experience palpitations or syncope. Another symptom with advanced heart failure may be what is termed "Cheyne-Stokes" respiration, which is characterized by alternating periods of slow breathing with pauses and periods of rapid, deep breathing.

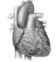

**HEALTHY HEART ♥ TIP**

*You've heard about the dangers of high blood pressure (hypertension). What about low blood pressure (hypotension)?*

*Most often lower is better—as long as you feel good. But if you're fainting, your systolic pressure (the top number in your blood pressure reading) may be too low. Aggressive high blood pressure treatment or a malfunction of your nervous system can cause hypotension. A very low diastolic pressure (the bottom number) may indicate a faulty heart valve or conditions that can lead to excessive blood flow through your arteries.*

*If your blood pressure drops too low, you may go into shock, indicated by confusion, clammy skin, poor breathing, low urine output and malfunctioning of other organs. Shock should be treated as a medical emergency.*

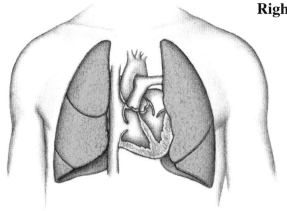

## Right and left heart failure

You may also hear doctors refer to right heart failure or left heart failure, depending on which side of the heart is most severely affected. In left heart failure, blood flow to the body is decreased and fluid accumulates in the lungs. These conditions develop because the left side of the heart becomes more like a dam, and the reservoir behind it is mainly the lungs. The congestion in the lungs is responsible for the sensation of breathlessness that is common in congestive heart failure.

Right heart failure also causes decreased blood flow, but the reservoir for the right side of the heart is mainly the rest of the body, so swelling occurs in the legs and abdominal organs, including the liver. Right heart failure can cause pain on the upper right side of the abdomen from liver engorgement, as well as loss of appetite, nausea, and bloating.

*If the left side of the heart functions inadequately as a pump, back pressure leads to congestion (**red**) of the lungs. Fluid accumulates in the lung tissue and air sacs, making breathing more difficult.*

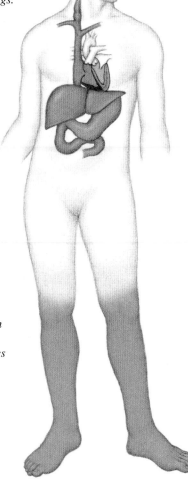

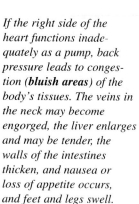

*If the right side of the heart functions inadequately as a pump, back pressure leads to congestion (**bluish areas**) of the body's tissues. The veins in the neck may become engorged, the liver enlarges and may be tender, the walls of the intestines thicken, and nausea or loss of appetite occurs, and feet and legs swell.*

## Low output failure

In some people the consequences of heart failure are related to inadequate blood flow rather than to accumulation of fluid (congestion). Doctors often refer to this as low output failure.

- If your kidneys do not receive enough blood flow, they do not produce enough urine; excess fluid and water accumulate in your body. This condition increases the swelling (edema).

- If your muscles do not receive enough blood flow, your endurance is reduced. The decreased endurance leads to early fatigue when you exert yourself.

- If your brain does not receive enough blood flow, you may become light-headed or confused.

## Heart failure due to cardiomyopathy

Loss of the pumping efficiency of the heart has many causes. These include a mechanical problem (congenital or valvular), prolonged high blood pressure (which increases the work load on the heart), damaged sections of muscle tissue in the heart from coronary artery disease (heart attack), and diseases directly affecting the entire heart muscle (cardiomyopathy).

Cardiomyopathy (cardio means "heart," myo means "muscle," pathy means "disease") is a disease of heart muscle. Cardiomyopathy can be further described by its cause (if known) or by the type of pumping defect that is present. For example, cardiomyopathy caused by alcohol use is called alcoholic cardiomyopathy. Although cardiomyopathy can be caused by a virus, in many cases the cause cannot be determined and the condition is then referred to as idiopathic cardiomyopathy (idiopathic means "self-diseased," that is, there's no identifiable cause).

Deaths from cardiomyopathy constitute about 1 percent of heart disease deaths in the United States. In general, men and blacks have the highest rates of death from cardiomyopathy.

## Types of cardiomyopathy

Cardiomyopathy is different from many other heart disorders. Although uncommon, affecting perhaps 50,000 Americans annually, the condition is a leading reason for heart transplantation. In all forms of cardiomyopathy, the heart rhythm may be disturbed, leading to irregular heartbeats or arrhythmia.

There are three basic types of cardiomyopathy, distinguished by the kind of muscle problem involved:

1. Dilated cardiomyopathy, in which the heart muscle becomes weak and the heart chambers subsequently enlarge (dilate). Dilated cardiomyopathy is the most common form. It occurs most often in middle-aged people, and more often in men than women. Still, the disease has been diagnosed in individuals of all ages, including children.

2. Hypertrophic (hyper means "over," trophic means "nourishment") cardiomyopathy, in which the heart muscle itself is much thicker than normal.

3. Restrictive cardiomyopathy, in which the heart becomes stiff and cannot fill efficiently during diastole, the period of the heartbeat when the chambers fill with blood.

### Dilated cardiomyopathy (weakened squeezing capacity)

*Charles is a 42-year-old commercial artist who recalls missing 2 days of work 4 months ago because of a "bad cold" with a runny nose, sore throat, and cough. Although these symptoms subsided, he never felt back to normal because he tended to be tired all the time. Six weeks ago he felt*

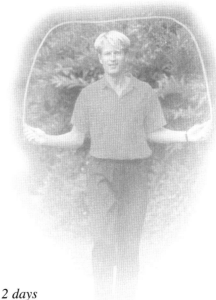

**Common causes of heart failure**

Coronary artery disease

Disease of the heart muscle (cardiomyopathy)

High blood pressure (hypertension)

Valvular heart disease

*distinctly short-winded during a softball game at a company picnic; he stopped playing early so he could sit and catch his breath. Since then he has noted shortness of breath when climbing one flight of stairs. One week ago he began waking up in the middle of the night feeling breathless, which he found he could minimize by propping himself up on three pillows. For the past 2 days his ankles have been conspicuously swollen. He was brought to the emergency room because he awoke gasping from an after-dinner nap and was unable to catch his breath. The doctor told him and his wife that his lungs are filled with fluid and his heart is enlarged. He was given an intravenous injection of a diuretic to increase elimination of fluid by the kidneys and was admitted to the hospital for evaluation.*

Dilated cardiomyopathy refers to overall enlargement (dilatation) of the heart chambers, especially the ventricles. Although this enlargement is a key part of dilated cardiomyopathy, it is not the initial problem but rather the heart's own response to a weakness of heart muscle and poor pumping ability. The weakness of the heart muscle in this condition is generalized ("global"); all parts of the myocardium are affected about equally. Enlargement of the heart is the heart's way of trying to compensate for the weakness of its muscle. This is called a compensatory mechanism.

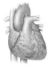

## HEALTHY HEART ♥ TIP

*Black people are at a disadvantage when it comes to high blood pressure (hypertension). For blacks, this disorder develops earlier in life and results in a higher heart disease mortality rate. They also have a higher rate of stroke-related deaths and 5 times the rate of hypertension-related, end-stage kidney disease.*

*That's why it's critical to have regular blood pressure checks. When treated early enough, black people can experience the same blood pressure declines as white people who receive the same treatment.*

If the heart muscle is weak, it is unable to pump out the same portion of blood that it could at normal strength. But our bodies have an impressive capability of adjusting to changes. Rather than simply "accepting" the limitations of decreased pumping ability, the heart and other organs of the body undergo compensatory changes to try to maximize their efforts.

Think of the heart chambers expanding and contracting like a soft plastic bottle being squeezed while being held under water. If your grip has become weakened, you cannot squeeze very much of the water out. Let's say that at normal strength you could squeeze out 60 percent of the water that flowed into the bottle when you let it expand under water. Similarly, a heart may pump out 60 percent of the blood it contained at the end of diastole.

With your weakened grip, however, you may be able to squeeze out only 20 percent of the water in the bottle. Likewise, weakened heart muscle may be able to pump only 20 percent of the blood it contains. Obviously, the volume of blood being pumped out of the heart with each beat would be much less.

However, if you got a bigger bottle, it would hold more water. Consequently, even with your weakened grip, if you squeezed out 20 percent of the water, that would be greater total volume than 20 percent of the smaller bottle.

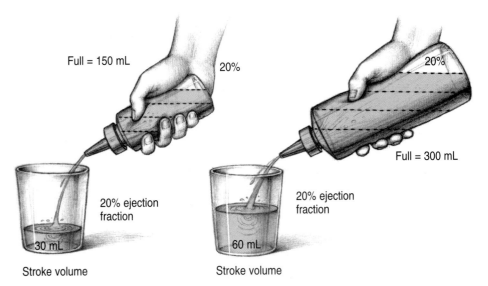

Full = 150 mL

20%

20%

Full = 300 mL

20% ejection
fraction

20% ejection
fraction

30 mL

60 mL

Stroke volume

Stroke volume

*The heart adapts to weakened pumping action by enlarging. The 150 mL squeeze bottle (**left**)*
*can squeeze only 20 percent of its fluid out. That's much less than the normal amount of about*
*60 percent. Thus its stroke volume is only 30 mL (mL, milliliters). The larger squeeze bottle holds*
*300 mL, so even with a reduced ejection fraction of 20 percent, it produces a stroke volume of 60*
*mL, which is an improvement.*

The same concept applies when the heart enlarges. There is a much larger
volume of blood in the chambers during diastole. Even if the heart pumps out only
20 percent of the blood it contains, the total volume pumped is larger.

Our bodies have other compensatory mechanisms, too. It is one of the basic
"laws of the heart" that the more you stretch heart muscle (up to a limit), the more
forcefully it will squeeze on the next beat (this is also known as Starling's law, after
one of its discoverers). When the heart enlarges, it stretches more to increase the
pumping force.

Other organs also attempt to compensate for a weak heart muscle. The kidneys
and various glands make hormones that increase the volume of blood and fluid.
Maintaining a high volume of blood in the heart is important for stretching the heart
muscle to maintain the amount of blood that is pumped with each stroke.

The heart rate may also increase in response to signals from your nervous
system. The heart tries to maintain its output by pumping faster.

However, all of these compensatory mechanisms can work only up to a point.
They eventually are unable to keep up as the heart increasingly weakens. Ironically,
in severe cardiomyopathy, the effects of the compensatory mechanisms lead to
many of the problems of heart failure.

For example, the hormonal and kidney adjustments that occur, to maintain or
increase blood and fluid volume, account in large part for the swelling in the legs
and abdomen and for the fluid in the lungs in heart failure. Elevated levels of certain
hormones, such as epinephrine (adrenaline), can cause constriction of blood vessels.

## Conditions that can lead to dilated cardiomyopathy

- High blood pressure
- Infections
- Toxic agents, especially alcohol and certain cancer treating drugs
- Heart valve defects
- Chronic (sustained) fast heart rate
- Nutritional deficiency
- Abnormalities of metabolism
- Blood diseases
- Neurologic disorders
- Pregnancy
- Hereditary (genetic) tendency
- Unknown (idiopathic) conditions

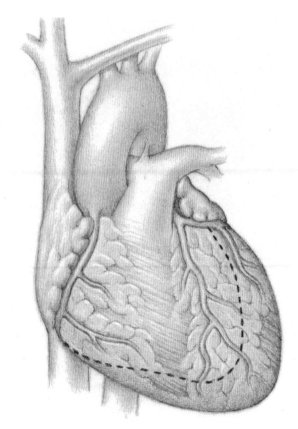

*Dotted lines indicate size of a normal heart. Dilated cardiomyopathy is an overall enlargement (dilation) of the heart chambers, especially the ventricles. The enlargement is the heart's response to a weakness of heart muscle and poor pumping ability.*

This increases the resistance and pressure against which the weakened heart must pump.

Ultimately, much of the treatment for heart failure may be to reverse some of the effects of these compensatory mechanisms.

Causes of dilated cardiomyopathy
**Idiopathic.** A major group of dilated cardiomyopathies are those that are caused by unknown factors. These are called idiopathic dilated cardiomyopathies. Many experts believe these idiopathic types are due to a viral infection of the heart (perhaps one that occurred in the past and is no longer detectable) that has left the heart weakened. Idiopathic dilated cardiomyopathy may occur at any age. It occurs more often in blacks than in whites, and in men more often than in women. Rarely, this type of cardiomyopathy develops in a woman during pregnancy and persists even afterward.

A key aspect of current research deals with the possibility that dilated cardiomyopathy is related to familial or genetic factors. Perhaps there is a genetic tendency toward the development of a cardiomyopathy after a viral infection, but this remains to be determined by current research.

**Toxins and drugs.** Many toxic substances can cause weakening of the heart muscle. Alcohol has a direct suppressant effect on the heart, and dilated cardiomyopathy can be caused by chronic, excessive consumption of alcohol, particularly in combination with dietary deficiencies. Toxins such as cobalt, which was once used in beers, for instance, may cause dilated cardiomyopathy. Drugs which are used to treat a different medical condition can also damage the heart and produce dilated cardiomyopathy. Examples include doxorubicin and daunorubicin, which are both used to treat cancer.

**Myocarditis.** Occasionally, a heart biopsy may show inflammation of the heart muscle, or myocarditis (itis means "inflammation"). Myocarditis is probably due to an active viral infection.

Signs and symptoms of myocarditis include fever, vague chest pain, joint pain, and an abnormally rapid heart rate. A person with myocarditis may improve as the inflammation goes away, but it is also possible that the myocarditis will leave the heart in a severely weakened condition.

One of the main goals of your doctor, of course, is to try to promote the healing of myocarditis successfully, and the means of doing this most effectively are still under careful study.

**Coronary artery disease.** Although coronary artery disease is the most common cause of weakened heart pumping, enlargement of the ventricles, and symptoms of heart failure, it does not cause a true dilated cardiomyopathy. Muscle damage resulting from coronary artery disease, such as heart attacks, sometimes referred to as "ischemic cardiomyopathy," should not be confused with dilated "congestive" cardiomyopathy, which is a form of nonischemic cardiomyopathy. Rather than causing generalized global damage of all heart muscle cells, coronary artery disease reduces the blood and oxygen supply to areas of heart muscle (myocardial ischemia) and damages zones of the heart. This regional damage then leads to inefficient pumping. The result is similar to what occurs in dilated cardiomyopathy, so some doctors refer to it as "ischemic cardiomyopathy" (related to an insufficient blood supply).

The most common problem occurs when the heart muscle is scarred and the heart is dilated because of a previous heart attack or heart attacks, in which case the damage is irreversible. However, less commonly, the weakened heart muscle is due to constant poor circulation to the heart without heart attacks; then there is some chance that pumping function can be improved if circulation is restored. This condition of reduced pumping function has been given the name " hibernating myocardium." Obviously, because one condition is reversible and the other is not, it is important to distinguish between the two. This may require sophisticated tests.

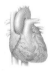

**HEALTHY HEART ♥ TIP**

*As many as 5 million to 7 million Americans have diabetes but don't realize it—which gives them at least double the risk for heart disease as everyone else. Are you among them?*

*Signs of type I diabetes usually appear suddenly:*

- *Thirstier than usual*
- *Increased amount and frequency of urination*
- *Weight loss despite increased appetite*
- *Exhaustion*

*Signs of type II diabetes generally develop gradually and may be subtle. They can include any of the above (except weight loss) and:*

- *Recurrent or slow-to-heal infections, especially vaginitis, skin or gum infections, or bladder infections*
- *Blurry vision*
- *Tingling or numbness in the hands or feet*

Symptoms of dilated cardiomyopathy. In some people, symptoms of dilated cardiomyopathy may develop gradually over months or years. In others, symptoms appear suddenly after a respiratory or flu-like illness.

You may get short of breath with activity, when you lie down, or during the night when you are sleeping. Your legs may swell, and you may have abdominal pain from congestion in your liver. About 10 percent of people with dilated cardiomyopathy have chest pain. In short, dilated cardiomyopathy causes the constellation of symptoms referred to as heart failure. In advanced stages, some people develop irregular heartbeats, which can be serious and even life-threatening.

How serious is dilated cardiomyopathy? In some studies, 50 percent of deaths due to dilated cardiomyopathy occurred within 2 years of diagnosis. But more recent studies are more encouraging. Some people have a milder form of the disease and can live for many years. Newer drugs have resulted in an improved outlook and quality of life.

When symptoms appear, the condition may be tentatively diagnosed by a physical examination and medical history. But a firm diagnosis usually requires an electrocardiogram and some measurement of left ventricular contraction by an echocardiogram or a radionuclide ventriculogram. Cardiac catheterization or a stress test may be required to exclude heart failure due to a blockage of the coronary artery.

### Hypertrophic cardiomyopathy (overgrowth of heart muscle)

*Rick is a 35-year-old teacher who has noticed the general development of breathlessness and chest heaviness during exertion. There is a family history of sudden death at age 45 in one of his uncles. His brother (age 26) is apparently healthy. At first these symptoms were very vague, so he's not sure when they started, although he thinks that they may have developed two years ago and that there has been some progression of severity during the last few months. Yesterday, he ran upstairs from his basement to answer the doorbell; when he reached the top of the stairs and opened the door, he almost passed out and had to lie down. After several minutes he felt better and was able to resume his normal activity.*

Hypertrophic cardiomyopathy is an overgrowth of heart muscle that causes symptoms by impeding blood flow both into and out of the heart. It's the second most common form of heart muscle disease. Although rare (occurring in no more than 0.2 percent of the U.S. population), it can affect men and women of all ages. Symptoms can appear in childhood or adulthood. This disease has been the focus of much medical interest due to advances in molecular genetics that have enabled physicians to define the hereditary nature of the disease.

*Below left: Normal heart. **Below right:** A heart with hypertrophic obstructive cardiomyopathy (previously called idiopathic hypertrophic subaortic stenosis). The wall (ventricular septum) between the left and right ventricles is thickened. The thickening makes the heart stiffer, so it relaxes less efficiently to let blood enter the ventricle. When the ventricle squeezes, the bulge may partially block blood flow through the aortic valve.*

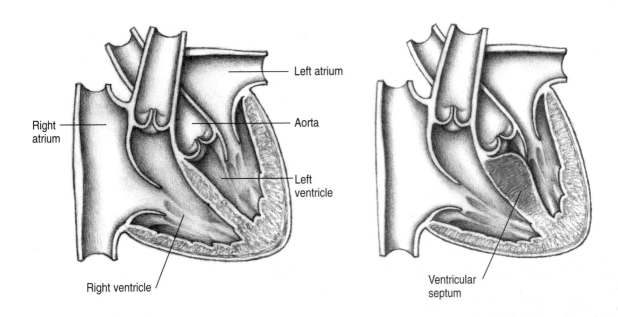

Left atrium

Aorta

Right atrium

Left ventricle

Right ventricle

Ventricular septum

Hypertrophic cardiomyopathy results from abnormal thickening of the heart wall for unknown reasons. The thickening can occur in several places throughout the ventricles. Most commonly it occurs in the septum between the two ventricles just beneath the aortic valve. The septum may be $1^1/_2$ or more times as thick as the outer wall of the heart. With a thicker muscle wall, the cavity of the ventricle may be smaller. Thus, the volume of blood in the ventricle may be normal or decreased.

The thicker wall develops abnormal relaxation, which in turn interferes with filling of the ventricle. The pump, therefore, despite normal strength, is unable to efficiently supply the circulation because it is inadequately "primed."

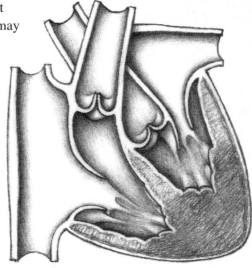

*Apical hypertrophic obstructive cardiomyopathy, yet another form of hypertrophic cardiomyopathy, is an excessive wall thickening (hypertrophy) limited to the tips of the ventricles.*

Hypertrophic cardiomyopathy was previously called idiopathic hypertrophic subaortic (beneath the aorta) stenosis, abbreviated IHSS. This overgrowth creates a bulge that protrudes into the ventricular chamber and impedes the flow of blood from your heart to the aorta and the rest of your body.

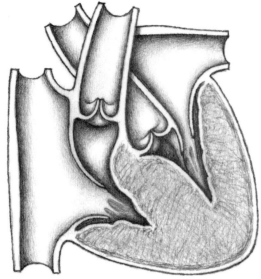

When this obstruction is present, the cardiomyopathy is also called hypertrophic obstructive cardiomyopathy (HOCM). In this condition, the problem is not that the heart muscle is weak but that the overgrown heart muscle impedes the flow of blood through and out of the heart. The thickened wall cannot relax normally, which causes an impairment in chamber filling.

If the example of the plastic bottle is used, the sides of the bottle have thickened, especially near the opening. The thickening decreases the space inside the bottle and gets in the way of the opening.

With HOCM, one of the leaflets of the mitral valve between the left atrium and the left ventricle moves forward during contraction, and this, along with the thicker septum between the ventricles, obstructs blood flow. Ironically, the obstruction to blood flow may worsen the harder the heart squeezes, because the thickened septum protrudes even farther into the pathway of the blood trying to flow out of the heart.

*Hypertrophy can also be widespread throughout the muscle of the ventricle. This type of condition may develop as a result of uncontrolled high blood pressure. High blood pressure is like weight-lifting for the heart—it results in bigger muscle. Unfortunately, hypertrophied heart muscle is less, rather than more, efficient. The result is that the ventricles do not fill with as much blood as they should for the next contraction.*

Hypertrophic cardiomyopathy does not always affect the area beneath the aortic valve. Sometimes the condition occurs down near the apex (tip) of the heart, and in other individuals the overgrowth is distributed more or less evenly throughout the heart muscle. These cases can be likened to the plastic walls of the bottle becoming thickened all over and making squeezing less effective. In those situations, the problem is not due to obstruction. The thickened muscle is simply inefficient at pumping and especially at relaxing. The blood flow can decrease because of this, and heart rhythms are a problem as well.

Causes of hypertrophic cardiomyopathy. True hypertrophic cardiomyopathy is of unknown cause (idiopathic). But genetic research is now pointing to an inherited change (mutation) in a specific gene as a common cause.

Mutations occur in genes that code for particular proteins making up the contractile apparatus of the heart muscle. It is likely that additional genetic mutations will be discovered in the near future and this will be particularly helpful in advising couples in family planning.

Better understanding of genetic mutations and the function of the genes involved will likely enable physicians to recognize the primary cause of hypertrophic cardiomyopathy in the near future.

Doctors also need to understand more clearly the role of nongenetic influences such as high blood pressure, physical activity, and body mass, which may play a role in determining who will or will not develop hypertrophic cardiomyopathy.

Similar conditions can arise from a long history of high blood pressure leading to overgrowth of heart muscle. The heart muscle builds up the same way a weight-lifter builds up the biceps with repeated weight-lifting, because high blood pressure imposes a high work load on the heart muscle. In a sense, the heart muscle is lifting a heavy load for a long time. Unfortunately, overgrowth of the heart muscle is not conducive to increased efficiency. Valve problems especially can lead to overgrowth (hypertrophy) of heart muscle.

Symptoms of hypertrophic cardiomyopathy. The three major symptoms of hypertrophic cardiomyopathy are shortness of breath, chest pain, and loss of consciousness with exertion, along with other symptoms of heart failure, including shortness of breath while lying down and palpitations. Some people may die suddenly.

Now that echocardiography is commonly performed, many cases of hypertrophic cardiomyopathy are being diagnosed, even when the condition is not causing symptoms.

Chest pain (angina) is a common symptom of hypertrophic cardiomyopathy; about three quarters of people with hypertrophic cardiomyopathy experience it. The angina is caused when the normal coronary arteries cannot provide the enlarged heart muscle with enough oxygen. Some people have chest pain that lasts longer than typical angina, and it often happens right after, not during, exercise.

Shortness of breath is present at some point in about 9 of 10 people with symptomatic hypertrophic cardiomyopathy.

Some people with hypertrophic cardiomyopathy experience light-headedness or loss of consciousness, because blood flow is so severely impaired that it is not sufficient for the rest of the body, including the brain. When you exert yourself, this is especially likely to happen. During exercise, the heart contracts harder and the overgrown bulge protrudes even farther into the already narrowed pathway.

The condition can be made even worse if the mitral valve contributes to the blocking action itself or allows blood to leak backward because of the high pressure in the ventricle. Some people with hypertrophic cardiomyopathy have syncope or sudden cardiac death because they are prone to heart rhythm abnormalities.

HEALTHY HEART ♥ TIP

*Long-distance travel can wreak havoc on your body, particularly when you have to sit nearly motionless for hours on an airplane. Here are some tips to keep from developing potentially dangerous blood clots:*

- *Wear comfortable, loose clothing and sensible shoes.*
- *Frequently stretch your legs, even while sitting.*
- *Do not cross your legs.*
- *Regularly squeeze and release the muscles of your stomach and buttocks.*
- *Periodically take slow, deep breaths.*
- *Get out of your seat and walk the aisle at least once an hour.*
- *Take aspirin if it's safe and appropriate for you.*
- *If you've had problems in the past, wear elastic support stockings.*
- *Avoid alcohol.*
- *Stay hydrated. Drink at least 1 glass or bottle of water each hour. By drinking you will also need to get up to urinate, which is good for your leg veins.*

Who is affected by hypertrophic cardiomyopathy? Hypertrophic cardiomyopathy can occasionally run in families. Symptoms of hypertrophic cardiomyopathy may occur at any age, but most start in the teens and 20s. In most people with hypertrophic cardiomyopathy who develop symptoms, the symptoms develop by age 35. Recently, families have been identified in whom the disease only becomes clinically evident when they reach their 50s.

Hypertrophic cardiomyopathy is present in 2 percent to 6 percent of people with cardiomyopathy and is more common in men than women and in blacks than whites.

**How serious is hypertrophic cardiomyopathy?** Most people with this condition do very well and can continue with a normal lifestyle. But the outlook does vary among individuals. You may have no symptoms at all or you could experience chest pain, shortness of breath and blackout attacks. Symptoms may appear gradually during teen years, or may appear later in life. Sudden death is rare.

Your doctor may prescribe a medication to relax your heart muscle. Betablockers can slow the pumping action of your heart. Calcium channel blockers relax the heart and reduce blood pressure. Antiarrhythmic drugs can help remedy irregular heart rhythms. Diuretics also may be used. Medications are mainly helpful in controlling symptoms and improving your lifestyle.

Surgery may also be an option. Your surgeon may remove a portion of the thickened septum to improve your heart's action. This procedure is called a myectomy.

Other treatments under investigation include placement of a pacemaker and the use of alcohol injection by means of a catheter that is threaded into a branch of the coronary artery supplying blood to the obstructive septum. Long-term results of these new procedures are not known. Genetic testing may also be an option some day in view of the fact that the disease is often inherited.

If you have hypertrophic cardiomyopathy, follow precautions for prevention of bacterial endocarditis (see page 71). Also, avoid nonprescription cold medications and drugs such as cocaine and methamphetamine, which can have disastrous consequences.

See your physician for instructions before you begin an exercise program, and avoid strenuous activity, such as competitive sports. Also, shun hot tubs and saunas.

### Restrictive cardiomyopathy (stiffness of the heart)

The least common type of cardiomyopathy, and probably the least understood, is restrictive cardiomyopathy. Restrictive cardiomyopathy is rare in the United States and in other industrial nations, but in certain parts of the world (Central Africa, for example) it is common.

Swelling of the legs caused by fluid retention is a particularly prominent and troublesome symptom. In this condition, the heart muscle is too stiff to allow enough blood in from the pulmonary veins. Blood has to get into the heart before it can be pumped out to the body. The heart cannot pump out blood that it does not receive.

In restrictive cardiomyopathy, filling of the ventricle is rapid but ends abruptly when the stiff heart stops expanding. As mentioned, restricted "inflow" is also part of the problem of hypertrophic cardiomyopathy in some people, because thick muscle does not relax as well as normal muscle.

Because the inflow of blood into the heart is compromised in restrictive cardiomyopathy, symptoms of heart failure can ensue.

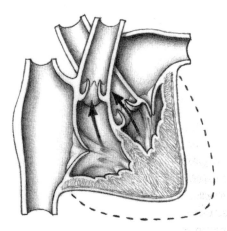 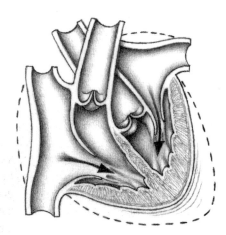

*Restrictive heart muscle disease results in problems during the relaxing phase of the heartbeat. The broken lines show how the heart should look when it is fully relaxed in diastole. During contraction (**left**), the heart squeezes normally. But during diastole (**right**), it does not relax efficiently. The result is that the ventricles do not fill with as much blood as they should for the next contraction.*

Causes of restrictive cardiomyopathy. In most cases, purely restrictive cardiomyopathy does not have a well-recognized cause, so it is idiopathic. But any condition that can cause extensive scarring in the myocardium or thickening of the endocardium can restrict filling of the ventricles. For example, your heart may have reactions to radiation or drugs for cancer, or to the cancer itself, which may result in stiffening of the muscle. Diseases that affect connective tissue throughout the body, such as progressive systemic sclerosis (scleroderma) and pseudoxanthoma elasticum, may also cause fibrosis or stiffening.

**Amyloidosis.** A recognized cause of restrictive cardiomyopathy is deposits of abnormal material into the heart muscle. One example of this is the condition known as amyloidosis, in which certain blood cells produce excessive protein material that deposits in the tissues. Sometimes the heart is the main tissue affected, and in this case the condition is called cardiac amyloidosis. In other conditions the heart is only one of several organs involved, including the kidneys, liver, skin, blood vessels, and intestinal tract. Amyloidosis can also lead to the dilated form of cardiomyopathy. Medical treatment for amyloidosis is not very effective.

**Hemochromatosis.** *Jerry is a 54-year-old county administrator. He has had diabetes for 2 years. One year ago he reported to his family physician that he had become unable to function sexually. He reports that over the past several months he has felt generally ill, tired, and short-winded. Now his ankles are beginning to swell and he has lost his appetite. His wife wonders why he has begun to look so "tan" even though he never goes outside. Jerry's physician obtains a test, which discloses a very excessive amount of iron in the blood.*

A defect in iron metabolism permits iron to build up in the body. This disorder is called hemochromatosis. Iron can build up in the heart muscle (as well as other organs) and cause stiffening.

Like amyloidosis, hemochromatosis can also lead to dilated cardiomyopathy. Hemochromatosis can occasionally be substantially helped by medications that leach the iron out of tissues and by repeated removal of pints of blood (the procedure for removing the blood is the same as that used when you donate blood). The removal of blood decreases the amount of iron, because the blood cells contain a large quantity of iron.

Symptoms of restrictive cardiomyopathy. With restrictive cardiomyopathy, typical symptoms are shortness of breath, and occasionally chest pain. These symptoms reflect the inability of the ventricle to fill during diastole and to provide an increase in blood flow when needed. Edema, right upper abdominal discomfort, nausea, bloating and loss of appetite are symptoms of reduced filling of the right ventricle.

Who is affected by restrictive cardiomyopathy? Men and women are equally affected by restrictive cardiomyopathy. The disease may occur at any adult age, but the average age at onset is in the 50s. Restrictive cardiomyopathy does not appear to be inherited. But some of the diseases that lead to this condition (such as amyloidosis and hemochromatosis) may be inherited.

How serious is restrictive cardiomyopathy? There is no specific treatment for restrictive cardiomyopathy. Often the underlying disease that causes the restriction (amyloidosis) may also be untreatable.

Medications commonly used to treat heart failure are ineffective. Surgery may be considered, but rarely.

The restrictive cardiomyopathies frequently cause heart block (see page 106), and a pacemaker may be required. Because heart failure or rhythm disturbances occur, long-term survival rates are disappointing. Transplantation may be an option.

## Looking ahead

Advances in the diagnosis and treatment of cardiomyopathies will depend upon a clearer understanding of the cause or causes of this disease. Widespread collaborative research should lead to a clear understanding of the basic causes of this disease and new therapies within the next five years.

# Congenital heart disease

Congenital heart disease refers to defects of the heart that are present at birth. About 6 to 8 babies out of every 1,000 who are born alive have a congenital heart defect.

When you consider that 3 weeks after conception the heart consists of a tiny tube that molds itself so that all of its basic structures are present by the eighth week of development, it is more amazing that things turn out right as often as they do.

If your child has a congenital heart defect, you probably have many questions. What exactly is wrong? How did it happen? How will it affect your child's life? What can be done about it? Your doctor will answer these questions specifically as they relate to your family, but this section provides a general background to help you understand the information.

## Continuing progress

The ability to stop the heart temporarily by using a machine to take over the function of the heart and lungs (cardiopulmonary bypass) led to spectacular advances in the treatment of congenital heart disease. At the Mayo Clinic, open heart surgery for congenital heart disease was first performed in 1955. More than 10,000 open heart operations, mostly for congenital heart disease, were performed during the next 15 years. Remarkable strides continue to be made in the detection, evaluation, and treatment of congenital heart disease. As a result, large numbers of people are alive and well who formerly would have died early in life (an estimated 11 million in the United States). Evidence of this progress is provided by the many girls who have surgery to repair congenital heart problems and then grow up to have children of their own.

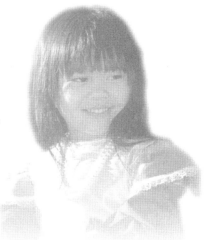

Progress is being made. Ultrasound examination can now detect some problems around the 18th week of gestation, well before the baby is born. This may allow increasing use of operations inside the uterus before birth. Because of these great strides, we can be more optimistic about the future for people with congenital heart disease.

## Classification of congenital defects

Any part of the cardiovascular system can be affected by congenital problems, and more than one defect can occur in the same heart. Some defects are mild enough to go unnoticed at birth. Others cause major problems shortly after the baby is born. Common defects include the following:

- Abnormally formed blood vessels that impede the flow of blood
- Valves that obstruct blood flow, allow backward leakage, or are missing
- Incorrect or reversed connections between the main arteries and the heart or between the main veins and the heart

- Defects in the partitions between the atria or the ventricles that allow blood to flow from the right side to the left side of the heart without going through the lungs, or from the left side to the right side without going through the rest of the body

Doctors often think of congenital defects in terms of whether they cause blueness of the skin (cyanosis). You have probably heard of "blue babies." Some of their blood circulates through their bodies without passing through the lungs to pick up more oxygen, and as a result their skin has a bluish tint.

## What causes congenital heart disease?

The exact cause of most congenital heart defects is rarely identified. Most experts believe that abnormal genes interact with environmental factors during the development of the embryo to produce congenital disease. Often an environmental cause, if any, cannot be detected. Most often, there are no easy answers.

Abnormalities in the chromosomes, including the one that causes Down syndrome, are associated with some heart defects. Infections such as German measles in the mother during early pregnancy increase the risk as well.

If you have a child or there is another person in your family with a congenital heart defect, you probably wonder what the chances are of problems in future children. Unless a specific chromosomal problem is identified, or a clear pattern of hereditary heart disease is seen in a family tree, most experts believe the risk of occurrence in your next baby is about 2 percent to 5 percent—less than 1 in 20. Or, put in a more positive framework, chances are 19 in 20 that your next baby will be fine.

## Management of congenital heart disease

Many types of congenital heart disease can cause major problems starting immediately or soon after birth. Some of them may even lead to irreversible changes that might prevent surgical correction later in life. Therefore, there has been a trend over the years to operate on children with congenital heart disease at earlier ages.

For example, an opening in the partition separating the ventricles (ventricular septal defect) can lead to an increase in blood flow to the lungs and hence to elevation of the blood pressure in the lungs. The high blood pressure can become an irreversible problem on its own. This complication, called Eisenmenger's complex, may occur in early childhood, or it can develop progressively over many years, depending on the severity of the defect. When Eisenmenger's complex develops, it is no longer helpful to close the ventricular septal defect.

## HEALTHY HEART ♥ TIP

*If your chest hurts after a bout of overexertion, you may be experiencing angina pectoris, the medical term for chest pain due to coronary heart disease. This condition can occur when the blood flow to the heart is adequate for your normal activities but not enough when the heart's needs increase.*

*Angina may occur during physical exercise, strong emotions or extreme temperatures. Some people, though, encounter angina when they're resting. In either case, treat it seriously; angina is a sign that you're at risk of heart attack.*

Most operations are reparative (or as close to a cure as possible), but continuing medical care generally is needed following the procedure.

Some operations are palliative. With palliative operations, the problem is not fixed, but adjustments are made to let the circulation work as well as possible under the circumstances. In some cases palliation is done at a young age to allow the heart and circulation to develop enough so a reparative operation can be done later. Sometimes a palliative operation is all that can be done.

One of the earliest palliative operations to be developed is the Blalock-Taussig procedure, which improves (palliates) the condition of patients with cyanotic heart disease. The operation was named after the surgeon and the pediatric cardiologist at the Johns Hopkins Hospital who developed it.

In cyanotic heart disease, not enough blood can flow through the lungs to pick up the needed oxygen to supply the body. The Blalock-Taussig operation increases the flow of blood through the lungs by making a connection (shunt) outside the heart between a large artery to one of the arms and a large artery to the lungs. Thus, the shunt operation does not correct the defects inside the heart that cause the severe reduction in blood flow through the lungs. Rather, it only relieves (palliates) the blueness and tiredness by increasing the flow of blood through the lungs.

The Blalock-Taussig operation may still be performed when complete repair is not feasible, or when the overall risks might be lessened by first doing a preparatory palliative shunt operation in anticipation of complete repair later on.

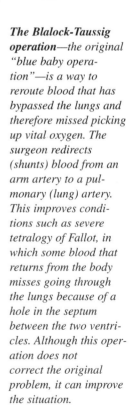

Shunt
(rerouted artery)

*The Blalock-Taussig operation—the original "blue baby operation"—is a way to reroute blood that has bypassed the lungs and therefore missed picking up vital oxygen. The surgeon redirects (shunts) blood from an arm artery to a pulmonary (lung) artery. This improves conditions such as severe tetralogy of Fallot, in which some blood that returns from the body misses going through the lungs because of a hole in the septum between the two ventricles. Although this operation does not correct the original problem, it can improve the situation.*

## What is the outlook?

As you might expect, congenital heart defects can result in the widest range of disabilities. They can be so severe that life cannot be maintained, or they can be so mild that trouble is not even suspected. A list of such minor defects would include an aortic valve that has only two cusps (bicuspid) instead of the normal three, mitral valve prolapse, or a small atrial septal defect.

Sometimes these abnormalities never do cause problems. Other times they become more abnormal with aging and then cause problems. For example, a child with a bicuspid aortic valve may have satisfactory function of the valve. As the child ages, the valve may thicken and calcify and lead to narrowing (stenosis), or it may retract and result in backward leakage (regurgitation). These changes may not produce symptoms until middle age or even later.

Many congenital heart defects can be surgically repaired at a young age, and your child can thus have a normal life. However, even after corrective surgery for congenital heart disease, residual problems can remain or crop up later, so your child will need continued medical observation. Heart rhythm disorders and endocarditis remain potential threats, even many years later.

Sometimes your doctor may recommend waiting for a time before repairing a defect. Reasons for this delay include the following:

- The problem will not get any worse if you wait for a limited time.
- The baby is too small. The operation will be easier at an older age.

In such cases, delaying an operation would be expected to have no adverse effect on the outcome for your child. In other cases, surgery may be delayed not by choice but because the problem was not found or the diagnosis was incorrect. Some congenital problems are very hard to diagnose without difficult, risky, and expensive tests, which are done only if there is a high suspicion of an abnormality. If the defect is not causing obvious problems, the likelihood increases that it might be overlooked at routine examinations.

With some congenital defects such as ventricular septal defect, if an operation to close the defect is postponed too long, the excess blood that shunts through the defect and through the lungs may damage the small end branches of the pulmonary artery. The damage might become so severe that an operation to close the septal defect would no longer be helpful. If the heart weakens because of the high lung (pulmonary) artery pressure, lung transplantation or special medicine to dilate the lung arteries will be needed.

## Examples of congenital heart disease

Some defects may occur by themselves. Others may occur in combination. Following are descriptions of just a few of the many types of congenital heart defects.

### Abnormal artery near the heart

#### *Patent ductus arteriosus*

The ductus arteriosus is an artery that allows blood in the fetus to bypass the lungs until the lungs expand at the time of birth. It normally closes soon after birth. When it remains open (patent), blood can flow from the aorta to the pulmonary artery. This defect overworks the heart, causes excess blood flow in the lungs, and can lead to heart failure. It is more common in infants whose mothers had German measles in early pregnancy and in infants who were born prematurely or at high altitude.

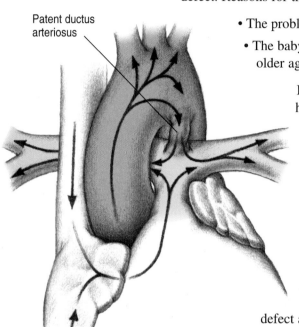

Patent ductus arteriosus

***Patent ductus arteriosus.*** *Instead of blood flowing out of the aorta to the body, some blood is directed back to the lungs through an opening that normally closes at birth. The heart is overworked because it must pump enough blood out of the left ventricle to supply the body with oxygen and allow for the amount that returns directly to the lungs.*

In premature babies, the patent ductus arteriosus often closes spontaneously within weeks or months after birth. If the duct remains open and heart failure does not respond to medical treatment, surgical closure may be required, even during infancy. Once the duct has closed, no further problems are typically encountered. New methods of closing the patent duct with a plug or "double umbrella" through a catheter (a tube passed through a major blood vessel to the heart) are currently being explored.

## Coarctation of the aorta

Coarctation (constriction) of the aorta is a narrowing that impedes blood flow from the heart to the lower part of the body and increases blood pressure. If heart failure develops, even during infancy, removal of the narrowed segment may be necessary. Experience is now accumulating with the technique of dilating the narrowed segment with an inflatable balloon catheter guided inside the narrowed zone of the aorta. Stents are also used. Even for children in whom heart failure has not yet developed, removal of the narrowed segment should not be delayed indefinitely, because the high blood pressure can become irreversible. Survival beyond age 50 is unusual in people who do not have the coarctation repaired; most die by the mid-30s.

Coarctation of the aorta accounts for 15 percent of congenital heart problems in adults. (More people with coarctation of the aorta are being identified in blood pressure screening programs.) Twice as many men have it as women.

## Incorrect connections of the main arteries and the heart

### Transposition of the great arteries

In this defect, the origins of the two arteries from the heart are reversed: The aorta comes from the right ventricle and the pulmonary artery emerges from the left ventricle. Thus, a portion of the person's blood recirculates through the right heart and lungs without ever passing through the rest of the body. Likewise, the remaining portion of the person's blood recirculates through the left heart and the body without passing through the lungs. If oxygen-carrying blood does not reach your body, you cannot live. For survival, there must be a connection between the two systems. The two systems may connect if there is an associated defect such as patent ductus arteriosus, atrial septal defect, or ventricular septal defect. If such a connection is not present, a palliative septal defect can be created between the two atria with a special catheter.

*Coarctation of the aorta. The aorta is narrowed (**arrow**), usually below the branches to the head and arms. The heart must work harder to pump blood, and blood pressure is often higher in the arms (above the narrowing) than in the legs (below the narrowing).*

***Transposition of the great arteries.*** *The great arteries (the aorta and the pulmonary artery) are in reversed positions (transposed). The aorta emerges from the right ventricle and the pulmonary artery comes from the left ventricle. Instead of a figure-8 circulation, the circulation is now two separate circles: Blood returning to the heart from the lungs (**shaded red**) is pumped right back to the lungs, and blood returning from the body (**shaded blue**) is pumped right back to the body. Unless the two circles are connected, for example by a ventricular septal defect, no oxygen can get into the blood going to the person's body—a fatal condition.*

Aorta

Pulmonary artery

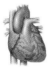

Although correction of this complicated condition proved challenging for a long while, several surgical procedures are now available to relieve this problem and help affected infants. Without treatment, 30 percent of these babies die in the first week of life. By the first year, 90 percent of the infants die if they do not have surgery.

### Truncus arteriosus

In truncus arteriosus, the pulmonary arteries (that go to the lungs), the aorta, and the coronary arteries all originate from a single large artery, or trunk (see page 66). Thus, all the blood, both oxygenated and poorly oxygenated, must mix together as it flows through the single exit valve and through the single truncus arteriosus (arterial trunk).

Truncus arteriosus is not common. It accounts for about 1 percent of all cases of congenital heart disease.

Surgery should be performed within the first 6 months of life. It involves sewing a flexible tube on the heart that carries blood from the right ventricle to the pulmonary arteries. This tube also contains a valve, made of animal tissue or artificial material, which substitutes for the deficient exit valve. Continued careful medical evaluation is required even after successful correction. Without correction, few children with this defect reach adulthood.

# Defects in valves

### Aortic or pulmonary valve stenosis

Narrowing of the aortic or pulmonary valves is among the most common congenital heart defects. These valve problems are described on pages 79 and 83.

### Ebstein's anomaly

This rare congenital heart defect accounts for less than 1 percent of all forms of congenital heart disease. It affects males and females equally.

Ebstein's anomaly involves abnormally developed tricuspid valve leaflets. (The tricuspid valve prevents backward blood flow from the right ventricle to the right atrium.) The leaflets are attached abnormally and have other related problems that produce back leakage of blood through the valve and make additional work for the heart. One in two individuals with Ebstein's anomaly has a hole in the heart (atrial septal defect) which allows mixing of atrial and venous blood. This mixing may cause blueness (cyanosis). Episodes of excessively fast heartbeats complicate Ebstein's anomaly in about one of four patients.

In some people with Ebstein's anomaly, symptoms develop gradually. Some live into their 60s and 70s, even in the presence of significant disease. Others die in infancy or early childhood.

Surgery is usually postponed until the onset of disability, because the long-term results are uncertain. But in people who have indications of increased risk, there are good results with surgical reconstruction or replacement of the tricuspid valve.

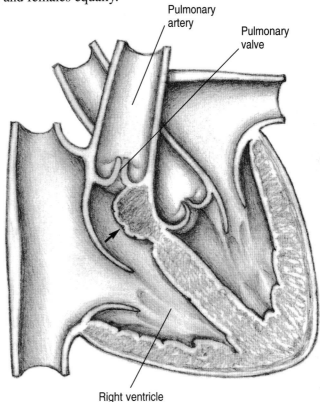

*Pulmonary valve stenosis* is a narrowing of the pulmonary valve at the origin of the pulmonary artery within the heart. There may also be thickening of the muscle of the right ventricle immediately below the valve (**arrow**), as is often seen with tetralogy of Fallot (see page 67).

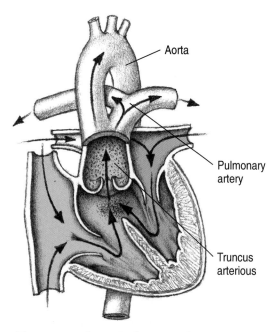

Aorta

Pulmonary
artery

Truncus
arterious

**Truncus arteriosus.** *In this unusual condition, the aorta and pulmonary artery emerge from the heart in a single tube (trunk) that gets blood flow from both the right and the left ventricles. The result is that some oxygenated blood returns directly to the lungs, and some deoxygenated blood returns to the body without going through the lungs first.*

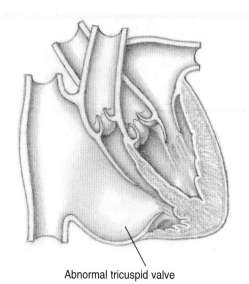

Abnormal tricuspid valve

**Ebstein's anomaly.** *The tricuspid valve is mis-shapen so that it does not properly prevent back leakage of the blood from the right ventricle to the right atrium.*

## Septal defects

### Atrial septal defect

This is a hole in the wall between the two atria (the upper chambers of the heart) that allows abnormal blood flow (see page 67). Girls with atrial septal defect outnumber boys 3 to 1.

The location and size of the hole are variable, but in all uncomplicated atrial septal defects, blood is shunted from the left to the right atrium during diastole (when the heart fills with blood), and blood flow to the lungs is increased. Often, the presence of an atrial septal defect is not recognized because symptoms may be nonexistent early in life and it is not easy to detect by physical examination alone. The defect may be found on a routine chest X-ray or when the doctor hears an abnormal pattern of blood flow during a routine checkup. It accounts for about 25 percent of congenital heart conditions detected in adults.

If the defect is recognized early, it is usually closed surgically between the ages of 1 and 6 years. The risks of surgery are low, and the long-term results are excellent. After surgery, a normal lifestyle with no restrictions is usually possible. Alternative methods to close the defect using catheter-based technologies and the avoidance of cardiac surgery are being evaluated and may prove to be effective alternatives to an operation.

The outlook for those who do not have the problem repaired is not encouraging. Most people die of heart failure before age 50.

### Ventricular septal defect

This is an opening between the ventricles (the pumping chambers of the heart) that increases blood flow, under high pressure, to the lungs (see page 67). Increased blood flow to the lungs overworks the heart; this may lead to high blood pressure in the lung arteries or congestive heart failure. If the defect is not repaired, eventually the blood shunts from the right to the left side of the heart, causing blueness from inadequate oxygen in the tissues.

Ventricular septal defect is a common heart malformation, accounting for 25 percent of the cases of congenital heart disease. Almost 50 percent of all ventricular septal defects close by themselves without an operation, mostly during the first few months after birth, because they are small.

Small ventricular septal defects that do not cause symptoms usually do not require surgery, but people with ventricular septal defects should receive preventive antibiotics before dental and certain surgical procedures.

In children with large defects, major problems, including heart failure, may develop in early infancy. Treatment for these babies is aimed at controlling the heart failure with drugs. If this is unsuccessful, surgery to close the defect is usually done before 1 year of age. After successful closure, a normal lifestyle is usual.

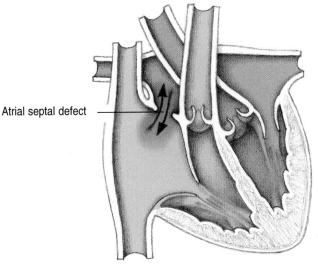

Atrial septal defect

*Atrial septal defect (right). A hole in the wall (septum) separating the two atria permits mixing of oxygenated blood and deoxygenated blood. Usually, the direction of blood flow through the hole is mainly from the left atrium to the right, and the result is excessive flow of blood through the lungs.*

Ventricular septal defect

*Ventricular septal defect (left). A hole in the wall (septum) separating the two ventricles permits mixing of oxygenated blood and deoxygenated blood. Initially, the direction of blood flow through the hole is mainly from the left ventricle to the right, and the result is excessive flow of blood through the lungs. With time, the blood pressure in the lungs becomes excessively high, forcing the direction of flow through the hole to reverse (this is called Eisenmenger's complex). Some deoxygenated blood now goes though the hole into the left ventricle and out to the body, causing a bluish tinge to the skin.*

## Combination of defects

### Tetralogy of Fallot

A French physician, Étienne-Louis Fallot, described this defect in 1888. Tetralogy of Fallot is really four defects in combination. First, the septum that divides the two ventricles is incomplete (so there is a ventricular septal defect), and oxygen-poor blood is thus allowed to mix with oxygen-rich blood. Second, the passageway from the right ventricle to the lungs is markedly narrowed. Third, the origin of the aorta is shifted toward the right side of the heart from the left. Fourth, the muscle in the wall of the right ventricle is thickened and stiffened. Only the first two of these defects cause significant trouble or require an operation. These defects result in decreased blood flow to the lungs and circulation of blue (unoxygenated) blood to the body tissues; both of these effects cause bluish skin (cyanosis), clubbing (bulging of the nailbeds) of the fingers and toes, and extreme fatigue.

Tetralogy of Fallot constitutes 10 percent of all congenital heart disease. It is the most common cyanotic heart defect; nearly 3,000 new cases a year occur in the United States. Infants may require palliative surgery (for example, the Blalock-Taussig shunt procedure) to improve blood flow to the lungs and decrease cyanosis. Once the child is past infancy, corrective open heart surgery is performed. The results of successful complete repair of tetralogy of Fallot are good: Cyanosis disappears, exercise tolerance improves, and people lead normal lives. Without an operation, only 30 percent of people with tetralogy of Fallot would survive to the age of 40 years. Surgery results in almost 90 percent of patients surviving for at least 25 years after surgery; generally, the results are best if the defect is corrected before the patient is 12 years old.

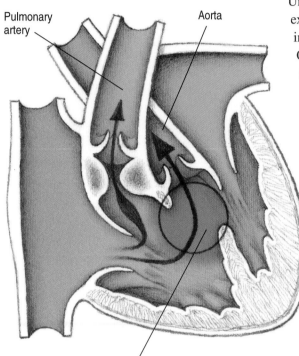

Pulmonary artery

Aorta

Ventricular septal defect

***Tetralogy of Fallot.*** *This heart defect is complex, but fairly common. Its features are ventricular septal defect, obstruction to blood flow beneath the pulmonary valve, an aorta that is shifted rightward, and a thickened right ventricular wall. The overall result is usually that some deoxygenated blood is shunted into the aorta. If the septal defect is small or the obstruction is mild, babies with this condition may be "pink" rather than "blue."*

## Defects in valves

The valves keep the blood flowing in one direction, like one-way gates. They open when the pressure of the blood pushes them in the forward direction, and they close when the pressure on the other side of the valve pushes them back. Diseased valves may be too stiff to open easily or they may fail to close completely. Each of the four valves (mitral and aortic on the left side of the heart, and tricuspid and pulmonary on the right side) may be subject to obstruction (stenosis) if they are too stiff and to back leakage (regurgitation) if they fail to close properly.

A valve opening can become narrowed and "tights" (stenotic), a condition that limits the blood flow through it and causes the blood and fluid behind it to back up as if behind a dam. The backup leads to symptoms of congestive heart failure, heart chamber enlargement, and overgrowth of heart muscle, which can lead to angina. Various heart rhythm disorders can also develop.

## Innocent heart murmurs

If your doctor tells you that your child has an "innocent" heart murmur, there is no need to worry. Innocent murmurs, by definition, do not cause problems.

Innocent murmurs are common in children. They may disappear and reappear, but they are harmless. Most innocent murmurs will disappear permanently when your child reaches adulthood.

Your child's doctor can hear innocent murmurs by listening to your child's heart through a stethoscope. Murmurs are sounds made by turbulent blood moving through the chambers and valves of the heart or through the blood vessels near the heart. Your doctor may also call them "functional murmurs" or "vibratory murmurs."

Your doctor may want to have your child undergo other tests to be sure that the murmur is innocent. Once they are done and if you are told that the murmur is innocent, you can relax. Your child does not have a heart problem. No restrictions or limitations in activity are necessary—your child is normal and healthy.

Valves may not close properly and therefore allow blood to leak back in the wrong direction (regurgitation). A "leaky" valve does not mean that blood leaks out of the heart, but that blood leaks backward through the valve. This causes the heart chambers to enlarge and pump blood inefficiently, because excess blood must be pumped forward to compensate for the amount that leaks back with each heartbeat. Again, this can lead to congestive heart failure, fatigue, and some rhythm disorders.

Causes of valve disease range from congenital defects to calcium deposits that accumulate on the valves as you age, and to infections.

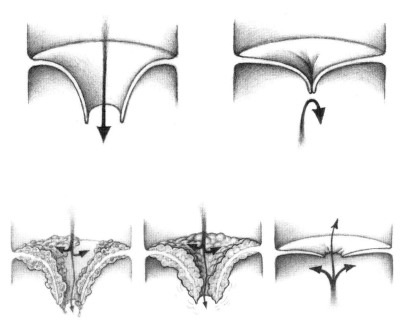

*Normal valves (**top two**) open widely to let blood easily flow forward, and close tightly to prevent blood from leaking backward.*

*In endocarditis (**bottom left**), vegetations consisting of bacteria, inflammatory cells, fibrin/platelet mesh and blood clots adhere to the valves, causing valve leakage. If they break off, they can spread the infection to arteries distant from the heart.*

*A valve with stenosis (**bottom middle**) is unable to open widely. Blood flow is partially obstructed. Thick deposits of calcium prevent the valve from opening very widely.*

*In valve regurgitation (**bottom right**), a valve is not closing well enough to prevent back leakage.*

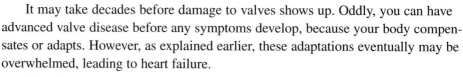

It may take decades before damage to valves shows up. Oddly, you can have advanced valve disease before any symptoms develop, because your body compensates or adapts. However, as explained earlier, these adaptations eventually may be overwhelmed, leading to heart failure.

Therefore, if you develop valve disease, it is important that the problem be treated before it becomes so advanced that repair or replacement of the valve is no longer possible. The timing of procedures to repair or replace the damaged valve is important, because your doctor has to weigh the potential risks of surgery against the possibility that the problem will become too advanced to remedy. (For information on heart valve disease caused by fen-phen, a weight-loss agent, see page 177.)

## Endocarditis

Damaged or weakened valves are vulnerable to a condition called endocarditis (see page 69). Endocarditis is an infection of the endocardium, the membrane that lines the inside of the four chambers and valves of your heart. Usually the inflammation is caused by actual infection of a valve with bacteria or other microorganisms.

Endocarditis can occur whenever bacteria circulate in the bloodstream. Certain bacteria (and other microorganisms) tend to settle, and multiply, on abnormal, damaged valves where blood flow is turbulent.

Although effective treatments are available, endocarditis is a major illness and can be fatal. It almost always results in a worse valve condition because of further destruction of the valve. Treatment of endocarditis may require 4 to 6 weeks or more of intravenous administration of antibiotics, often combined with surgical treatment.

Some organisms that cause endocarditis are becoming resistant to antibiotics, probably because of the overuse of antibiotics for minor infections and the widespread use of antibiotics in animal feed. Physicians are concerned about this trend, and work is under way on new medications.

### What causes endocarditis?

Endocarditis may be caused by certain bacteria that are often present in the mouth and upper respiratory tract. The organisms may enter your bloodstream during dental or surgical procedures such as getting a tooth pulled or having your tonsils removed. Still, most cases of endocarditis do not directly follow a surgical or dental procedure. More often they follow a minor gum injury or are caused by poor dental hygiene. Be sure to get regular, comprehensive dental care if you're at risk for endocarditis.

Bacteria in your intestinal tract, called enterococci, may also enter your bloodstream during an examination of or surgical procedure in the prostate, bladder, rectum, or female pelvic organs.

Endocarditis may also develop in people who abuse drugs and use contaminated needles to inject drugs into a vein.

In people with inadequate immunity to infection, endocarditis can develop from other organisms, such as fungi.

## Who is at risk for endocarditis?

If your heart is healthy and normal, you are unlikely to develop endocarditis. The organisms tend to adhere to and multiply in valves that are malformed or that have been damaged from rheumatic fever.

You are at risk for ineffective endocarditis if:

- You were born with a defect in your heart or heart valves
- Your heart valves have become scarred from rheumatic fever or other diseases
- You have an artificial heart valve

Severe mitral valve prolapse (with valve leakage) is the most common heart condition associated with endocarditis. Endocarditis may also occur with milder forms of prolapse.

## Precautions to take if you're at risk for endocarditis

### Dental procedures and oral or respiratory tract surgery

Before you undergo any procedure on your mouth (including routine cleaning at the dentist's office) or throat that may cause bleeding, your doctor or dentist will probably prescribe amoxicillin taken orally. You should take it 1 hour before the procedure.

If you are allergic to penicillin (amoxicillin is a type of penicillin), you can take another antibiotic such as cephalosporin, clindamycin or azithromycin. If you're at high risk, your physician may prescribe an injectable antibiotic.

### Urologic procedures, gastrointestinal surgery, or examination with instruments

Urologic procedures include bladder operations, transurethral resection of the prostate (TURP), and gynecologic procedures. Gastrointestinal procedures are, for example, hemorrhoid removal, polyp removal, or colon resection.

The germs in your intestine may be partially resistant to penicillin-type antibiotics when the risk of endocarditis is high. Your doctor may prescribe a combination of injectable antibiotics just before and again 8 hours after the procedure. For people at lower risk, antibiotics taken by mouth may suffice.

### Lung and skin infections

If you develop a lung or skin infection, your doctor may prescribe antibiotic treatment to prevent endocarditis.

### Think prevention

It is important to use good oral hygiene every day and to have regular professional dental care. This involves routinely brushing and flossing your teeth and gums and getting regular checkups.

Your dentist and each of your doctors should be aware that you are at risk for endocarditis. Many people use a handy card prepared by the American Heart Association for this purpose. To secure a copy, contact your local chapter.

Even if your heart condition has not caused you any symptoms, or even if the defect has been repaired and you are healthy, you may still be at risk for this serious infection. Your doctor is the best person to advise you about risk because your level of risk hinges on the particular defect that was repaired.

## How serious is endocarditis?

Endocarditis is a very dangerous disease that was nearly always fatal before the development of antibiotics. Although powerful antibiotics are now available, complications may occur, treatment can be difficult, and the results are not predictable. Therefore, doctors believe that prevention is the best approach.

## How can you prevent endocarditis?

Antibiotics can reduce your risk from infective endocarditis by destroying or controlling the harmful bacteria. Many experts advise using these drugs before procedures that may allow bacteria to enter your bloodstream, travel to your heart, and cause an infection.

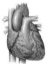

### HEALTHY HEART ♥ TIP

*What used to be bad may be getting better. Food manufacturers have begun introducing new, specially engineered product lines they call "functional foods." These new products, such as margarine, dried pasta, frozen entrees, bread, cereal, baked potato crisps and cookies, have ingredients that are intended to provide specific health benefits beyond basic nutrition. For one, manufacturers have developed foods they say will lower cholesterol, a contributing factor in cardiovascular disease, the leading cause of death in the United States and other industrialized countries.*

## Mitral valve prolapse and endocarditis

Mitral valve prolapse is a common condition in a small number of people predisposed to endocarditis. Mitral valve prolapse without regurgitation (valve leakage), heard by your physician as a murmur or seen on echocardiography, is not associated with endocarditis and does not require antibiotics before dental or surgical procedures. On the other hand, mitral valve prolapse with thickened leaflets or marked leakage (regurgitation) is a risk factor for endocarditis and requires prophylactic antibiotics.

## Rheumatic fever

In addition to congenital abnormalities and infections, valves may be damaged by rheumatic fever. Although rheumatic fever is not nearly as common in the United States as it was 40 years ago before the widespread use of penicillin, several outbreaks were reported in U.S. cities during the late 1980s. Rheumatic fever is still very common in underdeveloped countries.

Forty percent to 60 percent of people having a first attack of rheumatic fever have heart inflammation. The mitral valve is involved in about 85 percent of cases, the aortic valve is involved in about 44 percent of cases, the tricuspid valve is involved in 10 percent to 16 percent, and the pulmonary valve is rarely involved. More than one valve is frequently affected.

## Causes of rheumatic fever

Rheumatic fever seems to be the result of a reaction of your body to specific strains of the streptococcal bacteria. Symptoms of rheumatic fever generally appear about 2 to 4 weeks after an untreated "strep throat" infection. Thus, antibiotics to treat strep throat infections can prevent rheumatic fever. The damage to the heart valve seems to be related to antibodies the body produces to fight the throat infection, or to toxic substances produced by the bacteria. It is not caused by an actual infection of the valve.

Strep throat usually comes on suddenly, especially with painful swallowing, fever, and tender, swollen glands under the jaw. Laboratory tests (throat culture) are needed to confirm that the sore throat is due to a streptococcal infection.

## Symptoms of rheumatic fever

Symptoms of this disease include fever, rapid heartbeat, chills, joint pain that tends to migrate from one joint to another, a characteristic rash, fatigue, weakness, irritability, and occasional uncontrollable movement of the limbs. You may have raised, red patches on the skin or lumps under the skin.

## Who is affected by rheumatic fever?

Rheumatic fever usually occurs in young people age 5 to 15. It rarely affects adults. Once you have had it, you are more susceptible to another attack. Doctors may prescribe penicillin or another antibiotic continuously until adulthood after the first bout of rheumatic fever.

## How serious is rheumatic fever?

The heart inflammation from rheumatic fever does not always cause permanent damage. However, one or more of your valves may be scarred. The damage to your heart valves may take 10 to 30 years to show up. Serious complications may develop, and you may need surgery to repair or replace the damaged valves. In rare instances, the heart muscle itself can be severely inflamed, and this condition can lead to heart failure.

Most cases of strep throat do not lead to rheumatic fever. However, if you have step throat, take all of the medication your doctor prescribes, even if your sore throat is gone in a day or two. That approach is the best way to prevent rheumatic fever.

## Valve disease can be serious but subtle

Even in advanced stages of valve malfunction, you may not experience symptoms. One reason is that the heart and other parts of the body adapt to the problem and overcome it to some extent. But these adaptive or compensatory mechanisms can perform only up to a certain point. Then the problem becomes too overwhelming, and symptoms develop.

Sometimes you may not recognize symptoms because they develop so slowly. For example, intolerance of exercise may develop gradually. You may simply get used to it, so you do not recognize that you are restricted in any way.

Symptoms do not always correlate with the severity of the valve problem. Anyone with a valve problem must see a doctor regularly to monitor changes in the valves.

The problems brought on by valve disease vary depending on which valve is affected, whether it is too tight or too loose, and how advanced the disease is. Often, different types of valve problems occur together in the same person. For example, mitral stenosis and regurgitation can coexist, and treatment is frequently different from that for mitral stenosis alone.

Some combinations make the heart particularly inefficient. For example, with both aortic stenosis and mitral regurgitation, the blood not only has a hard time going forward during systole through the tight aortic valve but also is inclined to go backward through the leaky mitral valve. With these conditions, much of the blood will take the "easy path" and leak backward.

## Defects in valves on the left side of the heart

The most common valve problems involve the mitral and aortic valves on the left side of the heart (see page A7). The oxygen-rich blood from the lungs enters the left atrium, passes through the mitral valve into the left ventricle, and leaves the ventricle through the aortic valve on its way to the rest of the body. Both the mitral and aortic valves can have damage that leads to obstruction (stenosis) or back leakage (regurgitation).

### Mitral stenosis

*Ann, now a 39-year-old homemaker, missed several months of third grade due to rheumatic fever. She returned to good health, but during pregnancy with her third child at age 32 she experienced shortness of breath with congestion in her lungs. Her physician diagnosed a "valve problem," but no treatment was advised. One year ago, Ann suddenly became short of breath and went to the emergency room; the diagnosis was atrial fibrillation. Fortunately, a normal heart rhythm was restarted with an injection of medication. For the past 2 months, she has felt distinctly tired and notices breathlessness when she climbs the basement stairs. After a medical examination, she is told she has mitral stenosis.*

When the mitral valve is tight (stenotic), blood has a difficult time flowing from the left atrium to the left ventricle (see page 69). The result is that the pressure of blood in the left atrium increases. The left atrium may enlarge because of the back pressure. Eventually, that back pressure can cause leakage of fluid into the lungs (pulmonary edema) (see page 46). The left atrium is prone to develop rhythm irregularities (atrial fibrillation), which can further decrease the efficiency of the heart. You may suddenly experience symptoms, or mild symptoms may become worse.

Also, blood clots tend to form in the enlarged and fibrillating atrium. If a small fragment of blood clot breaks loose, it can travel to other parts of the body and lead to blockage in an artery. One of the most serious risks is a blood clot traveling to the brain and causing a stroke.

### Causes of mitral stenosis

Rheumatic fever in childhood is by far the most common cause of mitral stenosis. It can damage the heart valve and cause scarring, which results in problems later in life, usually in young adulthood (see page A7).

More rarely, mitral stenosis can occur from congenital heart disease or from calcium deposits that accumulate over years. Some experts speculate about a viral cause, but no proof has been found.

### Symptoms of mitral stenosis

You may not have any symptoms for years, even with significant mitral stenosis. When symptoms develop (commonly in the 30s), they include the symptoms of congestive heart failure. Inefficient circulation causes fatigue and shortness of breath (especially after exercise, at night, or when lying down). You may experience chest discomfort or palpitations. You may have frequent bouts of bronchitis. There is also the possibility of stroke.

### Who is affected by mitral stenosis?

Mitral stenosis is less common today than it was several decades ago, because the most common cause, rheumatic fever, has largely been eradicated in the United States. However, it remains a frequent problem in underdeveloped countries. It is more common in women than in men.

### How serious is mitral stenosis?

If you have mild mitral stenosis, you may remain well, or have only mild symptoms, for decades. Eventually, symptoms of fatigue and breathlessness may become problems if the deformityof the valve is severe. Mitral stenosis carries a risk of rhythm abnormalities (atrial fibrillation), in which the atrium beats in a rapid and uncoordinated manner. Atrial fibrillation can lead to the formation of dangerous blood clots.

In general, mitral stenosis does not need to be corrected until symptoms develop. Proper preventive measures against infective endocarditis are essential. Correction usually requires surgery, but balloon valulopasty may also be a treatment option (see page A8).

## Mitral regurgitation

*Martha is a 63-year-old lawyer who was told she had a heart murmur during a physical examination about 12 years ago. She was advised to take antibiotics at the time of dental appointments and to get regular medical checkups. Three years ago she was told her heart was enlarged, but in retrospect it was large on the chest X-ray from 9 years previously and had not changed much. Echocardiography was done, but no new treatment was prescribed. Now, her echocardiogram shows further heart enlargement and some decrease in pumping strength. The diagnosis (as before) is chronic mitral regurgitation. Martha feels she is wearing out a bit "from getting old," but otherwise feels all right. However, operation on the valve was recommended.*

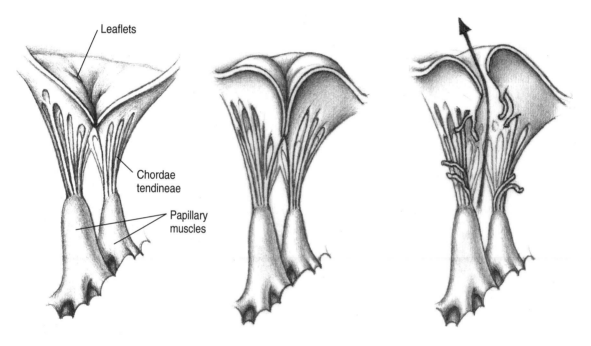

*Normally, the mitral valve (**left**) closes snugly to prevent back leakage of blood when the left ventricle contracts. The leaflets are tethered to the wall of the heart by stringlike chordae tendineae and papillary muscles.*

*In mitral valve prolapse (**center**), the valve leaflets bulge (prolapse) upward during closure. This is due to leaflets that are too large or chordae tendineae that are too long. The valve may prevent back leakage of blood anyway.*

*In uncommon cases, when some chordae tendineae break (**right**), the valve leaflets may "flail" and allow back leakage to develop.*

Mitral regurgitation is a much more common problem than mitral stenosis. In mitral regurgitation, the mitral valve leaflets do not close properly, so that the blood leaks back (regurgitates) into the atrium when the left ventricle contracts. The leakage decreases the blood flow to the rest of the body and increases the work load of the left side of the heart.

Closing the mitral valve and opening the aortic valve during systole (squeezing) should result in forward flow of blood. With mitral regurgitation, a portion of the blood in the ventricle is squeezed backward in addition to the portion that is squeezed forward through the aortic valve. This condition leads to inefficient functioning of the heart.

### Causes of mitral regurgitation

Mitral regurgitation can be caused by rheumatic fever, but this is a rare cause. The usual causes are mitral valve prolapse that has worsened, infection of the valve (endocarditis), heart attacks that involve the heart wall where the mitral valve leaflets are tethered for support, and deterioration of the valve with aging. Despite the fact that mitral valve prolapse is very common, only very few people with it ever develop a worrisome degree of mitral regurgitation.

### Symptoms of mitral regurgitation

If mitral regurgitation develops and progresses slowly (chronically), you may not notice any symptoms. However, some people experience symptoms of congestive heart failure (fatigue, weakness, shortness of breath with exercise or at night, swelling in the ankles) and irregular heart rhythms that may cause palpitations.

If severe mitral regurgitation develops rapidly (acutely), these symptoms can develop immediately and be very marked.

*Andrew is a 61-year-old accountant who has always been healthy. While doing yard work he suddenly became extremely short of breath and began gasping. He was able to walk slowly into the house, but if he lay on the couch he felt that he was smothering. His wife called the ambulance. In the emergency room a diagnosis of acute mitral regurgitation was established by listening with a stethoscope and viewing an echocardiogram. The problem was rupture of the chordae tendineae (cords that anchor and support the valve). Oxygen and injection of medication to remove fluid that had accumulated in the lungs helped while arrangements were made for urgent surgical repair of the valve.*

### How serious is mitral regurgitation?

You may not have any symptoms for 20 years or more with mitral regurgitation. Often symptoms appear in middle age or beyond.

Strange as it may seem, you may have very bad chronic mitral regurgitation and deteriorated pumping function and yet feel well. The cardiovascular system is generally very adept at counteracting deficiencies caused by the leaky valve. The problem is that if the valve is not fixed or replaced, the strength of the heart muscle may decline so far that even when the valve is operated on, the problem with the weakened pump remains. Thus, it is important to operate early enough.

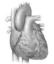

**HEALTHY HEART ♥ TIP**

*You may be too involved in your workout to stop and take your pulse, but still want to know how hard your heart is working. There's a simple way to find out.*

*If you can talk and walk at the same time, you're not working too hard. On the other hand, if you can sing and maintain your effort level, you're probably not working hard enough.*

*But be careful if you get out of breath quickly—especially if you actually have to stop and catch your breath. If this happens, you're most likely overdoing it.*

If you have severe mitral regurgitation but are in otherwise good health, mitral valve repair should be done as soon as possible to prevent damage to your heart (ventricle or atrium). (Enlargement of the atrium can lead to an irregular heart rhythm called atrial fibrillation.) With improved surgical techniques, this procedure now is done earlier than in the past. If your valve cannot be repaired, it can be replaced by an artificial valve.

Naturally, if you have mitral regurgitation, it is difficult for you to accept that a major operation may be advisable even though you feel well. However, this may be one of the most dramatic examples of "a stitch in time saves nine!"

## Mitral valve prolapse

Mitral valve prolapse is usually harmless. The condition may be present in as many as 1 in 10 Americans, although some experts believe that mitral valve prolapse is overdiagnosed.

In mitral valve prolapse, the leaflets of the mitral valve between the left atrium and left ventricle bulge (prolapse) into the left atrium like a parachute during the heart's contraction. This condition may keep the leaflets from closing tightly and may allow some blood to leak back into the atrium from the ventricle (see page A7).

Mitral valve prolapse is often called the "click-murmur syndrome" because your doctor may hear an extra clicking sound from the leaflets ballooning out and a murmur from the backward flow of blood (regurgitation).

### *Symptoms of mitral valve prolapse*

Most people with mitral valve prolapse do not have any symptoms. Some people may have brief episodes of rapid heartbeat (palpitation) or chest pain that is not typical of angina. A few may experience fatigue, shortness of breath, light-headedness, or loss of consciousness; an extremely rare occurrence is sudden death.

Many people with mitral valve prolapse suffer from undue anxiety. Perhaps this anxiety is in some ways explainable. Many people come to their doctors with otherwise inexplicable aches or pains or strange sensations. By default, in those who have mitral valve prolapse the condition becomes a scapegoat. Naturally, the patient becomes concerned. However, the mitral valve prolapse usually is not the source of all the problems.

### *Who is affected by mitral valve prolapse?*

Mitral valve prolapse is more common in women than men. It also occurs more often in women who have scoliosis or other skeletal abnormalities. It appears to occur more often in some families than others.

### *How serious is mitral valve prolapse?*

The vast majority of people with mitral valve prolapse have no problems. If you have mitral valve prolapse, you most likely have a normal life expectancy and do not have to make any changes in your activities.

About 15 percent of people with mitral valve prolapse may experience symptoms of valve leakage that are significant enough to require careful evaluation of the mitral valve and consideration of valve surgery. In rare individuals with mitral valve prolapse (like Andrew), sudden mitral regurgitation can develop from breakage of the chordae tendineae, which tether the valve leaflets. In these cases, symptoms (shortness of breath) can develop rapidly.

If your doctor diagnoses mitral valve prolapse, you may have a risk of infective endocarditis. Although it is a small risk, endocarditis is such a serious complication that you should take preventive antibiotics before and after dental and some surgical procedures if your doctor recommends them.

## Aortic stenosis

*Jacob is a 70-year-old retired librarian. Five years ago, an echocardiogram showed aortic stenosis that was "moderately severe." The aortic valve had heavy deposits of calcium on it. He was advised to use antibiotics at the time of dental examinations. He remained busy at work and home without difficulty. One year ago, an echocardiogram showed "severe" aortic stenosis, but he felt fine. During the past 6 weeks he has noticed chest tightness when working in his yard, and on one occasion he felt that he was about to black out. His doctor advised further evaluation and presented plans to replace his aortic valve with an artificial valve.*

The aortic valve controls blood flow from the left ventricle to the aorta and the rest of the body. It opens when the ventricle contracts and closes when the ventricle relaxes.

Aortic stenosis means the aortic valve has become narrowed (see page A7). The result is that the left ventricle must squeeze harder to get a sufficient amount of blood through the aortic valve with each beat. (Imagine trying to push the same amount of water through a small syringe needle as through a hose—it would take a lot more muscle power.) This increased work load makes the muscle of the left ventricle grow thicker (hypertrophy). Eventually the heart muscle cannot keep up with the work load and begins to fail.

### *Causes of aortic stenosis*

Aortic stenosis may be present at birth or may develop as a result of rheumatic fever or age-related valve degeneration (development of calcium deposits). Some people are born with an aortic valve that has only two cusps instead of three (bicuspid aortic valve). An abnormal valve may be more susceptible to calcium deposits that cause the valve to stiffen and narrow. Even a normal valve can become calcified with age.

### Symptoms of aortic stenosis

Aortic stenosis does not always cause symptoms immediately, even though the valve can be tight. When the heart begins to fail, symptoms of congestive heart failure can develop (fatigue, weakness, shortness of breath with exercise or at night, swelling in the ankles).

Other symptoms associated with aortic stenosis are angina and spells of passing out. Some of these spells may be due to rhythm abnormalities, but a more likely explanation is that the tight aortic valve does not allow enough blood to pass into the arteries of the body. The regulatory mechanisms of the body normally can adjust the blood flow to the various organs. If you needed increased blood flow—for example, to the muscles during exertion—the tight aortic valve could not let enough blood out to fill the blood vessels in the muscles, which have dilated to promote increased blood flow. The result is a drop in blood pressure that could deprive the brain of enough blood flow (and oxygen), and you would pass out.

Coronary artery disease makes aortic stenosis worse by depriving the enlarged and thickened, pressure-overloaded heart muscle of enough blood. If both conditions occur together, as they often do, a combined valve replacement and bypass coronary operation will be required.

### Who is affected by aortic stenosis?

Aortic stenosis can occur at any age (because the causes are different at different ages). People in their 20s and 30s may have murmurs, but symptoms might not occur until age 50 or 60. The condition is three times more common in men than women.

### How serious is aortic stenosis?

There is a long lag period in which you could have mild or moderate obstruction of blood flow and no symptoms (like Jacob). Your doctor may diagnose aortic stenosis by hearing a murmur at a checkup and confirming it with appropriate tests. You may have to limit strenuous physical activity to avoid overworking your heart. Even if you have no symptoms, you should be carefully monitored by your physician.

Once heart failure, angina, or passing out develops, survival is likely limited to 2 or 3 years or less unless you have surgery. This should be done without delay. After the operation, you will have no special limitations in activities.

If you have aortic stenosis, you are at risk for endocarditis and should take preventive antibiotics before and after dental and certain surgical procedures (see page 71).

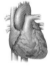

## HEALTHY HEART ♥ TIP

*Societal health risks from obesity are staggering. But consider what lies ahead: The number of overweight or obese children and teens in the United States has increased so sharply that many health officials now consider adolescent obesity a public health crisis.*

*Approximately 1 in five U.S. children between age 6 and 17 is overweight, more than double the number from 30 years ago. Being overweight can mean higher blood pressure and blood cholesterol levels, particularly in children genetically prone to these conditions. Obese children often become obese adults, which puts them at greater risk at a younger age for developing heart disease, diabetes, high blood pressure, high cholesterol levels, gallbladder disease, arthritis and certain cancers.*

# Aortic regurgitation

*Betty is a 55-year-old television network executive who was told that when she was 25 years old, she had a murmur. Eight years ago, an echocardiogram showed back leakage of blood through an aortic valve that had only two cusps instead of the normal three. Subsequent examinations and echocardiograms have shown gradual enlargement of the left ventricle, although it still has almost normal pumping function. She feels well and uses antibiotics for dental procedures. Her physician is recommending continued regular examinations for now.*

Aortic regurgitation is leakage of blood backward through the aortic valve, which controls the blood flow from the left ventricle into the aorta and the rest of the body (see page A7). The aortic valve should close tightly to prevent blood from leaking back from the aorta into the left ventricle.

When the aortic valve does not close efficiently, some blood leaks back during diastole, when the ventricle is relaxing. Thus, blood enters the ventricle from the left atrium through the mitral valve (as it should) and also flows back from the aorta through the leaking aortic valve. The heart has to work harder, which leads to enlargement of the left ventricle and inefficient functioning.

## Causes of aortic regurgitation

The usual causes of aortic regurgitation are degeneration of a valve that has two cusps instead of the normal three cusps, degeneration with aging, infection (endocarditis or rheumatic fever), and abnormal expansion of the aorta above the valve.

## Symptoms of aortic regurgitation

Symptoms of aortic regurgitation, when they develop, are usually those of congestive heart failure (fatigue, weakness, shortness of breath with exercise or at night, swelling in the ankles). You might also experience palpitations, night sweating, and angina.

## How serious is aortic regurgitation?

If you have aortic regurgitation, you can remain free of symptoms for a long time. If the aortic regurgitation is caused by rheumatic fever, symptoms may develop slowly over 10 to 30 years. If it is caused by endocarditis, symptoms may develop much more quickly and be more severe—even life-threatening.

*Paul is a 33-year-old manager of a fast-food franchise who has had a diagnosis of bicuspid aortic valve since age 19, when an echocardiogram was done to evaluate a murmur. Four weeks ago he had three cavities filled. For the past 2 weeks he has felt tired and had a fever on most days, often with chills. During the past 2 days, he has become short of breath and cannot lie flat without making the shortness of breath worse. Evaluation confirms the doctor's impression that he had an infection of the aortic valve and acute aortic regurgitation.*

Much of the decision-making difficulty associated with mitral regurgitation also applies to aortic regurgitation. You can have minimal symptoms and yet your pumping function can deteriorate to a point that even if the valve is replaced, you may not improve as much as you might have if an operation had been undertaken earlier. However, an operation for even very advanced aortic regurgitation is still likely to yield a good result.

## Defects in valves on the right side of the heart

The valves on the right side of the heart (tricuspid and pulmonary) are much less frequently affected by disease than those on the left side, and when they are, the disease is better tolerated in many cases.

Blood returning from the body flows into the right atrium, through the tricuspid valve, and into the right ventricle. From the right ventricle, the blood flows through the pulmonary valve to the pulmonary artery, which carries the blood to the lungs to receive oxygen. Both the tricuspid and the pulmonary valves can be affected by tightening (stenosis) or back leakage (regurgitation).

## Tricuspid stenosis

The tricuspid valve is the largest of the four valves in the heart. When it is affected by stenosis, it limits the blood flow from the right atrium to the right ventricle. Tricuspid stenosis is rare and usually occurs with other valve problems.

### *Causes of tricuspid stenosis*

Tricuspid stenosis is usually caused by rheumatic fever or congenital heart disease. Rarely, it can be caused by injury resulting from substances manufactured by a certain type of cancer cell called carcinoid.

### *Symptoms of tricuspid stenosis*

Symptoms of tricuspid stenosis include generalized weakness and discomfort in the upper right abdomen due to back pressure in the liver. In most cases the symptoms are related to associated disease in the mitral or aortic valve. These symptoms include fatigue, shortness of breath, and fluid retention.

### *How serious is tricuspid stenosis?*

Because tricuspid stenosis tends to occur along with other valve problems, the other valve problems determine the outcome more than the tricuspid stenosis. If the function of the valve has deteriorated badly, surgery may be necessary.

If you have tricuspid stenosis, you are at risk for endocarditis and should take preventive antibiotics before and after dental and certain surgical procedures.

## Tricuspid regurgitation

Tricuspid regurgitation allows blood to leak back into the right atrium from the right ventricle.

### Causes of tricuspid regurgitation

Tricuspid regurgitation is usually caused by congenital heart disease and rarely occurs by itself. It may also result from rheumatic fever or endocarditis, or when the pressure in the right side of the heart is high—a condition referred to as pulmonary hypertension.

Tricuspid regurgitation can occasionally be a result of blunt trauma to the chest, such as hitting the steering wheel in a car accident.

Prolapse of the tricuspid valve can occur, just as it does with the mitral valve. One rare but important cause of tricuspid regurgitation is deposits of a type of cancer cell called carcinoid.

### Symptoms of tricuspid regurgitation

If there is right-sided heart failure, you may feel fatigued and have swelling in the arms, legs and liver, along with nausea and vomiting (see page 46).

### How serious is tricuspid regurgitation?

Tricuspid disease is usually associated with other valve problems, and these will determine how serious the condition may be.

With the advent of sensitive tests that can assess blood flow in the heart, a small amount of tricuspid regurgitation can be seen in almost all normal individuals. Thus, although the valves normally work extremely well, they do not completely seal off a small amount of back leakage.

If you have tricuspid regurgitation caused by an abnormal tricuspid valve, you are at risk for endocarditis and should take preventive antibiotics before and after dental and certain surgical procedures (see page 71).

## Pulmonary valve stenosis

The pulmonary valve controls the flow of blood from the right ventricle to the pulmonary artery, which leads to the lungs. If the valve is tight, it limits the amount of blood that flows to the lungs (see illustration, page 65).

### Causes of pulmonary stenosis

When it occurs, pulmonary stenosis is almost always a congenital problem. Rarely, it is caused by rheumatic fever or deposits of carcinoid tumor cells on the valve. Sometimes a tumor or aneurysm may compress the valve.

### Symptoms of pulmonary stenosis

Symptoms occur only if the pulmonary stenosis is severe. They include fatigue, shortness of breath with exercise, light-headedness, and loss of consciousness. If the obstruction is severe, symptoms of right ventricular heart failure appear (swelling in arms, legs, and abdomen and a tender, enlarged liver). Bluish skin (cyanosis) may be present if the outflow of blood is substantially reduced or if there is associated shunting of blood from the right side of the heart to the left.

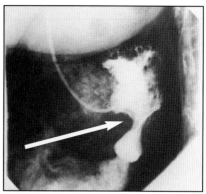 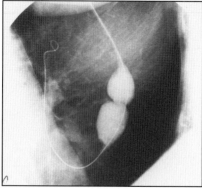 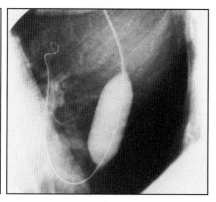

*Balloon valvotomy is used to open a stenotic pulmonary valve.* **Left:** *Tightened pulmonary valve* (**arrow**) *interrupts flow of blood to the lungs.* **Middle:** *As the balloon begins to inflate, the stenotic valve causes the center of the balloon to remain indented.* **Right:** *Fully inflated balloon opens the valve, allowing blood to flow freely to the lungs.*

### How serious is pulmonary stenosis?

Pulmonary stenosis, when severe, can lead to failure of the right ventricle and, ultimately, to death before 30 years of age. Thus, many people with pulmonary stenosis may require surgery or balloon dilatation using a catheter technique.

The traditional treatment for pulmonary stenosis was surgical pulmonary valvotomy, but this has largely been replaced by the catheter-based procedure known as balloon valvotomy, which avoids open heart surgery (see illustrations above).

If you have pulmonary stenosis, you are at risk for endocarditis and should take preventive antibiotics before and after dental and certain surgical procedures (see page 71).

## Pulmonary regurgitation

Pulmonary regurgitation allows some of the blood to leak back into the right ventricle from the pulmonary artery.

### Causes of pulmonary regurgitation

Pulmonary regurgitation can be caused by congenital disease or be a consequence of high blood pressure in the lungs. It is rarely caused by endocarditis.

### Symptoms of pulmonary regurgitation

People with pulmonary regurgitation usually have no symptoms unless severe regurgitation develops with right ventricular enlargement and heart failure. If these occur, you may feel generally tired and have shortness of breath with exercise, loss of appetite, nausea, vomiting, and discomfort in the upper right part of your abdomen (from liver congestion). You may also have swelling in the arms and legs.

*How serious is pulmonary regurgitation?*

Pulmonary regurgitation seems to be very well tolerated by the body. Indeed, there is evidence that some people can function perfectly well with the pulmonary valve removed.

If symptoms of right ventricular failure appear, surgery to repair or replace the valve may be done.

If you have significant pulmonary regurgitation due to structural abnormalities, take preventive antibiotics before and after dental and certain surgical procedures to prevent endocarditis.

## Coronary blockages and heart attack

Blockage of the coronary arteries supplying the heart muscle causes more deaths, disability, and economic loss than any other type of heart disease. More than 6 million Americans annually experience symptoms due to coronary artery disease, and many will seek emergency room evaluations for care. As many as 1,100,000 Americans will have heart attacks this year, and about one third of the attacks will be fatal. Coronary artery disease kills more than 350,000 women a year in the United States. Over 350,000 people in the United States develop angina pectoris each year.

Annually in the United States, more than 350,000 people undergo coronary artery bypass graft operations, and about 480,000 people will have percutaneous transluminal coronary angioplasty, to try to reroute or reopen clogged coronary arteries. Approximately 100,000 thrombolytic procedures are done each year to try to dissolve clots blocking coronary arteries in people having heart attacks. The American Heart Association estimates that in 1999, cardiovascular diseases and stroke cost the nation's economy $286.5 billion.

As dismal as these statistics sound, the past decade has seen dramatic declines in cardiovascular disease in this country and elsewhere. The death rate from coronary artery disease has decreased impressively since 1980.

Although no one can say exactly why this decline has occurred, it is likely that better control of risk factors has played a role. Beyond these factors, progress in the diagnosis and treatment of coronary artery disease has also had an impact.

*Coronary artery disease*

The coronary arteries are the heart's own circulatory system. They supply the heart itself with blood, oxygen, and nutrients. The heart uses this blood supply for energy to perform its continuous task of pumping.

HEALTHY
HEART ♥ TIP

*Of all the illegal drugs, cocaine has probably caused the most deaths from heart disease. The stimulant can be traced to other cardiovascular complications, too, such as chest-pain syndromes, heart attacks, strokes, fatal and nonfatal arrhythmias, myocarditis, endocarditis, pulmonary edema, vascular thrombosis and dilated cardiomyopathy.*

*Some of these potentially fatal complications can occur even in those who try the drug for the first time. Older individuals with abnormal coronary arteries and diseased cerebral vessels are at even greater risk, as are pregnant women and the fetuses they carry.*

Coronary artery disease can take many different forms (see page A10), but they all have the same effect: The heart muscle does not get enough blood and oxygen through the coronary arteries. Consequently, the heart's own demands for oxygen and nutrients are not met. This condition can be either temporary or permanent. When the heart muscle does not get enough blood and oxygen, it is said to be experiencing ischemia. Angina is the chest discomfort people experience during ischemia.

Most coronary artery disease is caused by atherosclerosis (commonly called hardening of the arteries). The term "atherosclerosis" comes from the Greek ather (meaning "porridge") and sklerosis (meaning "hardening"). Fatty deposits collect in and on the lining of the artery walls, primarily the large coronary arteries, producing narrowing. If the narrowing is severe, blood flow can be obstructed.

## Atherosclerosis (hardening and narrowing of arteries)

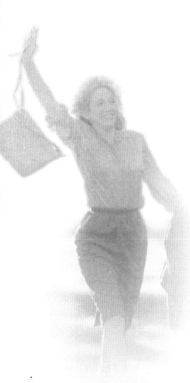

Healthy arteries are flexible, strong, and elastic. The inner layer of arteries is smooth, enabling blood to flow freely. As you age, your arteries normally become thicker and less elastic, and their calcium content increases. This hardening is believed to occur throughout the major artery system.

Atherosclerosis contrasts to this natural process, because it affects mainly the large arteries (including the coronary arteries). The inner layers of the artery walls become thick and irregular, and certain areas accumulate fats, cholesterol, and other materials. This gradual buildup of atherosclerotic plaque over a long time reduces the circulation of blood and increases the risk of heart attack, stroke, and other serious arterial diseases.

Initially the deposits are only streaks of fat-containing cells called fatty streaks. They are usually located at the points where arteries branch off. The fatty streaks can be found in the coronary arteries even as early as puberty. These streaks are common and have been found, incidentally, in teenagers who have died in motor

### Definitions

**Cardiovascular disease:** any disease that affects the heart or the blood vessels

**Coronary artery disease:** blockage in the coronary arteries

**Coronary heart disease:** coronary artery disease, plus its consequences (for example, scar tissue due to a heart attack caused by arterial blockage)

**Myocardial ischemia:** blockage of the coronary arteries resulting in insufficient blood and oxygen reaching the heart muscle

**Silent ischemia:** myocardial ischemia that causes no symptoms

**Angina:** chest pain or pressure that results from myocardial ischemia

**Myocardial infarction (heart attack):** myocardial ischemia that lasts long enough to cause tissue death in the area of the heart supplied by a blocked coronary artery

vehicle accidents. As the fatty streaks enlarge, they invade some of the deeper layers of the artery walls, causing scarring and calcium deposits. Larger accumulations are called atheromas or plaques.

In atherosclerosis, blood cells called platelets often clump at microscopic sites of injury to the inner wall of the artery. Fat deposits also collect at these sites.

The plaque consists of a firm "shell" that may contain calcium with areas of fatty material, and the center consists of soft cholesterol. The shell portion may crack or fissure, exposing the inner portion. When this happens, a blood clot tends to develop at that site. The clot may sufficiently reduce blood flow in the coronary arteries to cause angina (chest pain) or myocardial infarction (heart attack).

### Causes of atherosclerosis

The fatty streaks that are present very early in life do not necessarily grow into cholesterol-laden plaques. The mechanism that leads to the formation of blockages in the artery is still poorly understood. However, the risks of developing atherosclerosis are increased by certain identifiable factors, referred to as risk factors.

Some people are susceptible because of their genetic makeup or because they eat a high-fat diet. Other factors such as high blood pressure, high cholesterol levels in the blood, cigarette smoking, and diabetes can also promote the development of fatty arterial plaques.

### Who is affected by atherosclerosis?

Atherosclerosis occurs mostly in middle-aged and elderly people. Up to about age 50, women lag behind men in the severity of atherosclerosis. After that, however, they catch up quickly.

High blood pressure, high blood cholesterol levels, and smoking encourage the development of atherosclerosis. Older age, a family history of coronary artery disease, diabetes, obesity, and a sedentary lifestyle also make you more susceptible to atherosclerosis.

### How serious is atherosclerosis?

When atherosclerosis occurs in the coronary arteries, it can lead to myocardial ischemia. If the duration of ischemia is brief and your heart receives enough blood, oxygen and nutrients in time, the abnormalities caused by ischemia are reversible. However, if the duration of ischemia is longer than 40 to 60 minutes, significant irreversible injury may occur, and the parts of the heart muscle deprived of blood may become permanently damaged. This is a heart attack.

## Symptoms caused by coronary artery disease

Coronary artery disease can present as angina, myocardial infarction (heart attack), or sudden cardiac death. The most dramatic symptom of coronary artery disease is sudden death without prior warning. The most recognizable presentation of coronary artery disease is myocardial infarction, which can cause severe disability and death. At the other end of the spectrum is silent ischemia, which is significant coronary artery disease that causes no symptoms, at least for much of the time. Between those two ends of the spectrum is angina pectoris (chest pain).

## Angina pectoris

*Bob was late for his meeting. He grabbed his briefcase and headed for the elevator. When it didn't come within a few seconds, he decided it would be faster to run up the three flights of stairs. After the second flight, he stopped, put his hand on his chest, and took some deep breaths. He had a tight feeling behind his breastbone and seemed unusually short of breath. After he rested a few minutes, the discomfort faded away.*

Bob's description represents one of the most common patterns of symptoms in coronary artery disease—angina pectoris.

### Causes of angina pectoris

Angina is the symptom that results from myocardial ischemia. The degree of coronary narrowing can vary, ranging from partial blockage in one vessel to extensive clogging of many vessels.

### The discomfort of angina

When the heart muscle does not get enough oxygen and nutrients, the heart cells use their own stores of energy for pumping. However, this process can work for only a short time before the heart cells are permanently damaged.

Moreover, this process results in the buildup of by-products that cannot be removed efficiently because of the blocked blood flow, which caused the problem in the first place. This buildup of waste products (such as lactic acid) has been implicated as a cause of the pain in angina and heart attacks, just as the buildup of lactic acid in your other muscles causes pain when you overwork them.

### How serious is angina pectoris?

If angina occurs only after unusual physical exertion, no drastic change in lifestyle is required to prevent the pain. However, some people experience frequent bouts of angina during routine daily activities. They may change their daily routine so they do not have to do any strenuous exercise. Interestingly, the severity of symptoms does not relate directly to how many coronary arteries have blockages. A tight blockage in a small branch of a coronary artery can cause more discomfort in one person than severe narrowing of all three major coronary artery trunks in another person.

Some people with ischemia do not have typical anginal chest pain. Instead, they experience shortness of breath or, less commonly, fatigue or weakness as the only or main symptom of cardiac ischemia. Nevertheless, whatever the resulting symptoms, coronary artery disease represents ischemia in the heart muscle and should be monitored by your doctor.

### Who is affected by angina pectoris?

Angina is common, but only rarely occurs before age 30 in men and later in women. About 3 million people in the United States have angina, and 300,000 new cases develop each year.

### Types of angina

Angina related to blockage in the coronary arteries can be subdivided according to whether it has had a predictable pattern for a prolonged time (stable angina) or is new or increasing (unstable angina). A third type of angina, variant angina, has nothing to do with plaque buildup in the arteries. Instead, it is caused by spasm of the muscle encircling the coronary arteries.

Stable angina. When the pattern of chest pain has remained unchanged in terms of severity, frequency, and duration for several weeks or months, it is referred to as stable angina. The symptoms are relatively predictable and occur with fairly consistent amounts of exertion or stress.

The main problem in stable angina is a fixed blockage to blood flow through one or more coronary arteries, caused by an atherosclerotic plaque. This narrows the diameter of the coronary artery so that only a limited amount of blood, carrying oxygen and nutrients, can reach the heart muscle.

Bob should have known that he would have trouble with the stairs. He has had that same chest pain every time he has overexerted himself for the past year.

The blood flow may be adequate for the heart when it is at rest, but when you exert yourself, the blockage does not allow the blood flow to increase as the demands of the heart increase. The heart's demand for oxygen outstrips the supply. Myocardial ischemia results, causing the symptoms of angina. Treatment with medications may be sufficient for the management of stable angina.

Unstable angina. Unstable angina refers to a pattern of symptoms when angina is new, lasts longer, is more severe or frequent, is easier to provoke with less and less stress, occurs at rest, and responds less to medications that used to relieve the discomfort.

A month or so later, Bob started having his chest pain after only a few steps, and sometimes when he was just reading or watching television.

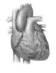

The presence of unstable angina implies that the underlying situation is fragile and worsening. Because this pattern often occurs before the development of a heart attack, it is sometimes called "preinfarction angina."

Researchers have not completely discovered what is happening during unstable angina. This is likely a phase of coronary artery disease in which the severity of the obstruction is intermittently getting worse and then better in a repeating cycle.

Some studies have shown that coronary arteries in people with stable angina have a smooth inner (endothelial) surface free of blood clots. People with worsening angina have ulceration and roughening of the endothelial lining, and people with unstable angina often have blood clots that form and dissolve sporadically.

When angina occurs at rest, the heart is not demanding extra oxygen, because there is no additional stress. Therefore, the problem must be a suddenly inadequate blood supply. This may be due to one of two things.

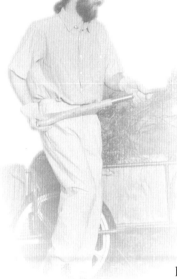

First, the coronary blood vessels, like all blood vessels, can dilate or constrict as a normal regulatory feature. When the nervous system signals an artery to constrict, and it is already severely blocked by atherosclerotic plaque, the blood flow—which is already inadequate—may be cut severely.

The second possible reason for inadequate blood supply is that the atherosclerotic plaque is at a point in the circulation where there is a great deal of turbulence (such as a bend in the artery) and the lining of the blood vessel (endothelium) is partly destroyed and malfunctioning. This damage leads to clumping of platelets on top of the atherosclerotic plaque. The additional clumping of debris impedes blood flow even further. After the platelets "pile up" to a certain point, the clump may dissolve or simply break up and move downstream, in which case blood flow can resume at its previous suboptimal level (see page A10).

Either of these mechanisms may account for the waxing and waning pattern of unstable angina. Because unstable angina is a serious development, your doctor frequently will recommend hospitalization for stabilization, assessment, and further treatment.

**Variant angina.** The muscle fibers encircling the coronary arteries may go into spasm in some individuals.

When that occurs, the lumen (the hollow part of the artery) at one point can severely narrow or even close off temporarily. Many problems can result, including silent ischemia, angina, and heart attack.

Variant angina (also called Prinzmetal's angina, after one of the first physicians to describe the pattern of symptoms) is different from the usual type of angina, in which demand for oxygen-rich blood outstrips supply. With variant angina, spasm can occur even in the absence of excess demand. In other words, the blood supply is cut off to a point less than the minimal requirements of the heart muscle even when it is at rest. Severe angina can occur with spasm, but some people experience no symptoms (silent ischemia).

The spasms may occur without apparent cause, but they also may result from strong emotional stress, exposure to cold, or inhaling cigarette smoke.

The symptoms of variant angina tend to be different from the pattern of stable or unstable angina. Variant angina is typically severe, lasts for a brief time, and frequently occurs at night, waking you from sleep. Abnormal rhythm disorders are common during the periods of blood flow cutoff, which can cause you to pass out.

### Is angina always painful?

Lack of oxygen to the heart—ischemia—can result in pain called angina. But ischemia can also be "silent," not causing any pain, even during a heart attack. One large study of residents of Framingham, Mass., found that 35 percent of heart attacks in women and 25 percent in men were not recognized by the affected individuals as heart attacks at all. About half of those studied reported feeling no symptoms, and half thought their symptoms were caused by another condition, such as indigestion.

Studies have also shown that as much as a 50 percent blockage in a coronary artery generally doesn't produce any symptoms at all. And severe ischemia caused by blockage in several coronary arteries can produce significant symptoms in some people but none at all in others. Ischemia may also be "silent" in some people because of differences in their perception of pain. For example, people who have diabetes may have a decreased sensation of pain due to nerve damage.

Some people may not be aware of a heart problem until they develop symptoms of congestive heart failure—extreme fatigue with exertion and shortness of breath, especially when lying down.

## Heart attack (myocardial infarction)

*Sam was just finishing breakfast when it hit: severe, intolerable pressure in his chest. He wanted to think it was indigestion and that it would go away if he waited a few minutes, but it didn't stop. He had a vague feeling of uneasiness. Should he tell his wife about it? When he started sweating profusely and feeling nauseated, he decided to tell his wife. He had a feeling of impending doom. His wife called 911. The doctors said it was lucky he came to the hospital: Sam was having a heart attack.*

Myocardial infarction (heart attack) can be thought of as the result of coronary artery blockage. An infarct is an area of tissue that has been permanently damaged because of starvation for oxygen and nutrients.

A heart attack occurs when a coronary artery is blocked permanently, or for longer than about 30 minutes to 2 hours. The region of the heart muscle (myocardium) supplied by that coronary artery is starved for oxygen and nutrition for so long that irreversible damage (necrosis) occurs.

A heart attack generally causes severe anginal pain for longer than 15 minutes, but it is also possible to have a "silent" heart attack in which no symptoms occur. The evidence of a silent heart attack may show up on an electrocardiogram or other tests on the heart, or it may be discovered during autopsy.

### *Causes of a heart attack*

Although physicians rarely have the chance to see coronary arteries at the exact moment of a heart attack (by doing coronary angiography), evidence indicates that a heart attack is caused by the sudden complete blockage of a coronary artery by a blood clot. The blood clot often forms at the site of a crack or rupture in an atherosclerotic plaque.

When angiography is done within several hours of a heart attack, a blood clot is frequently seen. If angiography is done later, however, there is less likelihood of seeing a blood clot. These angiographic findings suggest that blood clots tend to dissolve somewhat with time, although usually too late to prevent tissue necrosis.

Thus, one of the main treatments of heart attacks is the use of clot-dissolving medications (thrombolytic agents).

Most often, the clot that causes a heart attack forms in a coronary artery that has been narrowed by fatty deposits of atherosclerosis. Rarely, blood clots can develop inside the heart in conditions such as mitral stenosis or in people who have previous heart damage. Clots can break off and enter the circulation of the coronary arteries, causing a heart attack if the blood clot lodges in a coronary artery and prevents blood flow from reaching the heart muscle. (This is the same way that a stroke is caused by a blood clot lodging in an artery in the brain.)

### How serious is a heart attack?

A heart attack may lead to immediate death, either because so much of the heart dies that it can no longer function or because fatal rhythm disorders develop. However, many people survive a heart attack and are hospitalized.

If the area of damaged heart muscle (infarct) is small and the electrical system that controls your heart is not damaged, your chances of surviving a heart attack are good. The sooner you get to a hospital, the more can be done to limit the amount of heart muscle damage.

In general, damage to less than 10 percent of the ventricle muscle may lead to a decrease in the amount of blood that your heart can eject during each contraction. However, the reduction in heart function is mild, so a return to a reasonably normal lifestyle usually can be anticipated. If 25 percent or more of the heart muscle is damaged, your heart may enlarge and heart failure may develop. If 40 percent or more of the heart muscle is damaged, shock or death may occur. Any heart attack may lead to further complications.

The location of the tissue damage can also affect the outcome. If the heart attack involves the front (anterior) portion of the heart, the consequences are likely to be more serious than if the tissue damage is along the lower (inferior) part of the heart muscle. Anterior heart attacks are usually more extensive.

Most people who die of heart attacks have severe blockages of more than one coronary artery so that a large portion of the heart muscle is damaged. Also, the pumping function of the left ventricle is impaired, which is associated with fatal rhythm disturbances.

## Factors that improve your chance for a favorable outcome after a heart attack

- Younger age
- No prior heart attack
- No recurrence of pain
- No congestive heart failure
- No heart rhythm disorders
- Normal blood pressure
- No diabetes
- Normal weight
- Male sex

Most people who are still alive 2 hours after the heart attack started will survive. However, there are possible complications. Approximately 7 percent to 12 percent of people who have a heart attack die during their hospitalization, although these rates are declining with new treatment techniques. Of those who survive to leave the hospital, about 5 percent to 15 percent die in the first year after a heart attack. About the same percentage have another heart attack within the next year.

*Emergency signs and symptoms of a heart attack*

Not all of the signs and symptoms mentioned below are present in all cases of heart attack, and some people do not have any symptoms. The more symptoms you have, the higher the likelihood that you are having a heart attack. Get help if you have any combination of these symptoms:

- Intense, prolonged chest pain (often a feeling of heavy pressure)
- Pain radiating from the chest to the left shoulder and arm, back, and even jaw
- Prolonged pain in the upper abdomen
- Shortness of breath
- Fainting
- Nausea, vomiting, intense sweating
- Frequent angina attacks that are not caused by exertion

People sometimes think back and realize that they did have a few signs that things were not quite right before they had their heart attacks. A spouse or co-worker will often say the person looked older, paler, exhausted, or depressed before the heart attack. Unfortunately, only about one third of people with these symptoms consult the doctor. In elderly people, symptoms may be atypical, including vomiting of no known cause, unsteadiness, or confusion.

If you think you or some-one you are with is having a heart attack, find medical attention immediately and give a chewable aspirin. Fifteen percent of heart attack victims die suddenly within the first hour of symptoms. Sudden death can even be the first symptom of a heart attack. If you are with someone who stops breathing, begin cardiopulmonary resuscitation (CPR) immediately. After a person stops breathing, he or she can live only a few minutes without CPR. This limited time emphasizes the need for everyone to have training in CPR.

## Recognize a heart attack—you may save your life

Prompt, efficient treatment greatly improves your chances of surviving a heart attack. The first and most important step in treating a heart attack is your own recognition of what is occurring. The key to successful treatment is early treatment.

Unfortunately, too many people with heart attacks attribute the symptoms to something else or simply hope that the symptoms will disappear. They are putting themselves at an immediate disadvantage for effective treatment and survival. Of all people who die from their heart attacks, most of them (60 percent) die within the first hour after the onset of symptoms, before medical help is sought.

A heart attack is a medical emergency. It is important to reread the section on chest pain and recognize that if it lasts longer than 15 minutes and does not respond to nitroglycerin (if this medication has been prescribed for you), you must seek medical care at once.

Each year thousands of people die because they did not seek medical help in time. Don't worry about confusing a heart attack with indigestion or something else. Get immediate help. It may save your life.

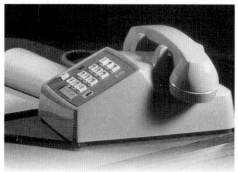

*Pick up the telephone.*

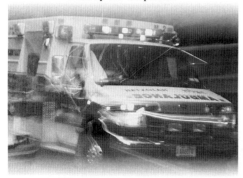

*Go to the emergency room.*

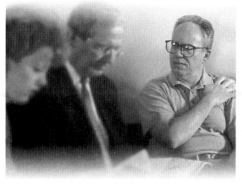

*Make your symptoms known
to hospital personnel.*

## Why people delay seeking help

- "I didn't think it was anything serious"
- "I thought the pain would go away"
- "I didn't think it was my heart"
- "I didn't want to inconvenience anyone"
- "I would be so embarrassed if I went to the hospital and they found nothing wrong"

Prompt treatment of a heart attack can make a big difference in the outcome. Medical attention within 1 hour is the goal, but treatment often is delayed by up to 4 hours. Indecision in seeking medical attention is the biggest factor, accounting for 62 percent of the typical delay. Transportation to the emergency room accounts for 9 percent, and delays within the hospital 29 percent.

If in doubt, wait no longer than 15 minutes before calling for help. Resist the temptation to delay calling based on the following factors:

- The tendency to attribute heart attack symptoms to less serious, noncardiac causes, such as indigestion
- The tendency to wait and see if symptoms will go away
- The tendency to self-medicate (take an antacid)
- The tendency to seek advice from family, friends or coworkers
- The tendency to call one's physician
- A reluctance to use the emergency medical services system

### Complications of a heart attack

The first problems associated with a heart attack—pain and discomfort, the risk of death, and permanent damage to the heart—may not be the last. Beyond these, a heart attack can lead to several other complications.

Congestive Heart Failure. After a heart attack, your heart may not pump as effectively, which may lead to symptoms of congestive heart failure. People with a severe decrease in blood flow and congestion in the lungs (pulmonary congestion) after a heart attack are at the highest risk of death.

Rhythm Abnormalities. Heart attacks can also lead to severe rhythm abnormalities. Rhythm disturbances account for more than one half of all deaths from heart attack.

The most lethal rhythm abnormality is ventricular fibrillation, in which the contractions of the ventricles are very rapid and uncoordinated. Actually, the movement of the heart is more quivering than contracting. Without regular contractions, your heart cannot pump blood to the vital organs, so this rhythm is life-threatening. It is often called "cardiac arrest," and it is the major mechanism for sudden cardiac death.

Other abnormalities in the sinus node (the heart's natural pacemaker, which initiates the heartbeat) and in the electrical system that conducts the heartbeat can result in a heartbeat that is too fast (tachycardia) or too slow (bradycardia).

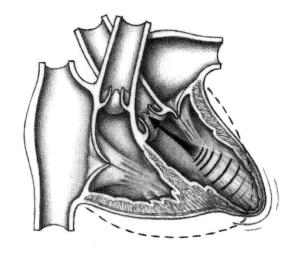

*A heart attack may weaken a portion of the heart wall, producing a bulge (aneurysm). When the ventricle contracts, the aneurysm may actually bulge out further.*

Ventricular septal defect. Tissue death and rupture of the muscular wall (septum) between the two ventricles lead to ventricular septal defect. Heart failure may develop suddenly in a previously stable person if the ventricular septum ruptures. If the problem is severe, immediate surgery to repair the septal defect is necessary.

Mitral valve regurgitation. A heart attack can destroy part of the mitral valve apparatus (such as a papillary muscle that supports the valve) and lead to severe, sudden regurgitation (back leakage) of blood from the left ventricle back into the left atrium. Severe congestive heart failure and death will follow shortly if the problem is not immediately recognized and treated.

Ventricular aneurysm. The section of heart muscle affected by the heart attack can expand and thin out like a weak portion on a bald tire. This bulge (or aneurysm) leads to ineffective pumping, rhythm disorders, and difficult-to-control chest pain. An aneurysm, especially early after the heart attack, is associated with a much higher risk of death, heart failure, arrhythmias, and blood clots.

Ventricular rupture. Because the damaged heart muscle is "mushy" until it forms a firm scar, the heart wall at the site of the myocardial infarction can actually tear (rupture). This catastrophic complication is like a blowout on a worn tire. Shock and circulatory collapse suddenly develop (because in this case the blood does flow out of the heart itself). Ventricular rupture almost always results in death. Fortunately, this complication is uncommon. When it does happen, it usually occurs within a week after the heart attack itself.

Some people may have an incomplete rupture of the wall of the heart. In this case, the pericardium and blood clots may seal the site of rupture. Death is not immediate in such cases. If the condition can be stabilized, surgical repair is possible.

Clot formation. Clots can form inside the ventricle, next to the muscle affected by the heart attack, especially when it becomes dilated or develops an aneurysm. Any clot that forms in the left ventricle can break loose and travel (embolize) to the blood vessels in the brain, causing a stroke. Medications that keep blood from clotting (anticoagulants) are essential.

Recurrence of angina. Around the zone of damaged muscle in the heart, there is usually a region of myocardial cells that survived the heart attack but are in danger

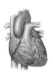

of permanent damage if any further ischemia occurs. If angina recurs after a heart attack, it may indicate that the heart attack is extending into this "area at risk." Such symptoms early after a heart attack should prompt an immediate aggressive attempt to limit further damage. This might include catheterization to determine whether blocked vessels can or should be opened up or bypassed.

Pericarditis. Inflammation of the pericardium (see page A16) develops in about 10 percent of people with heart attack. The inflammation is related to the death of the cells in the heart wall. The condition is usually brief and responds to anti-inflammatory drugs; only rarely is it a recurrent or persistent problem.

Cardiogenic shock. Cardiogenic shock results when the heart muscle is too weak to contract with enough force to maintain the blood pressure at a level that provides a sufficient amount of blood to the body and the heart muscle itself. A vicious circle develops. The coronary arteries do not get enough blood, which makes the heart weaker, which in turn further decreases the blood supply. This circle is fatal in most cases.

Cardiogenic shock is a complication during the first days after a heart attack in about 7 percent to 15 percent of people. Those who die of cardiogenic shock have infarction of 40 percent or more of the left ventricle. Most have severe disease in three of their coronary arteries.

New clot-dissolving medications or special catheterization techniques may help prevent this complication or decrease its severity.

### Silent ischemia

*At the age of 53 years, Ben was feeling great but was required by his company to have a medical examination before his promotion. His physical examination, chest X-ray, and blood test results were normal. His doctor told him, however, that his treadmill exercise test showed abnormalities consistent with ischemia, even though Ben had reached a good exercise level and had no symptoms other than getting normally breathless at the end.*

Ben's situation actually raises a number of complex and controversial issues. What conclusions should Ben and his doctor draw from his examination?

- Is the treadmill test incorrect? It is well recognized that it is not a perfect test and may occasionally yield a false result (see page 241).

- Is the test correct and does Ben have true ischemia even though it causes no symptoms?

- Is it necessary to do further testing to see whether the test is correct?

- If the test is correct, is treatment necessary? After all, Ben is not having any symptoms.

- Of course, the overriding question perhaps is: "Should Ben have had the screening treadmill test in the first place?"

The fact is that many of these questions cannot be answered with certainty for individual people. For now, it is important to recognize that coronary artery disease can be present and cause myocardial ischemia even in people who have no symptoms.

### Causes of silent ischemia

Silent ischemia, like all ischemia, is caused by a blockage in a coronary artery. Silent ischemia may be caused by brief or less severe blockage. Or ischemia may be "silent" because of a difference in pain perception in different people or in different circumstances.

Unrecognized ischemia may be discovered when a person undergoes any kind of stress test or is monitored with electrocardiography for an extended period of time. Although silent ischemia does not cause symptoms, it may be a warning sign of future problems.

### How serious is silent ischemia?

Ischemia can be entirely silent (without symptoms) and still be severe enough to cause a heart attack. In fact, one large study of the population of Framingham, Mass., showed that 35 percent of heart attacks in women and 25 percent in men are not recognized as heart attacks; about half were silent, and about half caused symptoms incorrectly attributed to another cause. Numerous people with typical heart attacks have had no prior "warning symptoms" despite having had coronary artery disease for some time. Even people with symptoms of angina are often found, upon examination with appropriate monitors, to also have had episodes of ischemia without angina.

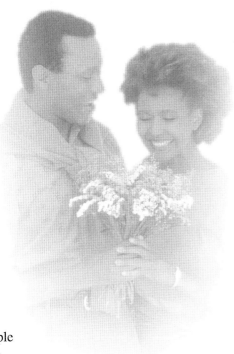

Growing evidence suggests that silent ischemia predicts a future course of events similar to that with typical symptoms—but this theory is hard to prove and is currently controversial. An educated guess based on several studies suggests that in the United States there are probably about 1 million men and women who have no idea that they have significant myocardial ischemia. Nevertheless, it is certainly not yet clear that looking for these people with expensive screening tests will have an overall benefit for them either individually or as a group.

## Kawasaki syndrome

Kawasaki syndrome is named for the Japanese doctor who, in 1967, described a newly recognized childhood illness. This syndrome is capable of producing coronary artery disease in children, and rarely it can cause heart attacks and death in this young age group. Since its discovery, the number of children affected by the illness has increased, and it is now one of the leading causes of acquired heart disease in children (as distinct from congenital heart disease)—a position once occupied by rheumatic fever.

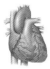

### HEALTHY HEART ♥ TIP

*Kawasaki disease is one of the leading causes of acquired heart disease in children in the United States.*

*Kids with Kawasaki experience fever, rash, swollen hands and feet, irritation and redness of the whites of the eyes, swollen lymph glands in the neck, and irritation and inflammation of the mouth, lips and throat. Doctors aren't sure what causes the syndrome, first discovered by Dr. Tomisaku Kawasaki, but believe it may be a virus. Death is rare, but nearly one fifth of those who have it experience some damage to the heart.*

*Doctors use aspirin to reduce fever, rash, joint inflammation and pain, and to help prevent blood clots from forming. When given early, intravenous gamma globulin can lower the risk of coronary abnormalities.*

### Causes of Kawasaki syndrome

No one is certain what causes Kawasaki syndrome. It is not considered contagious because no infectious agent has been identified, but it does tend to occur in outbreaks, especially in the winter and spring. Some experts suspect that an unusual virus or other germ may be the culprit, or toxic agents may be involved. Most of the hallmarks of Kawasaki syndrome are related to inflammation, and the damage that sometimes occurs in the coronary arteries or heart muscle may be due to the body's immune response.

### Symptoms of Kawasaki syndrome

Children who experience a lengthy (more than 5 days), high, spiking fever and any four of the following indicators may have Kawasaki syndrome, as long as there is nothing (such as a staphylococcal infection) to otherwise explain them:

Conjunctival infection (swollen, watery eyes)

Reddened, cracked, and swollen surfaces of the lips, tongue, mouth, and throat

Swollen, reddened hands and feet, followed by peeling of the skin in these areas

Measles-like rash

Swollen lymph glands of the neck

The feverish stage of the disease usually lasts 1 to 2 weeks, followed by improvement. It is during the phase of improvement that the heart can be affected. In about one out of five children with Kawasaki syndrome who are not treated, heart-related problems develop. The most common is expansion (aneurysm formation) of sections of coronary arteries. In some children, the aneurysm can become obstructed by clotted blood and cause a heart attack. Fortunately this is rare, especially with treatment.

### *How serious is Kawasaki syndrome?*

Although the illness can be harrowing, and despite its effect on the coronary arteries, Kawasaki syndrome is usually a self-limited illness. The death rate in treated children is well below 1 percent. Even among those in whom coronary problems develop, most have substantial resolution or improvement with time.

Treatment is designed to reduce inflammation and stave off damage to the heart and coronary arteries. This goal seems to be accomplished by high doses of aspirin (tablets) and injections of immunoglobulin (purified human antibodies).

### *Who is affected by Kawasaki syndrome?*

Four of every five people who get Kawasaki syndrome are less than 4 years old. People of Asian descent, even if they have lived in the United States for generations, are more susceptible. Some reports suggest that children with the syndrome had been exposed to recently shampooed carpets, but this finding has been inconsistent.

## Palpitations and passing out (arrhythmias)

Most likely you are entirely unaware of your heartbeat despite the continuous contraction and relaxation of your heart day in and day out. Like many things, your heartbeat remains unobtrusive as long as it is functioning smoothly and predictably. Unless you make some effort to detect your heartbeat by feeling the pulse at your wrist, you may never even appreciate the constant motion occurring inside you. You may become aware of the action of your heart only when normal circumstances are altered. If you lie on your left side in bed, with your ear pressed against the sheet, you may notice that you hear the sounds of your heart beating, transmitted through the mattress from your chest to your ear. Some people who notice this for the first time become concerned, but of course all they are hearing is the usual heartbeat.

The predictability of the heartbeat is what keeps the heart functioning "on schedule" and also lets you "get used to it" and ignore it. Although the normal heartbeat is predictable, it does not beat with clocklike precision. For one thing, your heart varies its rate of contraction during changes in your activities. It speeds up when you exercise, for the simple reason that by beating faster it can pump more blood to your laboring muscles. When your activity ceases, the rate of the heartbeat declines again to its normal resting level. If you exercise hard enough, your heart rate can accelerate to approximately 200 beats per minute.

The heart rate normally varies somewhat, even from one beat to the next. Heart rates from 50 to 100 beats per minute when you are inactive are normal, and you are seldom conscious of your heartbeat at those rates. This is called normal sinus rhythm. Disturbances of the heartbeat that cause it to go outside the limits of normal speeds or beyond the usual degree of variation may cause problems that range from the trivial (with no symptoms) to the very abnormal and deadly. The evaluation and treatment of abnormal heartbeats (called arrhythmias, meaning abnormal rhythms) constitute a major portion of the practice of cardiology.

The conduction system of your heart can be thought of as the electrical wiring that transmits impulses throughout the heart muscle and stimulates it to contract in an organized and regular way. It assures that your heart can carry out its task of pumping blood most efficiently. Problems with the electrical function of the heart account for the occurrence of arrhythmias.

## Symptoms of arrhythmias

The effect an arrhythmia has on you, in terms of symptoms and overall health, depends on several factors. To begin with, it depends on the specific type of arrhythmia. Sometimes, doctors can make educated guesses about what the arrhythmia is simply by observing (or hearing about) what has happened to you. Another factor is whether the arrhythmia is extremely abnormal or only a little abnormal. Not unexpectedly, the worse the arrhythmia (for example, very fast or very slow), the more severe will be the symptoms you experience.

Yet another consideration is the frequency with which an arrhythmia occurs. Does it occur daily? If so, it may cause major problems. If it occurs only once a year (or once in a lifetime), it might be considered a relatively minor problem. Of course, some arrhythmias are so serious that they need to occur only once to be devastating.

Another factor is how long the arrhythmia lasts when it occurs. Some arrhythmias last for only a single beat, although they may occur again in the next few seconds, minutes, or hours. Others last for hours or days or even throughout a person's life. Finally, the consequences of an arrhythmia depend on whether it is the only problem with the heart or whether there are additional problems such as cardiomyopathy or a recent heart attack. Usually, arrhythmias in the setting of other heart disease are more worrisome than if they occurred in an otherwise healthy heart.

## Diagnosis of arrhythmias

The evaluation of an arrhythmia may come about either because symptoms have occurred that might be due to a rhythm disorder or because an abnormality was discovered on an electrocardiogram during a routine checkup. Symptoms that may prompt a search for an arrhythmia include palpitations, fatigue, shortness of breath, light-headedness, syncope, or sudden death (and successful resuscitation, of course). The specific arrhythmias that may cause them are discussed in the following pages.

To treat an arrhythmia effectively (or, indeed, to determine whether treatment is even advisable) and overcome the symptoms it may be causing, the type of arrhythmia must be determined. An ECG shows the electrical component of the heartbeat most clearly. It would seem a simple matter to obtain an ECG, make a diagnosis, and start treatment.

Unfortunately, there are obstacles to this seemingly easy route. Just like clanking sounds beneath the hood of your car that go away as you drive into the mechanic's shop, arrhythmias and the symptoms they cause are notoriously hard to "catch." Several sophisticated tests have been devised to get around this obstacle, but it has not been eliminated. Once the arrhythmia is detected, other obstacles are the problems of deciding whether it is the cause of the symptoms and, if it is intermittent, whether it is likely to recur often enough or with serious enough consequences to warrant treatment.

## Classification of arrhythmias

Problems with the conduction system and rhythms fall into four general categories. The first category consists of abnormalities that are seen by the doctor on your ECG but do not directly cause an arrhythmia. In other words, you would not notice any unpredictable types of heartbeats by taking your pulse, nor would you experience any symptoms. This category is called "conduction system abnormalities." The second category is slow heartbeats (bradycardia). The third category might be termed irregular heartbeats. The fourth category is fast heartbeats (tachycardia).

Some specific arrhythmias overlap into different categories. For example, atrial fibrillation is usually both irregular and fast. The so-called sick sinus syndrome consists of both fast rhythms and slow rhythms at different times. Thus, not all arrhythmias fit neatly into one category, but all in all such a scheme helps to make sense of a very complicated topic.

## Conduction system abnormalities

*Bonnie is a 78-year-old retired credit union employee who has been entirely healthy throughout her life. A general medical examination this year disclosed a "bundle-branch block" on the ECG. Other than recommending her usual periodic physical examinations, her doctor does not recommend further action.*

Under normal circumstances, the electrical impulse that causes your heart to beat originates in the upper right atrial chamber, then moves through the middle of your heart to the lower chambers through special electrical conducting pathways. The rapid spread of this electrical impulse activates the lower chambers uniformly and allows your heart to effectively pump blood to your body and lungs. Slowing or interruption of conduction through this pathway is called a conduction system abnormality (see pages A12 and A13).

Not uncommonly, portions of the conduction system become defective and are unable to transmit the signal. Sometimes the signal is just slowed down as it travels down the defective portion of the circuit so that it is delayed in reaching its destination. In some cases the signal cannot get through that part of the conduction system at all; it is "blocked." The conduction system extends like branches from a tree trunk. If the block occurs in just one branch, the electrical impulse will have to take a different branch to reach its destination.

When the impulse takes an alternative branch, the rate and rhythm of the heart-beat are not affected, but the abnormal pathway the electrical impulse takes can be detected by your doctor on your ECG. There are several patterns that indicate where the block is located: The medical names of the main patterns are right bundle-branch block and left bundle-branch block. These can be further subdivided.

Another type of block that does not actually change the speed at which the heart beats occurs at the point where the impulse travels from the atria to the ventricles (the atrioventricular node). The impulse normally slows down here in order to coordinate the beating of the atria and ventricles. This slowing may become exaggerated, a fact that is recognizable only on the ECG; the slowing does not cause symptoms. It is referred to as "first-degree atrioventricular block." (You can probably guess that there are other degrees of atrioventricular block. You're right—they belong in other categories and are explained elsewhere.)

*An electrocardiogram shows the complete pattern of electrical impulses traveling throughout the heart during each heartbeat. When all parts of the conduction system are working properly, the electrocardiogram typically appears like this: A small "P wave" (atrial impulse) precedes a brief "PR segment" (as the impulse travels through the atrioventricular node), which is followed by a tall, narrow "QRS complex" (ventricular impulse). The circles (which do not actually appear on an electrocardiogram) show when the pulse from each heartbeat would be felt.*

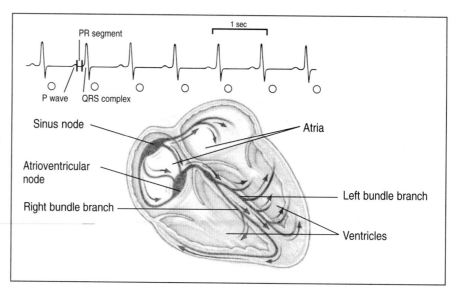

*In bundle-branch block (in this case, of the left bundle), the pattern of the electrocardiogram changes in characteristic ways. Because the impulse now has to take a more time-consuming and indirect route through the ventricle, the QRS complex becomes wide and abnormally shaped. However, the P wave, PR wave, PR interval, heart rate, and strength of the pulse are not affected.*

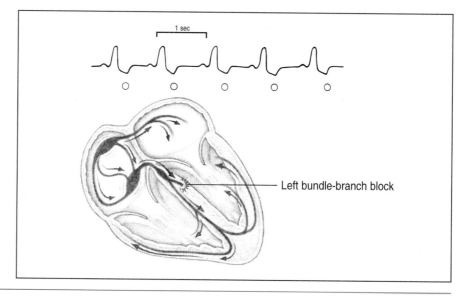

If these conduction abnormalities do not cause symptoms, are they a cause for concern? Although they almost never require treatment, they may be a subtle sign of other heart problems that may not have been recognized, or they may be a forewarning of more serious rhythm problems. For example, researchers have found that people with left bundle-branch block have a somewhat higher chance of developing coronary-artery-related problems, such as heart attacks, than people without left bundle-branch block. Left bundle-branch block may be the first sign of underlying heart muscle disease (such as dilated cardiomyopathy). Right bundle-branch block, however, is much less likely to be associated with coronary blockages or heart muscle disease.

There are a few exceptions to the benign nature of these conduction abnormalities. If left bundle-branch block develops during a heart attack, it is usually advisable to use a pacemaker temporarily, because left bundle-branch block in this fragile situation may indicate that a very slow heart rhythm may abruptly occur. Also, if a person with recurring fainting has no evidence of any problem except conduction system disease (even after a thorough evaluation), many doctors believe the cause of syncope is probably an intermittent, very slow heartbeat. A pacemaker might therefore be recommended.

### Slow heartbeats (bradycardia)

Any time the rate of heartbeats drops below 50 beats a minute, the rate is considered to be slow. However, the circumstances during which the bradycardia occurred must be taken into consideration. During sleep, for example, it is not unusual for the heart rate to descend into the 40s and even 30s in healthy individuals, and this should be considered a normal finding. Indeed, a slow heart rate, as long as the ECG and heart are otherwise normal, may be regarded as a sign of general fitness. Trained athletes often have resting heart rates of 40 to 50 beats a minute. Any slow heartbeat, regardless of cause, is referred to as bradycardia. Thus, slow heartbeats are called sinus bradycardia because the heartbeats still originate from the sinus node, your heart's natural pacemaker.

### Symptoms of bradycardia

*Megan is a 72-year-old retired professional flutist who began noticing sudden extreme fatigue about 2 weeks ago. Any of her routine activities caused her to be very tired and vaguely short of breath. She came to the doctor today because she suddenly "found herself on the kitchen floor" as she was preparing lunch. The office nurse takes her pulse: It is 32 beats per minute.*

Although slow heartbeats in athletes and during sleep may not be a cause for concern and are nonpathologic and not indicative of heart disease, other types of bradycardia are pathologic, or potentially so. Bradycardia in this sense means either a steady slowness of the heart over an extended time or pauses between heartbeats, either of which causes symptoms or poses a significant risk of causing future symptoms.

Typically, the symptoms produced by steady, slow heartbeats are fatigue, shortness of breath, or light-headedness (although these symptoms can also be due to many other causes). When your heart beats too slowly, it is not providing the rest of your body with sufficient blood supply to function efficiently.

Occasional pauses between heartbeats may cause no symptoms if they are brief (less than 3 seconds), especially if you are lying or sitting down when they occur. Pauses from 3 to 5 seconds will usually produce at least a passing sensation that you are about to black out. And pauses longer than 5 seconds will usually cause marked light-headedness or a blackout.

There is a marked variability in the effect of pauses on symptoms in that some people will abruptly lose consciousness after the 5-second pause, whereas others may be light-headed. The severity of the symptoms also depends on whether one is lying quietly or asleep at the time.

Classification of bradycardia. Bradycardia is differentiated on the basis of where the problem originates. There are three basic sites: the nerves that control the speed of the heartbeat (the autonomic nervous system), the sinus node that originates the heartbeat (it is the "spark plug" of the heart, so to speak), and the conduction system that distributes the electrical signal throughout the working muscle of the heart. Compromised function of any of these components may lead to a slow heartbeat.

**Problems with control by the nervous system.** Inappropriate function of the autonomic nervous system may cause abnormally slow heartbeats or, more often, pauses. The reflexes that automatically control the heartbeat temporarily seem to go awry in some people. One of these reflexes seems to have its basis in evolution: In certain animals, such as walruses, the heartbeats are known to slow down abruptly to an extraordinary degree when they dive into frigid waters. This decrease reduces the rate at which they use up energy and oxygen so they can remain submerged longer.

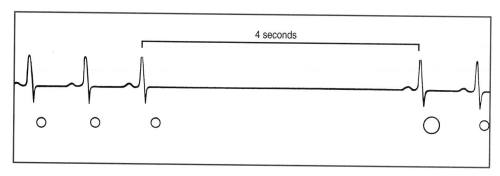

*This electrocardiogram shows a sudden pause in the electrical impulses produced by the sinus node. This results in a pause in the heartbeat, as depicted by the circles. In fact, you might feel a "stronger" heartbeat after the pause. This pause could produce light-headedness or even very brief loss of consciousness if you were standing up.*

Some people have pauses (and subsequent symptoms) because the part of the autonomic nervous system that promotes heart slowness suddenly does its job too well. Occasionally, this change can actually be provoked. For example, a tight necktie or collar may press on a region of the carotid artery in the neck called the carotid sinus. Nerves running through the neck at this point become activated by this pressure and may send a "slow down" message to the sinus node of the heart. (Don't confuse the carotid sinus and the sinus node—they are entirely different structures.) If you are too sensitive to the "slow down" signal, your heart may not just slow down a little (which would be normal), but it may actually stop for 5, 10, or even more seconds. The result is syncope. This type of syncope is called "carotid sinus hypersensitivity."

Other factors may activate the slowing part of the autonomic nervous system, such as straining at a bowel movement, urinating, gagging, or applying pressure to the eyeballs.

Doctors check for evidence of autonomic nervous system malfunction in people who report syncope by pressing on the (or massaging) carotid sinus while watching an electrocardiogram monitor. The doctor checks beforehand to make sure there is no evidence of blockage in the carotid artery, because the massage may aggravate it and precipitate a stroke.

Sometimes pain, fear, exhaustion, or low blood pressure can provoke bradycardia as well as further lowering of the blood pressure. When this happens, you may faint. "Simple fainting" (also referred to as vasovagal or neurocardiogenic syncope) can usually be distinguished from other more serious causes of loss of consciousness by the circumstances and by the associated symptoms. Typically, fainting is preceded by sweatiness, nausea, a prickly sensation in the skin, pallor, and at least a few seconds of "graying out" before the actual blackout occurs. Often it takes hours before you return to your normal state. This response is different from carotid sinus hypersensitivity or other types of syncope in which the passing out is characteristically abrupt, with little or no warning.

**Problems with the sinus node.** Sometimes the sinus node fails to perform adequately in its role as the heart's pacemaker. Despite proper signals from the autonomic nervous system, it simply initiates beats too slowly, pauses too long between beats, or simply stops producing beats. If it stops producing beats, a different part of the heart must take over the pacemaker function, which it usually does at a rate that is substantially slower than normal. The various ways the sinus node can malfunction are grouped under the term "sick sinus syndrome."

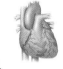

## HEALTHY HEART ♥ TIP

*When your heart's beating too fast, your doctor may decide to use radiofrequency ablation. This nonsurgical procedure is employed most often to treat supraventricular tachyarrhythmias, or rapid, uncoordinated heartbeats that start in the heart's upper chambers (atria) or AV node (the beginning of the heart's electrical system).*

*In radiofrequency ablation, your doctor pilots a catheter with an electrode tip to the area of heart muscle where there's an accessory pathway. Then she or he transmits mild radiofrequency to the site. This causes scarring that halts the extra impulses. With mild sedation and local anesthesia, the procedure has little or no discomfort. The success rate exceeds 90 percent.*

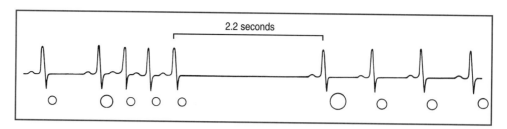

To complicate matters, sinus nodes that are "sick" also have a disconcerting tendency to beat too fast at times when they are not beating too slow. Thus, symptoms of sick sinus syndrome can be those associated with slow heartbeats (such as fatigue, light-headedness, and syncope) alternating with symptoms of fast heartbeats (such as palpitations). Either the slow or the fast rhythm can cause shortness of breath, light-headedness, syncope, or fatigue.

The fact that there is a slow and a fast component in many cases of sick sinus syndrome makes therapy complex. Sometimes a pacemaker may be required to prevent the slow heartbeats. But because a pacemaker cannot prevent fast heartbeats, additional medications to slow the heartbeat may be needed. Unfortunately, giving medications without the pacemaker may slow the heartbeats even more and lead to worse symptoms.

**Problems with the conduction system.** Bradycardia may occur when the electrical impulse generated by the properly functioning sinus node fails to get to the pumping chambers of the heart (the ventricles). This abnormal condition is referred to as atrioventricular block (AV block), because there is either intermittent or continuous block of the electrical signal between the atria, where the signal originates in the sinus node, and the ventricles. Again, do not confuse this "block" with coronary blockage, which is a problem with blood flow through the coronary arteries. Also, do not confuse it with bundle-branch block, which is blockage or delay of the electrical signal in only a branch of the conduction system. AV block is block of the one and only thoroughfare between the atria and the ventricles. AV block is occasionally simply referred to as "heart block."

Heartbeat
interrupted

*Heart block is an interruption in the path the electrical signal travels from the atria to the ventricles. As a result, the heartbeat starts in the ventricles.*

Heartbeat
starts

AV block occurs with varying degrees of severity. First-degree AV block does not cause bradycardia. Second-degree AV block may be more serious. It occurs when there is an intermittent block of impulses traveling from the atria to the ventricles. The block may be frequent (every other beat), less frequent (every third, fourth, or fifth beat), or very rare. If it is frequent, it results in an overall slowing of the heartbeat. The sinus node may be issuing signals for the heart to beat at a rate of 80 beats per minute, but if every other signal is blocked, the heart will contract at a rate of only 40 beats per minute.

However, if the block occurs infrequently, the overall heartbeat will not be slowed that much. Nevertheless, there will be occasional small pauses between the heartbeats when the signal does not get through. Thus, second-degree AV block can also be considered a type of irregular rhythm.

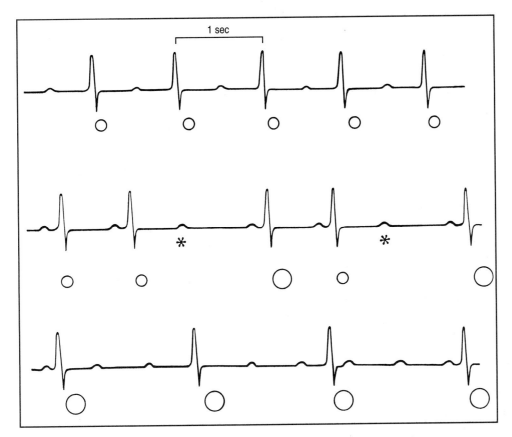

*Problems with conduction of electrical impulses through the atrioventricular node range in severity:*

**Top:** *The mildest form is first-degree atrioventricular block: The impulse is slowed down as it passes through the atrioventricular node, causing a PR segment that is longer than normal.*

**Middle:** *Second-degree atrioventricular block occurs when some impulses originating from the sinus node do not get through the atrioventricular node. On the electrocardiogram, this is seen as some P waves (\*) that are not followed by a QRS complex.*

**Bottom:** *The most severe form is third-degree atrioventricular block, also called complete heart block. In this situation, none of the impulses get through the atrioventricular node. On the electrocardiogram, none of the P waves are followed by a QRS complex. Instead, other parts of the conduction system may take over and produce a heartbeat, but at a much slower rate. You can see that the P waves and the QRS complexes are going at separate rates, unrelated to one another.*

*The circles indicate that some heartbeats may feel stronger (the large circles) and more rapid (the circles that are close together) than normal.*

Third-degree AV block is the most serious type of AV block, often resulting in severe and symptomatic bradycardia. In this case, no signal from the sinus node gets through to the ventricles. Another name for third-degree AV block is complete heart block. Fortunately, most of the time the conduction system in the ventricles or the ventricular muscle itself can initiate impulses, so the heart does not stop entirely. But these substitute pacemakers are too slow to allow the cardiovascular system to function efficiently. They are only backup systems to permit survival. However, they are not always reliable, and if they should fail, the consequences could be fatal. So third-degree AV block is usually a medical emergency requiring treatment with a pacemaker in most cases. The only exceptions are in rare individuals who are born with third-degree AV block (congenital complete heart block). They may do well until early adulthood, at which time a pacemaker is usually advisable.

### Irregular heartbeats

Irregular heartbeats can take several forms. One is described on page 106: second-degree AV block. More common types of irregular rhythms are those related to the occurrence of extra heartbeats and those related to atrial fibrillation. Remember that even a perfectly normal heartbeat may have some irregularity to it, but this does not cause symptoms and is of no concern even when it is obvious on an electrocardiogram.

**Symptoms of irregular heartbeats.** Irregular heartbeats, if they cause any symptom at all, produce palpitations. As a result of awareness of palpitations, some people also develop anxiety and even fatigue from worry. Occasionally there may be associated unusual pains. By and large, however, irregular rhythms produce only palpitations, and many people with very irregular rhythms remain totally unaware of them.

**Types of irregular rhythms.** *Andre is a 51-year-old corporate lawyer who has noted "thumps" in his chest for several years. These have become more frequent in the past several weeks, which he notes have also been a stressful time professionally. They do not really bother him, but he is concerned about their implications.*

**Extra beats.** Andre is likely experiencing extra beats, the most common type of irregular rhythm. In fact, everyone has occasional extra beats even if they are unaware of them. Thus, extra beats in themselves probably should not be considered abnormal because they are so common. They are abnormal when they occur frequently or in certain patterns or when they cause symptoms (palpitations). Palpitations in association with extra beats (ectopy) may not necessarily imply an abnormality requiring treatment. Extra beats can often increase, or be more noticeable, under stressful circumstances.

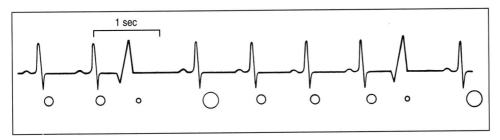

*The heart can occasionally produce an early (premature) beat. The premature beats shown here originate in the ventricle. Premature beats sometimes are called "skipped beats" because it feels as if the heart is "missing" a beat. Actually, the premature beat produces only a very small pulse, as shown by the smallest circles, because the heart has not had time to fill after the previous beat. The beat after the premature beat, however, is stronger than usual because the heart has had time for extra filling after the premature beat.*

Extra beats are exactly what the name describes. (The technical term is "extrasystoles.") They are beats that are "inserted" between normal beats. In effect, they just occur too early, and therefore they beat the next normal beat to the punch. Thus, another term for them is "premature beats or contractions." Oddly enough, despite the presence of an extra beat, most people perceive a sensation of a small skip (thus the term "skipped beats") between heartbeats followed by a "thump." The reason for this is that the premature beat is so early that it makes the heart contract before it has really had a chance to expand and fill with blood. So it is like firing a blank charge—no effective pulse is generated. After the premature beat, the heart usually has a little extra time for filling so the next normal beat enthusiastically pushes out a lot of blood with a rather big thump.

Premature beats can originate from the ventricles (ventricular premature contractions) or from above the ventricles (supraventricular premature contractions). Their only direct significance is the discomfort they may cause, especially if the palpitations are frequent. If ventricular premature beats are extremely frequent or occur in series of several in a row, and if they are associated with certain types of heart disease, they may be a warning sign of worse rhythms in the future. Under these circumstances, further evaluation and treatment may be appropriate.

*Sara is a 54-year-old magazine editor in whom rapid pounding of her heart developed yesterday afternoon. She says her heart feels that it is racing and "out of sync." These symptoms do not seem to make her feel bad, but she is troubled by the constant "bumping around" in her chest and "fullness" in her throat. Her doctor takes her pulse: It is 128 beats per minute and irregular. The doctor makes a diagnosis of atrial fibrillation, and this is confirmed by an ECG. The findings on the rest of Sara's medical examination are satisfactory, although she tells the doctor she drinks 10 or 12 cups of regular coffee daily.*

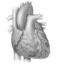

## HEALTHY HEART ♥ TIP

*Just because you're trying to lower your saturated fat intake doesn't mean you must forgo meat altogether. You can take some simple steps to significantly reduce your saturated fat count.*

*First, take meat off center stage by limiting your meat, poultry and fish to 6 ounces daily. Choose lean cuts with the least marbling, usually marked "select." Also, trim the fat before you cook to prevent fat from seeping into the meat or poultry.*

**Atrial fibrillation.** Atrial fibrillation is a chaotic beating of the heart. It occurs when the right and left upper chambers (atria) cease to have effective, orderly contractions and begin beating chaotically at a rate of 300-400 times a minute.

This heart problem is common. More than 2 million Americans suffer from this rhythm abnormality, with 160,000 new cases occurring annually.

Atrial fibrillation occurs more frequently with age. Although less than 1 percent of people in their 50s have this problem, around 10 percent will experience the disorder in their 80s. Changes that occur in the electrical and structural properties of the upper chambers with aging probably contribute to the disorganization of the normal atrial rhythm.

The activity of the sinus node is shut off, and the fibrillation takes over the rhythm of the heart. Because the atria are experiencing a continuous electrical impulse traveling through them, this impulse is directed down through the atrioventricular node.

The atrioventricular node functions like an electrical gate or relay station, preventing a continuous flow of impulses into the pumping chambers. But many impulses get through at irregular intervals. The result is a very irregular rhythm with varying intervals between heartbeats.

The pulse at rest usually ranges from 60 to 150 beats a minute but may be faster (a form of tachycardia). There also tends to be a fast heartbeat, so atrial fibrillation is considered a form of tachycardia. The heartbeat is so irregular that doctors refer to it as "irregularly irregular" to distinguish the cadence of the pulse from the patterned variations caused by second-degree AV block or premature beats.

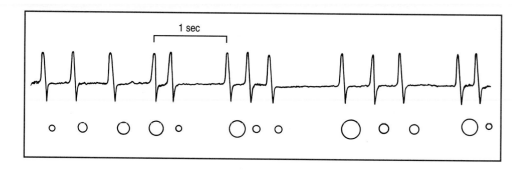

*This electrocardiogram shows atrial fibrillation. The atria are twitching chaotically, so no P waves are visible. Electrical impulses go through the atrioventricular node at irregular intervals and cause an irregular heart beat. As with premature contractions, the pulse (shown again by circles on the figure) caused by early heartbeats is weaker than the pulse after a longer interval.*

Atrial fibrillation is prone to cause palpitations, and if it is exceedingly fast it may cause chest pain, shortness of breath, light-headedness, or fatigue. Without atrial contractions, the heart beats less efficiently; in individuals who may have weakened heart muscle to begin with, congestive heart failure may develop.

After long periods of rapid heartbeat due to atrial fibrillation, the heart muscle may weaken and develop dilated cardiomyopathy. Perhaps the most serious consequence of atrial fibrillation is the risk of a blood clot forming in an atrium. Because the atria are not actively contracting, blood may not be propelled normally through the atria. This lack of normal propulsion motion predisposes to clotting. If a clot dislodges and travels to the brain, a stroke can occur. If it blocks an artery in some other region, the interrupted blood flow can lead to damage elsewhere, such as the kidneys.

Fortunately, atrial fibrillation does not always lead to clots. People under 65 with atrial fibrillation—who do not have high blood pressure, diabetes, a prior stroke, atrial chamber enlargement or a weakened lower heart chamber (ventricle), or other heart valve abnormalities—are at low risk for stroke even if atrial fibrillation persists. Still, a blood-thinning medication may be advised to prevent a stroke, and to prevent clots from forming in the atria.

If you have atrial fibrillation, the initial goal of treatment may be to slow the pulse rate and regain normal sinus rhythm, either with medication or shock treatment (cardioversion). Caffeine and alcohol have been implicated as culprits in promoting the occurrence of fast rhythms in the atria, and they should be avoided once a normal rhythm is restored. Avoid smoking. Also, your doctor will order blood tests to determine whether the atrial fibrillation is due to an overactive thyroid, which would require specific treatment, or some alternative approach.

If cardioversion is unsuccessful, or if atrial fibrillation recurs despite treatment with medications, the goal is to keep the rate of ventricular contractions at an acceptably slow pace, although it will still be irregular.

People with fast heart rates during atrial fibrillation are generally treated with drugs that decrease electrical conduction or transmission of the impulse through the AV node to the ventricle. The mainstay of treatment is drugs such as beta-blockers, calcium channel blockers and digitalis. Most people get used to the irregularity as long as the heart rate is not too fast.

Some people don't respond to long-term drug therapy or cardioversion. If you have persistent, unacceptable symptoms or rapid heart rates despite treatment, your doctor may recommend nondrug therapy.

The most common nondrug approach is radiofrequency catheter ablation, an interruption (ablation) of the AV conduction system. It blocks transmission of electrical impulses between the upper and lower chambers of the heart. Your heart rate is then controlled by an implanted pacemaker. The atria remain in fibrillation following ablation so that long-term use of a blood-thinning drug is still required.

In radiofrequency ablation, a specially designed catheter is positioned near the AV node and a special form of energy is delivered to the heart tissue (see page 112). The energy heals and scars the tissue, thereby blocking transmission of electrical impulses. Most often catheter ablation is effective. When it is not, there are alternative treatments such as the Maze procedure, which requires open heart surgery today but may someday be available by means of a catheter.

Other techniques under investigation include the use of implantable atrial defibrillators and various atrial-pacing techniques.

### *Fast heartbeats (tachycardia)*

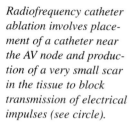

*Radiofrequency catheter ablation involves placement of a catheter near the AV node and production of a very small scar in the tissue to block transmission of electrical impulses (see circle).*

Tachycardia is a major problem for a large number of people. New techniques for assessing and treating tachycardia offer relief of symptoms and a better long-term outlook for people who have some of these rhythm disorders.

**Symptoms of tachycardia.** Regardless of the specific type, tachycardia causes various symptoms, including palpitations, shortness of breath, angina, light-headedness, and syncope. Some types of tachycardia cause immediate symptoms (which may be bad enough) but also pose a risk of catastrophe, including death.

**Classification of tachycardia.** Tachycardia, like extra beats, can originate either from a ventricle (ventricular) or above a ventricle (supraventricular). Indeed, most types of tachycardia start from an extra beat at one of these sites. Different types of tachycardia can be present at either of these locations. In general, fast ventricular rhythms have more dire consequences because they make the heart function especially inefficiently, tend to cause more severe symptoms, and have a greater potential to result in death.

**Types of supraventricular tachycardia.** *Atrial flutter.* Like atrial fibrillation, atrial flutter is also a very rapid, ineffective beating of the atria, but it is somewhat more coordinated and regular. Atrial flutter causes the atria to beat about 300 times per minute. If the ventricles were also to beat at that rate, blood would not circulate efficiently. Luckily, the atrioventricular node usually performs its gating function and prevents at least every other atrial beat from being transmitted to the ventricles. Consequently, if you have atrial flutter, your pulse rate is usually about 150 beats per minute.

Sometimes the atrioventricular node lets only every third or every fourth beat through, in which case your heart rate would be 100 beats or 75 beats per minute, respectively.

The symptoms of atrial flutter are those of any tachycardia, namely, palpitations, chest pain, shortness of breath, or light-headedness.

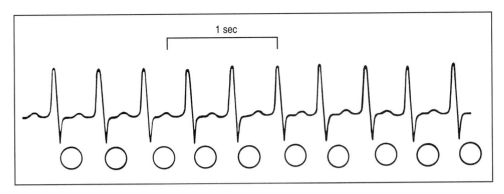

*A fast heartbeat can originate in the atria, such as shown in this electrocardiogram of a supraventricular tachycardia. Notice that about 2½ heartbeats occur every second, so this person's heart rate is 150 beats per minute.*

*Paroxysmal supraventricular tachycardia.* This term applies to bursts (paroxysms) of rapid heartbeats originating above the ventricles. Supraventricular tachycardia may occur when an extra pathway exists in the atria, in the AV node or between the atria and the ventricles (Wolff-Parkinson-White syndrome). The rapid heartbeats are usually all transmitted to the ventricles but occasionally may be blocked. The bursts usually begin suddenly and end just as suddenly, sometimes with a pause that actually causes symptoms as well. The episodes can last seconds to hours or days, if not treated. The heart rate during supraventricular tachycardia can range from 140 to 240 beats per minute, and the degree of tachycardia symptoms depends in part on how fast the heart is going.

The most common form of supraventricular tachycardia is AV nodal reentry tachycardia. In this condition an extra pathway exists in, or near, the AV node. If an electrical impulse enters this pathway, it may start traveling in a circular pattern and can cause the heart to contract with each cycle. This may result in a rapid heartbeat.

Supraventricular tachycardia is seldom life-threatening, but it can certainly produce bothersome symptoms. Conservative measures to reduce its frequency should be undertaken, such as avoiding caffeine, smoking or excess alcohol. Some people can break a spell of this type of rapid heartbeat by doing certain maneuvers that slow the heart rate. These include bearing down (as though straining at a bowel movement), gagging (by tickling the back of the throat), or splashing cold water on their faces. Numerous medications are available to help treat this rhythm disorder. Catheter

*An extra pathway exists in, or near, the AV node in AV nodal reentry tachycardia. Impulses that enter this pathway may travel in a circular pattern and can lead to a rapid heartbeat.*

Extra pathway

ablation techniques, as well as some operations, can cure people of most of these arrhythmias.

*Wolff-Parkinson-White syndrome.* In Wolff-Parkinson-White (WPW) syndrome, an abnormal "bridge" of tissue connects the atria and ventricles. This extra pathway, called an accessory pathway, makes it possible for electrical impulses to travel from the atria to the ventricles without going through the AV node.

In people with WPW, an arrhythmia can get started when an impulse travels down the AV node to the ventricles, and then up through the accessory pathway to the atria. If the impulse continues to travel in a circular pattern, it may cause the heart to contract with each cycle and may result in a very rapid heartbeat. Because it tends to conduct impulses rapidly, an accessory pathway may also allow extremely rapid and potentially serious rhythms to occur.

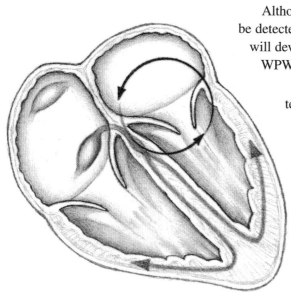

Although the presence of accessory pathways sometimes can be detected on an ECG, not everyone with an accessory pathway will develop tachycardia or require special treatment. While WPW is not common, it is certainly not rare either.

WPW syndrome can be cured by the nonsurgical technique of catheter ablation, which disrupts (destroys) parts of the abnormal electrical pathway causing the arrhythmia. In WPW syndrome, doctors first determine the exact location of the accessory pathway by "mapping" electrical signals during the tachycardia and by pacing the heart. If it is determined that the extra pathway causing the rapid heartbeat is in or next to the AV node, that pathway can also be ablated without destroying the AV node itself. Success rates are around 98 percent for this procedure

*An arrhythmia can start when an impulse travels down the AV node to the ventricles, and then up through the accessory pathway to the atria. If the impulse continues to travel in a circular pattern, it may cause a rapid heartbeat and potentially serious rhythms. This is called Wolff-Parkinson-White syndrome.*

**Types of ventricular tachycardia.** *Ventricular tachycardia.* When used as a specific diagnosis, this term refers to a rapid, regular heartbeat originating from a site in one of the ventricles. The rate can be anywhere from 100 to 250 beats per minute.

Unlike paroxysmal supraventricular tachycardia, many episodes of ventricular tachycardia (called VT or V tach) do not stop spontaneously. Worse, there is a predisposition for VT to deteriorate into ventricular fibrillation. Thus, VT is usually a medical emergency, even if the symptoms it is causing are rather slight.

Most VT is associated with other serious heart disease, such as coronary artery blockage, cardiomyopathy, or congenital or valvular heart disease. But several other forms can occur in younger people without underlying heart disease, and are generally triggered by exertion. Although perhaps less serious, they do require medical attention.

Treatment is directed first to ending the bout of VT. If intravenously administered medications do not produce immediate results, a shock to the chest is usually required. The next step is to prevent the VT from returning; options are medications, correction of an underlying problem such as myocardial ischemia, use of an implantable cardioverter-defibrillator, or surgical or catheter procedures to eliminate the site in the ventricle that is causing the VT.

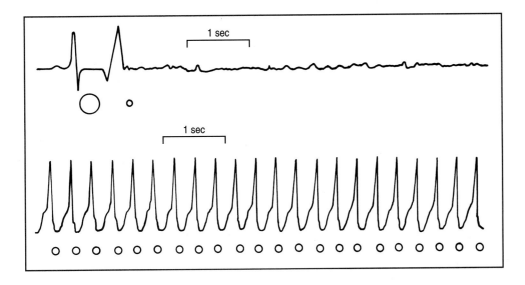

*Top:* Ventricular fibrillation is seen on this electrocardiogram after a normal beat and a ventricular premature beat. This chaotic twitching of the ventricles does not pump blood, so there is no pulse. Without cardiopulmonary resuscitation and defibrillation, this person would die.

*Bottom:* Ventricular tachycardia is a fast heartbeat originating in the ventricular muscle of the heart. In this example the heart rate is 180 beats per minute.

*Ventricular fibrillation.* The absolutely worst heart rhythm you can have is ventricular fibrillation (VF). In this condition there is no effective heartbeat—only useless quivering of the ventricular muscle. As far as circulation of blood is concerned, the heart is stopped. Do not confuse VF with atrial fibrillation. VF is the rhythm that is almost always the cause of "cardiac arrest" or "sudden cardiac death." Unless someone is nearby who can administer cardiopulmonary resuscitation (CPR) when you go into VF, you will die. There are seldom second chances otherwise; this urgency underscores the importance of knowing CPR.

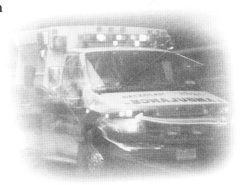

VF seldom occurs in the absence of other substantial problems with the heart, although rarely it may.

# Diseases of the arteries and veins

On its journey from the heart to all the tissues in your body, your blood travels through the vascular system (see pages A2 and A3). The vascular system consists of the blood vessels—the arteries and veins. The vessels connected to the heart are the biggest in your body, with a diameter similar to that of a garden hose. The arteries branch into smaller vessels as they travel to your tissues, finally becoming capillaries that allow the passage of only one blood cell at a time.

In healthy persons, blood flow is regulated so that various parts of your body receive exactly the amount of blood they need. When you exercise, more blood goes to your muscles, and when you eat, more blood goes to your stomach and intestines. When you get hot, more blood flows to the outer layers of your skin to help dissipate the heat. When you are cold, blood is routed to deeper vessels away from your skin to help conserve heat.

The arteries function to carry oxygen and nutrients to the brain, other organs, and muscles. Veins function predominantly as conduits to carry the deoxygenated blood back to the heart.

To accomplish these tasks, arteries and veins are structurally different. Arteries have muscle in their walls that enables them to expand or contract and actually helps route the blood to various parts of the body. Because veins carry blood back from the organs and body to the heart, they function under conditions of much lower pressures. Veins are thin and work more passively than arteries. They do not have the ability to squeeze or constrict as arteries do. Either the arteries or the veins, or both, can be affected by diseases but, in general, the diseases of these two different types of blood vessels are also different. In addition, the arteries of the lungs can be affected by disease.

## Diseases of the arteries

### Atherosclerosis

The higher pressures that arteries work under make them susceptible to atherosclerosis. A degree of atherosclerosis eventually develops in almost everyone. As you age, the elastic fibers and smooth-muscle cells of your arteries degenerate and are partially replaced by fibrous tissue. The arteries normally become thicker and less elastic, and the inner lining becomes abnormal.

#### Causes of atherosclerosis

In some people, the degeneration of the lining and walls of the arteries may be accelerated. The lining (endothelium) may be damaged. Blood platelets stick to the site of injury, and a chemical signal is activated that promotes an influx of cholesterol. Cholesterol and other substances such as calcium build up in the artery wall. Eventually, a plaque forms that bulges into the bloodstream and impedes blood flow through the artery.

Your risk of developing atherosclerosis increases if you smoke or have a family history of atherosclerosis. Diabetes, high blood pressure, and high levels of cholesterol in the blood increase your risk as well.

Many times the blockages are incomplete and develop over time, gradually narrowing the artery until the blood flow is nearly stopped. Sometimes the body can compensate for these narrowings by developing small branches, called collaterals, that bypass the narrowed sections or blockages. The collaterals, although helpful, are not always enough to restore circulation to an affected region of the body.

### Symptoms of atherosclerosis

Symptoms usually develop gradually. As arteries become increasingly blocked, progressive symptoms frequently develop. The specific symptoms depend on which artery or arteries are obstructed. If the leg arteries are affected, then the symptoms are usually numbness, fatigue, or pain in the leg (claudication). Leg pain is associated with exertion such as walking.

Atherosclerotic obstruction of the coronary arteries may lead to symptoms of angina or even a heart attack. Other commonly affected arteries include the carotid arteries in the neck (a situation that predisposes to stroke) and the abdominal aorta (which may become partially obstructed and cause claudication or become weakened and lead to expansion (aneurysm) (see page A15).

Symptoms caused by progressive atherosclerotic narrowing of an artery are more likely to occur during exercise than at rest, at least initially. Early symptoms may occur only after great exertion, but as the narrowing worsens, less and less activity is required. The symptoms develop during exertion because your arteries cannot supply your muscles with enough oxygen and nutrients. The more severe the blockage, the less exertion it takes to surpass the ability of the artery to supply adequate blood. When you stop and rest, the discomfort resolves in a few minutes. However, blockages can be so severe that even resting muscle does not get enough blood flow, and you may experience symptoms, such as claudication or angina, with minimal exertion.

If you have atherosclerosis of your lower extremities and pain in your leg even when resting, see your doctor right away. This is a serious sign needing prompt intervention to prevent possible loss of the limb.

Indeed, it is the symptoms caused by inadequate blood flow to a part of the body that may bring you to a physician, who then attempts to discover the cause. Atherosclerosis is the cause of chronic obstruction of the arteries in 95 percent of cases, but other causes are important to know about.

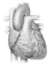

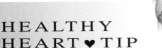
**HEALTHY HEART ♥ TIP**

*People who spend most of the day sitting are probably not fit. If you feel tired most of the time, are unable to keep up with others your age, and avoid activity because you tire quickly, you fall into this category.*

*It doesn't take much to get active. Thirty minutes or more of low to moderately intense physical activity on most days of the week should improve fitness. Low-intensity exercise can come from walking for pleasure, gardening, yard work, housework and social dancing. Moderately intense exercise includes brisk walking, hiking, stair-climbing, aerobic dancing, jogging, bicycling, rowing and swimming.*

## Arterial thrombosis and arterial embolism

Sometimes clotting of blood (thrombosis) inside an artery results in a blockage. A blood clot that forms and stays at its place of origin inside a blood vessel (or the heart) is called a thrombus. A thrombus can partially or totally obstruct the artery and prevent sufficient blood flow.

When a blood clot forms in one place but breaks off and travels through the blood vessels to another point in the circulation where it lodges, the resulting problem is referred to as thromboembolism.

The actual blood clot is a thromboembolus and is often referred to simply as an embolus. Emboli can also originate from infected cells in the circulation (septic emboli) from cancer cells that enter the circulation (tumor emboli), or from fat cells that enter the bloodstream (fat emboli), especially after major bone fractures.

A sudden blockage (occlusion) may occur when an embolus lodges in one of your arteries. Blood clots can originate from the chambers of the heart or can develop in large arteries and lodge in smaller arteries after they break loose. This process often occurs where arteries branch or divide.

### Symptoms of embolism

When arteries are suddenly blocked, there is no time for collateral arteries to develop, and the blood flow to the tissues beyond the blockage literally stops. This blockage results in pain, whiteness, weakness, tingling, numbness, or coldness below a blockage in an artery to one of your limbs. If an embolus lodges in an artery to the brain, a stroke results. A coronary artery embolus may produce a myocardial infarction (heart attack).

## Living with claudication—what can help?

Although intermittent claudication does not affect your life expectancy, it may affect your lifestyle. Treatment options include a walking program, medication, and correction of the arterial obstruction by surgery or angioplasty.

If it hurts to walk, why might your doctor recommend a regular walking program? The answer is that regular walking for periods of 30 minutes (stopping to rest as necessary) 5 days a week may increase your ability to walk, climb stairs, or complete other physical tasks of everyday living. Regular walking promotes the development of collateral vessels, as well as blood flow to the affected muscles. This may result in an actual improvement in blood flow and may slow progression of the disease.

Medications that decrease blood viscosity, in a sense making it easier for the blood to flow through narrowed vessels, may improve your comfort while walking.

Surgery or angioplasty (dilating the narrowed site of an artery with a balloon catheter) is often elective (optional); it depends on your need or desire to walk farther. If you have a nonhealing skin ulcer or pain at rest due to severe obstruction of arterial blood flow, then improving blood flow by angioplasty or surgery is recommended to relieve symptoms and lessen the risk of amputation.

### How serious is embolism?

If the blood supply is cut off to a limb, finger, or toe for more than a few hours, the muscle and skin in an affected limb may become gangrenous. If the blockage is not removed or dissolved promptly, the tissue below the blockage may die and require amputation.

## Stroke: A neurologic condition related to cardiovascular disease

Stroke refers to a brain injury that is caused by an inadequate supply of blood (ischemia) to the brain. Transient ischemic attacks (TIAs) are temporary episodes that resemble a stroke. They are regarded as serious warning signs that a stroke may occur in the future.

Because the brain is the organ affected by strokes, if you have a stroke you will be attended to by a neurologist. However, strokes are closely related to cardiovascular disease and therefore are mentioned here.

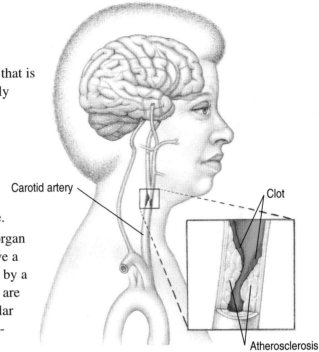

Carotid artery

Clot

Atherosclerosis

*Atherosclerosis partially blocks this carotid artery, and a thrombus (clot, purple) has also formed. If any of the clot breaks free, it would travel up to a branch of an artery in the brain and completely block blood flow. The result would be a stroke.*

### Causes of stroke

Many strokes are caused by a small bit of clot or cholesterol debris breaking off from its site of formation in the carotid arteries in the neck. The clot travels up in the bloodstream through smaller branches of the artery until it becomes wedged into a small branch in the brain and blocks further blood flow. This is called a cerebral embolism.

Clot or debris can also form in the aorta upstream from the branches of the carotid arteries or in the left side of the heart such as the left atrium, left ventricle, and artificial valves in the aortic or mitral position. The clot can break off and travel to the brain, where it causes a stroke.

Atherosclerosis or a blood clot that forms and stays in the carotid or cerebral artery (arteries in the neck and brain) can block blood flow enough to cause TIAs or a stroke. This condition, called cerebral thrombosis, differs from cerebral embolism in that the clot has not moved from its site of origin.

A less common but important cause of stroke is formation and release of a blood clot from a vein in the legs (an event that in itself is not rare) that travels to the heart. The clot crosses from the right side of the heart to the left side of the heart through an abnormal opening in the septum (partition that divides the atria and ventricles). From the left side of the heart, the clot then proceeds through the arterial circulation into the brain, where it causes a stroke. This event is occasionally the first sign that there is a hole in the wall separating the two sides of the heart (septal defect).

Not all strokes are caused by clots or obstruction. Other causes of stroke include bleeding into the brain (cerebral hemorrhage) or around the surface of the brain (subarachnoid hemorrhage) and other disorders of blood clotting.

### Symptoms of stroke

The symptoms of stroke can be extremely varied, because they depend on which area of the brain was affected. Symptoms can include paralysis or weakness of a limb, abnormalities of sensation (such as numbness of a limb), and defects of speech, comprehension, or vision.

### How serious is stroke?

Depending on the severity and location of the stroke, it is often possible for the person to improve with physical therapy or by relearning skills that were lost, but there is a residual defect in half the people who survive. Each year, of the 500,000 people in the United States who have a stroke about one quarter of them die.

## Aneurysms

Sometimes atherosclerosis can damage the walls of blood vessels and lead to a situation in which the arteries, including the aorta, develop abnormally widened areas called aneurysms (see page A15).

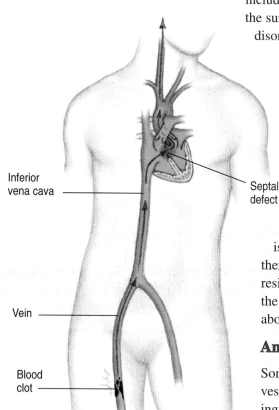

Inferior
vena cava

Septal
defect

Vein

Blood
clot

*Rarely, a stroke can be caused by a blood clot that forms in a leg vein, breaks away and crosses through to the left side of the heart (by way of a septal defect), and then proceeds into an artery of the brain.*

Aneurysms can occur in virtually any artery, but the segment of the aorta that runs through the abdomen is the most common site of localized ballooning. Other sites of aneurysm are the aorta in the chest and the arteries in the thigh and behind the knee.

### Causes of aneurysm

More than 90 percent of abdominal aortic aneurysms are associated with atherosclerosis. The weakness in the wall that gives rise to an abdominal aortic aneurysm is usually caused by an accumulation of cholesterol containing fatty deposits (atherosclerotic plaques). Smoking and high blood pressure can also be predisposing factors, as can inheritance.

### Symptoms of aneurysm

Most abdominal aortic aneurysms do not produce symptoms, but some people feel a pulsating sensation in the abdomen. These silent (asymptomatic) aneurysms are often recognized by careful physical examination, chest X-ray, and ultrasonography. When aneurysms do not cause symptoms and are small, they can be safely watched and do not require surgery. It is important, however, to have periodic evaluations. When aneurysms become larger, the chance of sudden rupture is greater, and these should be surgically repaired.

### Who is affected by aneurysm?

Abdominal aortic aneurysm is most likely to occur in people older than 60 years. It affects men more often than women and is more common in people who have a family history of aneurysm. It's more frequent in smokers and in people with high blood pressure.

### How serious is an aneurysm?

The main risk of an abdominal aortic aneurysm is that, like a balloon that is blown up too far, it may rupture. Rupture results in life-threatening internal bleeding (hemorrhage). The larger the aneurysm gets, the more likely it is to rupture. Approximately 15,000 Americans die each year from a ruptured aortic aneurysm. When detected in time, this condition can usually be repaired with surgery.

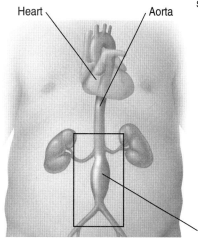

Heart    Aorta

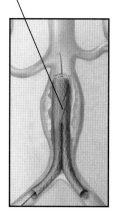

Graft with stent

Aortic aneurysm

*An aortic aneurysm occurs when the wall of the aorta becomes weak or damaged, allowing a section to slowly enlarge. Surgery to repair or prevent aneurysm rupture involves inserting a synthetic tube—a graft with or without a stent— that strengthens the artery.*

Surgery usually is warranted only when the aorta (which normally has a diameter of less than 1 inch) enlarges to about 2 inches, because the likelihood of rupture increases at that point. A 2-inch-wide aneurysm has a 1 in 25 chance of rupturing within 1 year. An aneurysm that is $2^3/4$ inches across has a 1 in 5 chance of rupturing in the next year. Aneurysms usually grow about 1/8 to 1/4 inch per year, but this rate can be highly variable.

Surgical correction often involves replacing a part of the diseased artery with a graft or tube made from synthetic materials.

## Endovascular surgery

An exciting new but still investigational technique is designed to allow placement of the graft but without the need for an extensive surgical incision. In this procedure, a synthetic graft is attached to the end of a catheter. The catheter is threaded upstream to the aorta and used to position the graft at the site of the aneurysm.

Once in place, the graft is expanded and attached to the vessel with metal stents, which are small hooks or pins. It remains to be seen whether this form of treatment will be effective in the long term.

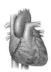

### Berry aneurysm

Important, but less common, types of aneurysm are not related to atherosclerosis. Berry aneurysms are bulges in the walls of arteries within the brain. As the name implies, they appear like little berries attached to a blood vessel, usually at a point of branching. They usually do not cause symptoms unless they rupture, in which case they may cause stroke or coma or be fatal.

Aneurysms can develop in any blood vessel anywhere in your body. The majority occur in large blood vessels, especially the aorta. Although more than three quarters involve the abdominal aorta, the rest occur in that part of the aorta that runs through the upper chest, in which case they are called thoracic aneurysms. Most of these are diagnosed before there are symptoms, often as an incidental finding on a routine chest X-ray.

## Aortic dissection

Dissection is a catastrophic form of arterial disease. It usually involves the aorta or a portion of it (aortic dissection). Dissection means that layers of the wall of the aorta separate. The inner layer peels off from the remainder of the vessel, so that blood can be forced between the layers, extending the dissection along the involved artery.

### Causes of dissection

Aortic dissection tends to occur in persons with high blood pressure. There is also some association with diseases that cause general defects in the structural tissue of the body such as a hereditary syndrome called Marfan's syndrome, abnormalities of the blood vessel walls such as cystic medial necrosis, certain types of atherosclerotic plaques that burrow into the heart vessel wall, certain types of arteritis (inflammation of arteries), bicuspid aortic valve (two cusps instead of the normal three), and pregnancy.

### Symptoms of dissection

Dissection of the aorta typically causes sharp and tearing chest and back pain. Often the pain is focused in the back between the shoulder blades, although it may descend into the lower back as well or feel as if it is boring into the chest. Typically the pain is severe and comes on suddenly. At other times it can be vague, or like angina. Sometimes it's misinterpreted as a heart attack. Occasionally it occurs with no symptoms.

### Who is affected by dissection?

Dissection of the aorta is two to three times more common in men than in women. It usually occurs between ages 40 and 70.

### *How serious is dissection?*

This is a medical-surgical emergency. If blood erupts outside the aorta, the condition is often fatal. The dissection can extend into or block branch vessels of the aorta, such as the carotid arteries to the brain and arteries to the arms, kidneys, legs, or spinal cord. The result is decreased or absent blood flow to these organs. Dissection of the aorta may require urgent surgery, depending on the areas of the aorta that are involved. Even before surgery, though, the first goals of management are to reduce blood pressure to the lowest acceptable level and to determine the portion of the aorta involved by the tear.

The aorta may be ruptured in crushing injuries or with sudden deceleration such as in automobile accidents or falls. With sudden deceleration, aortic rupture usually occurs in the chest and is usually fatal. Aortic injury due to penetrating wounds usually results in life-threatening hemorrhage (bleeding).

## Inflammation of arteries

In some diseases, arteries become inflamed. The inflammation can result in narrowing of the opening (bore or lumen) of the vessels. The medical term for inflammation of the artery is arteritis. If the inflammation persists, the vessel may become permanently scarred and narrow. There are many different types of arteritis. Although each type has different symptoms and can affect different arteries, the primary goal of treatment is to reduce the inflammation and prevent scarring of the arteries.

Typically, arteritis is part of a generalized illness with disease in other organs.

Examples of arteritis include:

- Takayasu's disease
- Temporal arteritis
- Buerger's disease
- Polyarteritis nodosa

### *Takayasu's disease*

This is also called "pulseless disease," because some pulses usually present are absent. Takayasu's disease is rare and occurs mostly in women younger than 40 years. It occurs in women nine times more often than in men.

It is an inflammatory process that most commonly produces marked thickening of the aorta and its main branches, eventually blocking the major branches of the arteries. The blockage reduces the pulse downstream, for example, at the wrist if the artery to the arm is involved.

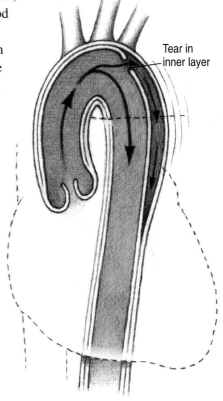

Tear in
inner layer

*An aortic dissection occurs when blood pushes forcefully into a tear in the inner layer of the aortic wall and splits the inner layer away from the outer layer.*

### Temporal arteritis

Temporal arteritis is also called cranial arteritis or giant-cell arteritis. People who have temporal arteritis are almost always older than 55. It is twice as common in women as in men.

In this disease, the inflammation may involve one or both temporal arteries on the side of the head. Headache and a tender, red, inflamed artery in the temple are clues to the diagnosis, which can be verified by removing a tiny sample (biopsy) of the affected artery. Prompt diagnosis and treatment of temporal arteritis is essential, since blindness can be a complication.

Treatment with corticosteroids controls this disease and prevents complications such as blindness. Long-term follow-up is necessary to detect delayed complications of aneurysms involving the thoracic aorta.

### Buerger's disease

One particularly severe form of vessel inflammation is thromboangiitis obliterans, also called Buerger's disease. In this disease, inflammation obliterates small and medium-sized arteries. It occurs most commonly in men younger than 30 years who use tobacco. Redness and tenderness of superficial veins of the feet or legs and pain in the arch of the foot or calf when walking suggest Buerger's disease.

Progression of Buerger's disease can be thwarted by abstaining from tobacco use. People in whom the disease continues are usually those who continue to smoke.

### Polyarteritis nodosa

As the name suggests, polyarteritis involves inflammation (itis) of many (poly) arteries. Areas at greatest risk are the skin, intestines, kidneys, and heart, although any area of your body can be involved.

Symptoms are often vague: unexplained weight loss, progressive fatigue, weakness, and fever. The diagnosis is confirmed by removing a tiny sample (biopsy) of the involved part of the body for microscopic evaluation of the arteries. Treatment is a prolonged course of corticosteroids, often supplemented by other medications.

### Fibromuscular dysplasia (overgrowth of muscle in artery walls)

Another cause of obstruction in the blood vessels is overgrowth of the muscle in the wall of the artery, which is called fibromuscular dysplasia. The arteries to the kidneys are most vulnerable. Renal (kidney) arteries can also develop atherosclerotic blockages.

Regardless of cause, when blood flow is diminished to the kidneys, your blood pressure tends to increase. Here's why: When your kidneys get inadequate blood flow, they react as though blood pressure were low all over the body. This response triggers the kidneys to release hormone "messengers" that increase blood pressure. This process is similar to blowing cold air on a thermostat: The thermostat responds by increasing the heat in the whole house. Artery blockage in the kidneys can also lead to a decrease in their ability to eliminate waste products.

## Arterial spasm

Spasm of the arteries is a rare cause of arterial blockage. Often it is associated with taking medications that provoke spasm, especially ergots (which are in some medications used to treat migraine headaches).

## Raynaud's phenomenon

Raynaud's phenomenon is an exaggerated response to the normal reflex mechanism that causes blood vessels in the hands and feet to narrow (spasm) in the cold or with emotion. It affects 1 in 20 Americans to some degree, mostly women between the ages of 15-40. In men it occurs later in life.

If you experience Raynaud's phenomenon, your fingers or toes (and in some people, ears and nose) turn chalky white when you are exposed to cold or strong emotions. They also sting or become cold and numb. The entire episode may last less than a minute or may persist for hours. Your skin may turn blue or bright red upon return to a warmer environment before normal color returns.

## Diseases of the veins

### Venous thrombosis

Diseases of the veins are different from those of the arteries because of the structural differences. Blockages can occur in the veins, but these are usually caused by blood clots (thrombi) and not by atherosclerosis. When a thrombus forms in a vein, blood is prevented from traveling back toward the heart. The collection of blood results in increased pressure and often leads to swelling and tenderness. For example, a blood clot in the deep vein of the calf will cause the calf and foot to become swollen and tender. This condition is referred to as deep-vein thrombosis. The leg is still getting enough oxygen and nutrients from the arteries, so it is not threatened, but the back pressure of unreturned blood and the resulting seepage of fluid into the surrounding tissues (edema) can be uncomfortable. Clotting of blood in the veins tends to occur whenever the blood flow in the vein is slow or becomes stagnant. Typically this occurs in the legs when you are still, as in a long ride in a car or plane, when you are constantly in bed because of illness or surgery, or after an injury to the leg.

## Tips for preventing blood clots during travel

You're packed into a crowded airplane, bracing yourself for the 7-hour ride to your vacation or business destination. If you remain motionless in your seat for the duration, you increase your risk for the development of potentially dangerous blood clots.

Blood clots interfere with blood flow and can break loose and travel to an artery in one of your lungs. Clots can form while you sit for extended periods in cramped quarters. This problem can happen during any form of travel, but it is more common on long airline flights, especially if you are sitting in the coach section. Doctors therefore have coined the term "economy class syndrome."

Despite its name, economy class syndrome can develop regardless of whether you sit in first class or in the coach section. On long-distance flights or rides, follow these tips:

Wear loose, comfortable clothing and shoes. Airlines often provide customers in the first-class cabin with bootie socks. It is easy to bring your own. They help keep your feet warm and are not as tight or confining as shoes.

Stretch your legs occasionally, even while remaining in your seat, and move your feet up and down.

Tighten and then loosen the muscles of your abdomen and buttocks from time to time.

Take slow, deep breaths periodically.

Get out of your seat and walk the aisle at least once an hour.

Ask your doctor whether it is appropriate to use aspirin when you travel. Small doses of aspirin may help prevent clots from occurring. Remember to check with your doctor first. Aspirin is not recommended for everyone.

If you have had problems with thrombophlebitis in the past, wear elastic support stockings when prolonged sitting is unavoidable. This may require a prescription for extra-strong support hose. Elastic support stockings are available for both men and women.

Avoid dehydration. It can increase your risk of blood clots in leg veins and can also lead to other conditions, such as vasovagal or vasopressor syncope and renal colic due to kidney stones. Use alcoholic beverages minimally if at all. They are a prominent cause of dehydration. Regular intake of nonalcoholic fluids serves the dual purpose of preventing dehydration and encouraging motion in the form of trips to the restroom.

The main risk of blood clots forming and causing deep-vein thrombosis is that the blood clot can enlarge and extend up the vein. If a piece breaks off, it can travel upstream and lodge in the heart or lungs. Just as in the arterial circulation, this disorder is called thromboembolism. A thrombus that dislodges from a vein in the leg will travel through larger and larger veins until it reaches the right side of the heart. From there it will enter the pulmonary artery and lodge in a branch, at which point it blocks blood flow to part of the lung. A clot in the lung circulation is a pulmonary embolus.

Treatment with anticoagulants ("blood thinners") in the early stages of deep-vein thrombosis can prevent enlargement of the clot and lessen the likelihood of pulmonary embolism.

### Thrombophlebitis

Thrombophlebitis means clotting of blood (thrombus) and inflammation (itis) in a vein, most commonly in the legs. It is often just called phlebitis. It can affect either the deep or surface (superficial) veins.

### Symptoms of thrombophlebitis

When the deep veins are involved, your leg may become tender, painful, and swollen. You may also have a fever. When a superficial vein is involved, a red, hard, and tender bump or cord may be present under the surface of the skin.

### Who is affected by thrombophlebitis?

Your risk for thrombophlebitis increases if you are confined or immobile for prolonged periods. Thrombophlebitis commonly occurs after surgery, heart attack, hip or leg fracture, or prolonged bed rest or inactivity (such as sitting for a long time in a plane or car). Cancer patients also have a higher risk, as do people who are overweight, who use oral contraceptives, or whose blood has an abnormally high tendency to clot.

### How serious is thrombophlebitis?

If the thrombophlebitis is in a superficial vein lying just under the skin, serious complications are generally rare. An exception is thrombophlebitis of surface veins near the groin.

If the clotting is in a deep vein, the valves in the veins may be damaged, and this damage leads to future problems of swelling of the leg. If a portion of the thrombus is dislodged, it may travel to the lung and cause pulmonary embolism.

If the thrombophlebitis is in a superficial vein, your doctor may recommend applying heat to the sore area, elevating the leg, and using an anti-inflammatory drug. If your thrombophlebitis is in a deep vein, treatment probably will require

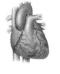

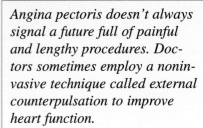

**HEALTHY HEART ♥ TIP**

*Angina pectoris doesn't always signal a future full of painful and lengthy procedures. Doctors sometimes employ a noninvasive technique called external counterpulsation to improve heart function.*

*This method, still under evaluation, uses sequences of pressure cuff inflations on the legs to lower the pressure the heart must pump against. This increases the amount of blood and oxygen going into the coronary arteries, decreasing the work of the heart as it beats.*

hospitalization, especially if the swelling is severe. Occasionally thrombophlebitis can be dealt with on an outpatient basis with low-molecular-weight heparin, a blood thinner.

If you're hospitalized, your leg will be elevated and an anticoagulant drug will be administered intravenously. If for some reason a blood thinner cannot be given, it may be necessary to insert a "filter" into the inferior vena cava (the vein that carries blood back to the heart) to prevent the clot from traveling to your lungs. The filter can be inserted either with a catheter or a surgical procedure.

## Pulmonary embolism

Sometimes with thrombosis or thrombophlebitis of a deep vein, a portion of the thrombus becomes detached and travels through the veins to the right side of the heart and is then pumped into the lung circulation, where it blocks an artery in the lung. This is called pulmonary embolism. It is a serious condition requiring hospitalization.

### Symptoms of pulmonary embolism

Depending on the size of the pulmonary embolus, it can cause chest pain, painful breathing (pleurisy), shortness of breath, cough (that may produce blood-streaked sputum) or fever. In extreme cases, loss of consciousness or even sudden death may occur.

Pulmonary embolism is not always considered when doctors evaluate these symptoms, especially if the person already has heart and lung disease. Prompt diagnosis is critical, because about 10 percent of people with pulmonary embolism die within the first hour.

### Who is affected by pulmonary embolism?

Your risk of having a pulmonary embolus increases if you are confined or immobile for prolonged periods, in other words, the same conditions that are likely to cause deep-vein thrombosis or thrombophlebitis. The most likely times for pulmonary embolism to occur are after surgery, stroke, heart attack, hip or leg fracture, or prolonged bed rest or inactivity (such as sitting for a long time in a plane or car). Your risk is also higher if you are overweight or if your blood has an abnormally high tendency to clot.

### How serious is pulmonary embolism?

With appropriate diagnosis and treatment, the outlook is good for people who survive the immediate event. Blood thinners (anticoagulant drugs) can keep the thrombus in the vein from enlarging and prevent further thrombi in other veins from forming. Surgery to remove

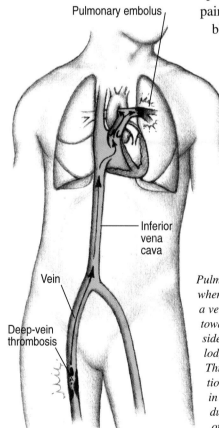

Pulmonary embolus

Inferior vena cava

Vein

Deep-vein thrombosis

*Pulmonary embolism occurs when a blood clot (thrombus) in a vein breaks loose and travels toward and through the right side of the heart, until it finally lodges in a pulmonary artery. This blocks blood flow to a portion of the lung and may result in pain, shortness of breath due to inadequate oxygenation of blood, reduced overall blood flow and blood pressure, and even death.*

the blood clot or treatment with agents to dissolve thrombi or thromboemboli (thrombolytic drugs ) is sometimes necessary for massive pulmonary embolism.

Unless you have other problems, you should be back to normal within a few weeks. Typically, you will be treated with an orally administered anticoagulant (warfarin) for about 6 months after you leave the hospital. You should make a point to be as active as possible and avoid long periods of sitting without moving around. Elevating your legs and wearing specially prescribed support stockings will also help prevent the blood from pooling and clotting in your legs. Some people, particularly those at high risk for with recurring pulmonary embolism, may have to take anticoagulant drugs indefinitely.

## Destruction of vein valves from thrombophlebitis (chronic venous insufficiency)

Another consequence of thrombophlebitis, especially in the deep veins of the legs, is damage of the valves in the affected veins. These valves prevent backward (downward) flow of blood in the veins when you stand up. Because veins do not have muscle in their walls to help "pump" the blood back to the heart, they are affected by gravity and the gentle squeezing provided by the surrounding skeletal muscle. To improve the flow of blood back to the heart, veins have valves. These valves work like safety cogs on mountain trains, which prevent them from rolling backward if they lose power while climbing up a steep mountain slope. In much the same way, the valves in the veins prevent the blood from flowing back as it is gradually pushed uphill toward the heart.

When the valves in the veins do not work properly, several problems can occur. The pooling of blood can lead to ballooning of the vein, resulting in varicose veins. In some cases the pooling gets so bad that the leg swells. This condition is commonly referred to as venous insufficiency. With chronic swelling and the associated increase in pressure on the skin, discoloration called stasis pigmentation can develop in some people, and in severe cases, actual skin ulceration can develop.

## Varicose veins

The term "varicose veins" refers to veins that are abnormally dilated. When the veins close to the surface of the legs become varicose, you can see them as soft, bluish, curving bulges under the skin.

### Causes of varicose veins

Conditions that may lead to varicose veins include pregnancy (because the uterus can press on veins in the abdomen and cause back pressure to build up in the leg veins), previous thrombophlebitis, or obesity. All of these problems elevate the pressure in the leg veins or damage the valves of the veins or both. Frequently these problems are inherited.

Some people are born without venous valves or without an adequate number of valves. These people frequently get large varicose veins at an early age.

### Symptoms of varicose veins

Besides the unsightly appearance, varicose veins may cause aching and swelling in the legs, and also hemorrhage, particularly after an injury.

### Who is affected by varicose veins?

One in 10 Americans has varicose veins. Women are twice as likely to have them as men, because of the effect of pregnancy.

### How serious are varicose veins?

For many people they are only a cosmetic annoyance. Still others have minor symptoms of mild swelling and a feeling of heaviness or aching in the legs at the end of the day. In some cases, varicose veins are serious enough to lead to chronic skin thickening or ulceration. For many people, support or elastic stockings to help counteract the increased pressure in the veins are extremely helpful for limiting swelling and other more serious complications.

Over time, varicose veins tend to become more prominent. You can help slow progression of your varicose veins by using elastic support stockings, by not standing for too long, and by not being too sedentary.

If you are overweight, it is important to lose weight. Also, discuss with your physician any medications you're taking. Some drugs can aggravate edema. Switching to a different drug may result in considerable improvement.

Move around as much as possible, but periodically lie down and elevate your legs above the level of your heart ("toes above the nose") at the end of the day to help relieve swelling. Regular exercise will also decrease the pressure in the veins.

Surgery to strip or remove the varicose veins can be performed in severe cases. In one study, 85 percent of people who had surgery had no recurrence of the varicose veins during the next 10 years. If you have small and less severe varicose veins, you might be best treated with injection of the veins or with a laser. (Surgery cannot be performed if there's leakage of a deep, as opposed to a superficial, vein.)

Laser therapy may be used on very small, superficial blood vessels, but injection therapy (sclerotherapy) is usually best if the blood vessels are large enough for the procedure to be performed. Sclerotherapy may be helpful alone or in combination with surgery. Sclerotherapy is done on an outpatient basis. The physician slowly injects a solution into one or several of the visible veins while you are standing. Then, a small bandage is wrapped snugly over the veins for 24 hours. It may take more than one treatment session to achieve optimal results.

Sclerotherapy collapses the veins, and blood is then prevented from flowing into them, and the discoloration is eliminated within about a month. The treatment has no significant effect on circulation in the leg. In about one third of people who have sclerotherapy, a yellow-brown discoloration may appear in the area and can take weeks, months, or even longer to fade.

## Diseases of the pulmonary arteries

Atherosclerosis can be present in pulmonary arteries, but it seldom if ever produces symptoms or other problems. Also, the pulmonary arteries are the "target" of emboli that may form in the deep veins of the legs, and they may also be involved in inflammatory conditions. The pulmonary arteries, however, are subject to some problems that are different from those affecting the arteries that serve the rest of the body or from problems with the veins.

## Pulmonary hypertension

The condition that most commonly affects the pulmonary circulation is pulmonary hypertension. This general term refers to conditions that raise the blood pressure in the arteries to the lungs but not in other arteries.

### Causes of pulmonary hypertension

In most cases of pulmonary embolism in which the initial event is survived, there are no subsequent problems with the pulmonary arteries. However, in rare cases the embolus does not dissolve and instead remains as an obstruction to blood flow through the lungs. The final result may be pulmonary hypertension.

Congenital heart conditions in which there is excessive blood flow through the pulmonary blood vessels may also lead to a condition of severe pulmonary hypertension known as Eisenmenger's complex.

Any situation that continuously lowers the amount of oxygen getting into the bloodstream, whether it is due to constant living at a very high altitude or to emphysema, may elevate pulmonary blood pressure.

Finally, pulmonary hypertension can exist in the absence of any apparent cause. This is called primary pulmonary hypertension, to indicate that it is the main problem rather than secondary to another problem.

### Symptoms of pulmonary hypertension

The earliest symptoms are usually tiredness and shortness of breath that become progressively worse with time. Other symptoms include angina (chest pain), passing out spells ( syncope), and blueness of the skin (cyanosis). In the later stages of the disease, the right ventricle can no longer pump blood effectively, and symptoms of right ventricular failure develop: swelling of the legs, enlargement and pain in the abdomen, loss of appetite, and bulging of the jugular veins in the neck.

**HEALTHY HEART ♥ TIP**

*An important element in your blood lipids is triglycerides, the chemicals in which most fat exists in food as well as in your body.*

*Your body converts calories it doesn't need immediately to triglycerides and transports them to fat cells for storage. Later, hormones regulate the release of the triglycerides to meet your energy needs between meals.*

*If your blood reading shows an excess of triglycerides (a condition called hypertriglyceridemia), it may be because of other diseases, such as untreated diabetes mellitus, but it's also linked to the occurrence of coronary artery disease in some people.*

### Who is affected by pulmonary hypertension?

Individuals with previous pulmonary embolism, chronic emphysema, and certain types of congenital heart disease are at higher risk for the development of pulmonary hypertension. Primary pulmonary hypertension is rare; it occurs most often in young adults, but it can occur at any age. It affects about twice as many women as men.

### How serious is pulmonary hypertension?

Pulmonary hypertension is usually a very debilitating and often fatal problem; however, the symptoms and life expectancy are extremely variable, even for people with the same degree of pulmonary blood pressure elevation. People with Eisenmenger's complex seem to be able to endure very severe pulmonary hypertension for years, although they may be limited in their activities. In people with primary pulmonary hypertension, symptoms tend to develop more rapidly and life expectancy is shorter.

## Diseases of both the arteries and veins

An uncommon problem with blood vessels is a malformation in which arteries and veins are directly connected, instead of being joined by capillaries. This can take two general forms: arteriovenous malformation, which is a congenital condition, and arteriovenous fistula, which is usually the result of trauma.

Arteriovenous malformations are "tangles" of small arterial vessels that are intertwined with small veins. The blood from the arteries flows directly into the veins. These malformations can be present anywhere in the body and in any organ. The consequences of having an arteriovenous malformation depend on their location and size. A small one in the brain may produce more problems than a larger one in the liver, for example.

A fistula can be thought of as a window or conduit that directly connects a large artery with a large vein. This might occur if a person receives a puncture wound that penetrates an artery and a vein that lie next to each other. Even after the healing process occurs, a connecting pathway between the two vessels may remain. Some blood from the artery may be diverted (shunted) directly into the vein before it goes to the capillaries. If a fistula (or arteriovenous malformation) is large, the blood flow through it may be very high. If so, the heart works excessively hard to keep up with the needs of the body.

Some arteriovenous malformations can be fixed by blocking the artery from which they branch. This can occasionally be done by inserting a special small balloon or other material directly into the artery with a catheter.

# Pericardial disease

The pericardium is the sac that surrounds the heart and portions of the great vessels. It anchors the heart in place in your chest, protects it from nearby inflammation, and reduces the friction that is caused by your heart's beating.

The pericardium can be a site of disease caused by inflammation, fluid accumulation (effusion), or stiffness (constriction). These forms may occur singly or in combination.

## Inflammation of the pericardium

Inflammation of the pericardium is called pericarditis. It occurs most often in men between ages 20 and 50 years, sometimes after a respiratory infection.

### Causes of inflammation

Causes of inflammation of the pericardium include infection, usually from a virus, or widespread inflammatory diseases such as lupus (systemic lupus erythematosus). Pericarditis may result from cancer or radiation to treat some types of cancer. However, in most cases the cause is unknown.

### Symptoms of inflammation

Inflammation of the pericardium produces a fairly characteristic set of symptoms and findings on examination. The main symptom is chest pain, but usually it is very different from angina. Typically, it is a sharp, piercing pain over the center or left side of the chest. The pain can extend up to the left shoulder and worsen when you take a deep breath. It can be lessened somewhat by sitting up and leaning forward and worsened by lying down.

Although this is the classic pattern, the pain can also be insidious or dull. You may have a low-grade fever, and in general you just feel sick. Some people have pain with swallowing.

### How serious is inflammation of the pericardium?

Acute inflammatory pericarditis usually lasts 2 to 6 weeks and does not lead to any further problems. About one in five people has a recurrence within months or, rarely, within years. Each recurrence tends to be less severe, until the episodes finally stop.

## Pericardial effusion

Pericardial effusion means that there is a collection of fluid around the heart within the pericardial sac (see page A16). The type of fluid in the pericardial sac depends on the underlying cause. An infection may produce a collection of pus. A tumor that has extended into the pericardium or a rupture of the heart after a heart attack with leakage of blood can produce bloody pericardial effusions.

Pericardial effusions may or may not press on the heart enough to limit its movement within the sac. If the fluid accumulates slowly so that the pericardial sac can distend, it may not compress the heart. However, if the fluid accumulates fast enough or reaches a large enough volume, it can compress the heart and reduce its efficiency.

In this case the heart cannot expand enough during diastole to fill sufficiently, so there is less blood to be pumped out on the next beat. When the heart is affected in this way, the condition is called cardiac tamponade.

### Causes of pericardial effusion

Pericardial effusion can be caused by inflammatory pericarditis as well as other factors. These include heart attacks, cancer extending into the pericardium, and kidney failure.

Cardiac tamponade may occur when there is bleeding after heart surgery, infections, tuberculosis, radiation treatments for some kinds of cancer, and trauma.

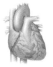

### HEALTHY HEART ♥ TIP

*Women with a history of heart disease, heart murmur, rheumatic fever, or high blood pressure should take extra precautions when they decide to become pregnant. It is especially important both before and during pregnancy to schedule frequent visits to your health care provider.*

*In addition, women with congenital heart disease show an increased risk of having babies with some types of heart defect. You may need to have diagnostic tests done, such as a fetal ultrasound test, and you'll need to consider what may be involved in caring for your child later.*

### Symptoms of pericardial effusion

If the heart is not compressed by the collection of fluid, there may be no symptoms.

Cardiac tamponade produces symptoms of inadequate heart function, because the heart is unable to pump blood effectively to the lungs and body. People with tamponade are obviously ill. Their skin may have a bluish discoloration because of lack of oxygen. They may be short of breath, anxious, light-headed, or dizzy, and they may go into shock.

### Pericardial constriction (stiffness)

One of the after effects of some cases of pericarditis is the development of a very stiff pericardium.

It is similar to the result of soaking your leather shoes in the rain—the leather becomes stiff. The stiff pericardium decreases the ability of the heart muscle to expand between contractions and fill with blood. It occurs in all age groups, but it is more common after age 30.

### Causes of pericardial constriction

Pericarditis that was originally caused by infectious agents (such as in tuberculosis), by radiation exposure during treatment of cancers in the chest, or by inflammatory conditions is most likely to lead to pericardial constriction.

### Symptoms of pericardial constriction

Pericardial constriction involves both ventricles, but the most prominent symptoms are usually those of right-sided heart failure such as swelling of the abdomen and legs. Shortness of breath and fatigue are also common and usually precede the swelling.

### How serious is pericardial constriction?

In cases of heart failure, the pericardium may need to be removed surgically. If this happens, you do not need to worry. You can get along fine without your pericardium, just as you can get along without your appendix or gallbladder.

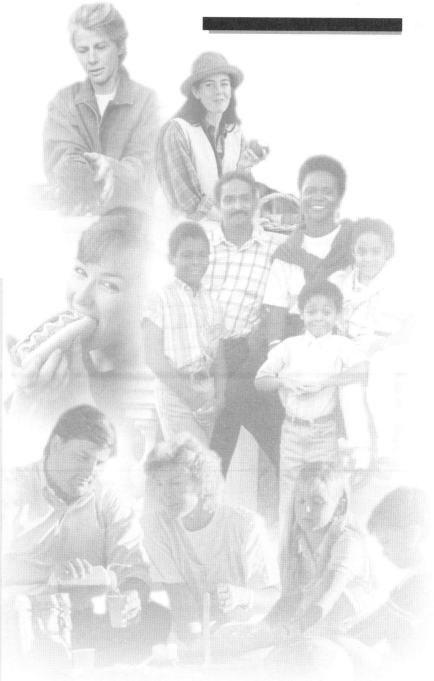

# Part 3

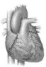

136

# Dealing with the risks
# of coronary artery disease

Y ou may not want to live forever, but you would certainly like to be healthy for as long as you possibly can. Since your lifestyle affects your health, developing good habits and avoiding harmful ones can positively influence not only the length but also the quality of your life.

## Chapter

# Chapter

# 8

# Understanding your risks

Y ou can control some risk factors. But others are beyond your control. That's why it's important to understand the risk factors, know whether they pertain to you, and see how you can eliminate or modify any that may affect you.

Risk factors you can't alter include sex, age and heredity. Although unchangeable, these risk factors are nonetheless very important. In fact, the presence of one or more of them may provide added incentive to do something about the factors that you can influence, because the uncontrollable risk factors can interact with those that are controllable—the harmful effect may be additive. Risk factors over which you have at least some control include high blood pressure, high blood cholesterol, smoking, diabetes, excess weight, improper diet, physical inactivity, and your response to stress. Using certain drugs—cocaine, for example—also increases your risk of having a heart attack.

## Risk factors for coronary artery disease

High blood pressure

High blood cholesterol

Smoking

Excess weight

Diabetes

Physical inactivity

Stress and your reaction to it

Certain drugs (cocaine, oral
  contraceptives for women who smoke)

Family history of coronary artery disease

Increased age

Male sex

Menopause

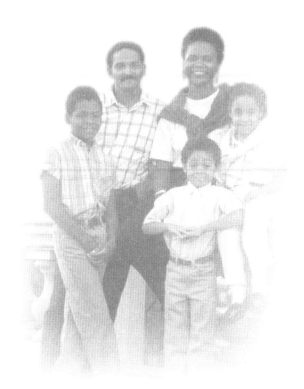

When considering your health, risk refers to the odds or chances that something will occur. It does not mean that it is inevitable. There are no guarantees. Although risk factors affect your odds of developing coronary artery disease, having one or more risk factors does not make it inevitable that you will develop this disease. Similarly, the absence of risk factors doesn't guarantee that you'll avoid coronary artery disease.

If you drive a car 10,000 miles a year, you are more likely to have a car accident than someone who drives only 500 miles a year. However, the high-mileage driver may never have an accident. Conversely, a truck may hit as someone leaves the driveway.

Yes, you occasionally hear of someone who smokes two packs of cigarettes a day and lives to a ripe old age. Meanwhile, a vigorous person with a seemingly healthful lifestyle may die early. These observations strongly suggest that there are many other risk factors and genetic traits that influence health and life span. Within the next few years we will certainly learn a great deal about genes and disease, but the important lesson for the present is to modify those risk factors that we already know so much about.

## How risk factors interact

Risk factors interact with each other in important ways. If you have two risk factors—high cholesterol and a smoking habit, for example—your odds of having coronary artery disease are much higher than if you had either risk factor alone, especially if you add in a family history of heart disease.

In fact, the total risk, when you have multiple factors, may be greater than you may anticipate by simply adding the risks together. Some factors are actually magnified in combination with others.

Once you understand the risk factors, you can make responsible decisions about your lifestyle. Your decisions revolve around the value you place on your health in relation to the risks that may compromise it in the future.

It's like many games of chance. You can plot a strategy based on the odds (your risk factors) and the stakes. With coronary artery disease, the stakes are your health and your life span—items that are probably high on your list of priorities. Yet, for a variety of reasons, you may take great risks that increase your likelihood of having coronary artery disease.

Why do you take these risks? Perhaps you believe or hope that risky behavior won't actually affect you. Or you may be faced with a conflicting priority that temporarily causes you to choose something above your health. Some risky activities are fun, glamorous, carefree or sociable—at the time, at least. Like many people, you may take your health for granted, especially if you've never been deprived of good health. And finally, the consequences of your decisions about many risk factors don't show up immediately, but occur later in life—beyond the normal planning period of most young people.

Understanding why you take risks is an important first step in learning to deal with your risks constructively. Modifying your risk factors often means depriving yourself of a pleasure in the short term—smoking a cigarette or eating fast food, for example—in favor of a more abstract benefit over the longer term.

## Risk factors you're given

Risk factors for heart disease that you cannot change include heredity (your family history), age and sex. While you can't affect them, they're factors you need to take into account when considering your risk of coronary artery disease.

### Your heredity

If one or both of your parents or another close blood relative (first-degree relative) had a heart attack at an early age, your risk for developing coronary artery disease is higher than someone whose family has no members with heart disease. Your risk is above average if your father or brother developed coronary artery disease before age 55—or if your mother or sister developed it before age 65. Even if you eliminate risks not recognized a generation ago—smoking or high blood cholesterol, for example—the fact that your father died of a heart attack at age 50 makes your risk somewhat higher than that of someone who does not have this family history.

The most significant genetic risk is a predisposition for dangerously high cholesterol levels (familial hypercholesterolemia). Other factors you may have inherited from your parents include the tendency toward moderately high cholesterol levels, high blood pressure, obesity or diabetes.

Although, strictly speaking, it's not heredity, your early environment and experiences also affect your risk factors. Your family may strongly influence the types of food you eat, your exercise habits, and whether you smoke. And even if you don't smoke, exposure to tobacco smoke in your home or work place is an additional health risk.

But your heredity and background neither doom you to nor fully protect you from the risk of heart disease. Knowing that your heredity contributes to your risk of coronary artery disease can provide an extra incentive for you to develop more healthful habits. Clearly, you can make a big difference by evaluating and controlling other risk factors—especially smoking, high blood pressure and high blood cholesterol.

### Your age

As you age, the risk of developing many health problems increases. Men over age 45 and women over age 55 are at increased risk of coronary artery disease. But you can slow some of the natural effects of aging by controlling your weight and diet, getting regular and appropriate exercise, and controlling your blood pressure and cholesterol levels.

The sooner you tackle your risk factors for coronary artery disease the better. Sometimes, habits developed in early childhood encourage cardiovascular disease to develop gradually. The sooner you can minimize risk factors that contribute to a build-up of fatty deposits in the lining of your arteries (atherosclerosis), the likelier you'll be to avoid angina and heart attack later in life.

## Your sex

Coronary artery disease is the leading cause of death for both men and women. It's hard to evaluate the role of sex apart from other factors, such as smoking, high blood pressure and high blood cholesterol. Whether you're a man or a woman, you're at a higher risk of heart disease if you have high blood pressure or elevated blood cholesterol levels.

Before a woman reaches menopause, given only the difference of sex, a man is much more likely than a woman to have coronary artery disease. After menopause the difference in risk levels shrinks.

However, this does not mean that a woman is immune from heart disease (see page 378). In fact, 47 percent of Americans who have fatal heart attacks are women. On average, a woman develops coronary artery disease about 10 years later in life than a man does.

Researchers aren't sure why this is the case. The female hormone estrogen may be one protective factor against heart disease. After menopause, estrogen levels decline and a woman's risk increases.

Although evidence points in a favorable direction, scientists are not yet certain whether using estrogen after menopause (hormone replacement therapy) reduces a woman's risk of heart disease. Incidentally, estrogen replacement may also help a woman avoid osteoporosis. However, this therapy may slightly increase the risk of breast cancer or cancer in the lining of the uterus (endometrial cancer). Smoking appears to reduce a woman's estrogen levels and hasten menopause—additional reasons to consider smoking an important risk factor for heart disease.

Until recently, most research relating to coronary artery disease focused on men. Now studies are under way to determine whether the findings of previous research on men apply to women as well.

## Risk factors you can control

You have some control over many risk factors for coronary artery disease. Since risk factors often occur in clusters and relate to one another, moderate changes in one factor can reduce several others at the same time. For example, by gradually working into a regular exercise program, you may lower your blood pressure, help control your weight, and increase good (HDL) cholesterol.

Some risk factors are obvious without a medical examination, including smoking, being overweight and being physically inactive. Other risk factors—including high blood cholesterol levels, high blood sugar levels (diabetes), and high blood pressure—usually show up only during a medical examination.

One of the main purposes of a medical check-up is to help you identify risk factors or early evidence of disease of your heart or other organs, so that you can tackle those risk factors that you can change—as soon as possible.

How often should you have a general medical evaluation? Most doctors agree that you should have a check-up every 3 to 5 years until age 40 if you are apparently healthy. During your 40s you should see your doctor four times, and during the decade of your 50s you should have five general examinations. After age 60, it's advisable to have an annual examination.

If you have one or more risk factors for coronary artery disease, your doctor may recommend further diagnostic testing, even if you have no symptoms. Then you can take measures necessary to reduce the risk factors you can control.

## Is prevention worth the effort?

The purpose of identifying and controlling your cardiovascular risk factors is to prevent a heart attack, early disability, and death. Although it's difficult to pick one risk factor as the greatest predictor of coronary artery disease, most doctors would probably agree that the most important risk factors are smoking, elevated lipids (cholesterol) in your blood, high blood pressure, excess weight, a sedentary life style, and diabetes.

Millions of Americans have learned about these risk factors and, with help from health professionals, have tried to modify their risk. You can drastically reduce your risk of coronary artery disease by controlling your high blood pressure, stopping smoking, and lowering your cholesterol level.

If you doubt that you can make a difference in your risk of developing coronary artery disease, consider the following: The average cholesterol level of the American population has decreased during the past 25 years, probably because many people have altered their diets and are getting more physical activity. Experts believe that these changes have contributed to the declining death rate from heart disease in the United States.

*Primary prevention* is treating or correcting a risk factor in order to prevent coronary artery disease from occurring. You can think of it as preventive maintenance, taking steps to reduce your risk factors before coronary artery disease develops. About half of all deaths from heart disease occur before there is time to start treatment—despite great improvements in treatment methods that are saving more lives. Waiting to treat coronary artery disease until after it develops is not the ideal way to reduce deaths from heart disease. The best way to save lives is to prevent heart attacks by eliminating or reducing risk factors.

*Secondary prevention* is the attempt to reduce risk factors after you show documented coronary artery disease or have a heart attack. Even in this case, you can still reduce your chances of further complications by reducing your risk factors. Aggressively treating risk factors can actually decrease atherosclerosis. If you give up smoking, exercise regularly and develop healthful eating, living and work habits, you can diminish the effects of existing cardiovascular disease. This is the aim of a cardiovascular rehabilitation program after you've had a heart attack. The goal is to help you reduce the risk of a second heart attack, compensate for the damage to your heart, decrease the extent of atherosclerosis or prevent its progression, and resume as normal a lifestyle as possible.

## Should you take aspirin?

Aspirin's ability to inhibit the activity of platelets (a blood component that contributes to clotting) is well known. By doing this, aspirin reduces the tendency of blood to clot. Thus it may help reduce or prevent narrowing of your blood vessels due to atherosclerosis. Your doctor may recommend using aspirin in these situations:

- *To avoid the recurrence of conditions caused by blood clotting or atherosclerosis (secondary prevention).*

  If you've already had a heart attack, stroke, warning signs of a stroke (transient ischemic attack) or unstable angina, you may benefit by taking medications, such as aspirin, that inhibit the activity of platelets. In fact, taking aspirin can reduce your risk of death by 15 percent and the risk of complications (such as a nonfatal heart attack or stroke) by 25 to 30 percent. Medical researchers estimate that if 100 people with cardiovascular disease took aspirin for 2 years, they could avoid one death and two major nonfatal events—seemingly small numbers that become important when applied worldwide to the total number of people with cardiovascular disease.

  If you've had a coronary artery bypass operation, aspirin may reduce the likelihood that the bypass grafts will be blocked by a blood clot or atherosclerosis.

- *To prevent the initial occurrence of a blood clot or other complication related to atherosclerosis (primary prevention).*

- *To reduce the effects of a heart attack (myocardial infarction).*

  If you think you're having a heart attack, first call for emergency help. Then immediately chew an adult aspirin or crush and drink it dissolved in water for faster absorption. Aspirin may help restore some blood flow through your clogged arteries.

Aspirin in low doses is inexpensive, generally safe and easy to take. Most doctors recommend it as an effective measure to reduce future risk in people who already have one problem. So why not just treat everyone with aspirin and reduce the incidence of heart attack and stroke?

If you don't have heart disease, it's not clear that aspirin offers any cardiovascular benefits and, although uncommon, aspirin can cause stomach irritation and gastrointestinal bleeding. While a study of 22,000 American male doctors revealed that those who took one aspirin every other day had 44 fewer heart attacks,

they did not have fewer strokes or deaths attributable to cardiovascular disease. A similar British study did not reveal fewer heart attacks with aspirin.

The main benefit of preventive use of aspirin seems to begin at age 50. It's also unclear whether aspirin benefits women. One study of more than 80,000 female nurses suggested that women who take one to six aspirin weekly have less chance of a heart attack. However, the benefit was small, and the study was not designed to produce a solid recommendation.

When doctors recommend aspirin for preventing complications of a blood clot, low doses are sufficient. You can substantially reduce the ability of your platelets to clot by taking less than one aspirin a day. In fact, one baby aspirin (equivalent to one fourth of a regular-strength adult aspirin) is sufficient. Avoid taking aspirin if you're allergic to it, if you have bleeding problems, stomach ulcers or irritation, or if you are already taking an anticoagulant (such as warfarin).

- *To avoid blood clot formation if you have atrial fibrillation, which predisposes you to abnormal clotting in your heart (see page 111).*

If you have atrial fibrillation, you are at increased risk for a stroke. This is due to the greater likelihood that blood clots will form in your left atrium, break off and travel to a blood vessel in your brain. One study showed that aspirin effectively reduced stroke in some people with atrial fibrillation, but warfarin is even more effective. Three major studies established that low doses of warfarin reduced the likelihood of stroke by about 70 percent. Neither aspirin nor low doses of warfarin produce bleeding problems in most people with atrial fibrillation.

If you have atrial fibrillation—even if you have no evidence of other types of heart disease—you should take either aspirin or warfarin. If you're young and have no evidence of other cardiovascular problems, 325 mg of aspirin a day may be sufficient. If you have any other evidence of heart disease—including high blood pressure, congestive heart failure, past problems related to blood clots, reduced pumping function of your left ventricle, enlargement of your left atrium, or valve abnormalities—you should probably take warfarin, unless another condition, such as a tendency to bleed, makes the use of warfarin dangerous.

If you are considering taking a regular, preventive dose of aspirin, discuss it first with your doctor.

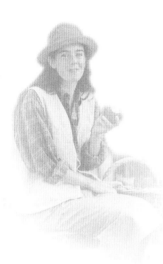

Whether or not you have coronary artery disease, it's worth making an effort to reduce your risk factors. Of course, it may not be easy to change habits you have lived with for many years. This part of the book describes each risk factor, discusses how it's evaluated, and explains why each is harmful.

## Smoking

Smoking is the leading cause of preventable illness and death in the United States. Smoking causes more than 400,000 deaths in the United States every year. At least a third of these deaths are related to cardiovascular disease. Smoking kills more people each year than AIDS, alcohol (including driving while intoxicated), cocaine, other drug abuse and accidents—combined! In fact, the Surgeon General estimates that nearly 20 percent of all deaths in the United States are related to smoking.

All members of society—whether smokers or nonsmokers—bear the immense cost of this human tragedy through higher health insurance costs, lower productivity and higher taxes. Nationally, smoking places a financial burden on Americans of more than $50 billion per year. This provides a tremendous incentive—both individually and as a nation—to reduce tobacco use.

### Why is smoking harmful?

Tobacco smoke contains more than 4,000 different substances. Many of these substances, such as tar, nitrosamines and polycyclic aromatic hydrocarbons, produce adverse health effects. No one is exactly sure whether nicotine by itself is quite so harmful or whether its toxicity results from its combination with other substances.

The main risks you incur by smoking are developing atherosclerosis in your blood vessels, and lung cancer, or cancer at other sites within your body. Smoking also causes your blood to clot more readily—an effect that some experts believe may even be more important than the effect of smoking on atherosclerosis. The mechanisms by which this occurs remain elusive, despite the clear statistical association with tobacco use. Researchers have identified several potential links. For example: smoking reduces the proportion of "good" HDL cholesterol to "bad" LDL cholesterol in your blood. Smoking also increases the tendency for blood to clot inside your blood vessels and obstruct the flow of blood. Furthermore, components of tobacco smoke may directly damage the internal protective lining of your blood vessels (endothelium).

Inhaling tobacco smoke produces several adverse effects on your heart and blood vessels—effects that are serious enough to provoke a heart attack or other major event. Nicotine in the smoke increases your blood pressure and heart rate. Carbon monoxide, a by-product of tobacco smoke (and the same gas in your car's exhaust that's lethal in an enclosed space), gets into your blood, where it reduces the amount of oxygen that your blood can carry to your heart and throughout your body. It also causes arteries in your arms and legs to constrict.

By temporarily decreasing the diameter of the arteries that feed your heart, smoking can deprive your heart muscle of the blood and oxygen it needs to function properly. If your arteries are already narrowed by atherosclerosis, this additional constriction may be enough to cause angina or a heart attack.

If you are a smoker and have angina, you will get chest pain more quickly when you exert yourself, since smoking reduces the amount of oxygen that's carried to your heart and makes your heart beat faster. Ironically, as your heart's demand for oxygen increases, the supply of oxygen to your heart decreases. Not only does smoking block the increased blood flow that normally occurs when you exercise, but it also reduces the effectiveness of some drugs that treat angina.

Even if you have no symptoms, studies show that smoking deprives your heart muscle of the oxygen it needs to function properly. Sometimes smoking even causes coronary arteries that are not blocked by atherosclerosis to go into spasm and become narrow enough to cut off the flow of blood to your heart muscle.

Smoking also causes other damage to your cardiovascular system. It's a major risk factor in the narrowing of vessels that carry blood to your arm and leg muscles (peripheral vascular disease). Consequences of this condition may range from leg pain that occurs with exertion (claudication) to the actual destruction of skin or muscle tissue that your arteries are unable to serve sufficiently. When this condition is severe it may require vascular surgery or even amputation. If you are a woman who smokes and takes birth control pills, you're also at a higher risk for another serious vascular problem—stroke.

Furthermore, smoking is the main cause of chronic lung diseases such as bronchitis, emphysema, and lung cancer.

## Who smokes—and why?

The percentage of Americans who smoke has gradually declined during the past two decades. This is probably due to increased awareness of the health consequences of smoking, more vocal nonsmokers, the social stigma attached to smoking and increased restrictions on smoking in public places.

However, more than one fourth of all men and women were regular smokers in 1999. And a recent and alarming increase in smoking among young people may reverse the decline in overall smoking rates that has occurred for two decades. A very large number of people will continue to smoke into the next millennium.

Why do people expose themselves to all the risks that smoking brings? Although most smokers are well aware of the known hazards to their health, they develop a physical need or addiction to the constituents of tobacco, especially nicotine, in order to function comfortably and avoid nicotine withdrawal. Their repetitive smoking behavior is triggered by many cues, including stress, meals, and conversations on the telephone. However, smokers can overcome these addictive behavior patterns.

Although the dangers of smoking are well known, every day about 3,000 children take their first smoke. It's likely that tobacco ultimately will kill more of these people than will alcohol or drugs. Unfortunately, it's difficult to convince young people of the reality of their future health problems.

## How high is the risk?

If you smoke, your risk of cardiovascular disease is at least twice that of a non-smoker. The risk increases with the amount you smoke each day. If you smoke one pack of cigarettes a day, your risk is twice as high as that of someone who never smoked. If you smoke two or more packs a day, your risk is three times as high as that of a person who never smoked.

A recent study of men in the United States, Europe and Japan showed that, even among men who smoked fewer than 10 cigarettes a day, the death rate from heart disease or lung cancer was 30 percent higher than among men of the same age who didn't smoke. If you smoke two packs of cigarettes per day, your risk of death from heart disease alone (disregarding death from other causes or other health problems short of death) is twice what it would be if you had never smoked.

The earlier you begin using tobacco, the greater the risk to your health. Of every 10 smokers, eight begin before age 18. Thus, the risk and damage accumulate over a large portion of their lives. Diseases related to smoking don't usually kill you rapidly, but slowly rob you of your vitality over a period of years.

Young people start smoking for a variety of reasons: peer group acceptance, rebellion against authority, susceptibility to the tobacco industry's targeted advertising, and a perception that smoking imparts an image of someone willing to take risks. Recent studies also indicate that some young people smoke to control weight or to cope with stress or depression. Some people consider smoking an expression of individual rights. Advertising has capitalized on all of these attitudes.

But attitudes about smoking are changing. Increasingly, people see smoking for what it really is—an annoying, dangerous addiction. They are concerned about the implications of rising smoking rates among teenagers and college students for the future health of our population.

## What about second-hand smoke?

Not everyone who smokes does so voluntarily. Environmental tobacco smoke, termed "a major preventable cause of cardiovascular disease and death" by the American Heart Association, causes heart disease and cancer.

The risk of second-hand smoking increases as your exposure increases. Experts estimate that environmental tobacco smoke is directly responsible for more than 50,000 deaths from cardiovascular disease and 3,000 to 5,000 lung cancer deaths each year. There is no threshold below which environmental tobacco smoke is free of risk.

## Does it lower your risk to smoke cigarettes with lower tar and nicotine levels?

Smoking in any form is hazardous to your health. No cigarettes are safe. There is no research to support the theory that smoking cigarettes with less tar or nicotine reduces your risk of coronary artery disease or cancer.

People who smoke cigarettes with lower tar and nicotine levels often inhale more deeply, hold their breath after inhaling, and smoke more cigarettes in an unwitting effort to maintain the nicotine levels to which their bodies are addicted. Thus, they not only fail to reduce their nicotine exposure as they may have hoped, but they also inhale more of the other toxic substances contained in the smoke.

## Health benefits of quitting

From a health perspective, it's most beneficial never to begin smoking in the first place. However, if you do smoke, you can gain a lot by stopping.

After you quit smoking, the risk of heart disease caused by smoking drops greatly within about 2 years. After about 10 years of not smoking, your risk of having a heart attack is about as low as if you had never smoked.

Even if you're relatively older, there is an excellent advantage to discontinuing smoking. Recent studies have shown that smokers older than age 60 could add 5 to 7 years to their lives by quitting. It's never too late to quit.

## High blood pressure

High blood pressure is called the silent killer. You can have it and not even know it, because high blood pressure seldom causes symptoms that warn you of a problem.

However, high blood pressure, or hypertension, is the most common cardiovascular disease. It affects about one of every four Americans—one of every three black people. Every year there are 2 million new cases. One in six office visits to health care providers is made for the purpose of managing high blood pressure.

### It's a serious matter

High blood pressure is a serious condition. It can damage components of your circulatory system, including the blood vessels of your heart, brain, eyes and kidneys. The higher the pressure or the longer it goes undiagnosed or uncontrolled, the worse the outlook.

However, high blood pressure is often not given the serious attention it deserves. Nearly a third of the 50 million Americans with this condition don't even know they have it. Only about half are receiving treatment, and only about one in four is controlled at a goal level of blood pressure. Up to a fifth of the patients undergoing treatment for high blood pressure aren't even aware that they have high blood pressure and are being treated for it.

### Not a natural result of aging

If you live in the United States, your chances of having high blood pressure increase as you age. However, although you have a one in two chance of developing high blood pressure by the time you reach 60 years of age, it's not a normal part of aging. Many people do not get hypertension. In some parts of the world aging does not bring an increase in hypertension levels. Therefore, it's reasonable to assume that you can prevent high blood pressure with lifestyle changes.

Despite the current situation, there has been a significant reduction in deaths from stroke (almost 60 percent) and coronary heart disease (more than 50 percent) in the past 30 years. However, this remarkable trend is slowing, as the number of

## What you can gain by quitting smoking

*Immediate*

Cleaner, less smelly house, clothes, hair, breath, car

Easier breathing, improved exercise tolerance

Less offense to others

An end to exposing family and friends to risky second-hand smoke

Better-tasting food

No more smoker's cough

Less dental staining

Reduced fire hazard

Increased spending money

Insurance discounts

Positive example for your children

Reduced heartburn

*Ultimate*

Reduced risk of cardiovascular disease

Reduced risk of emphysema and bronchitis

Reduced risk of lung, esophageal and other types of cancer

Increased life span and quality of life

Americans with their blood pressure under control is not increasing as it had in earlier decades. This is occurring despite the fact that hypertension is easy to detect and steps can be taken to lower your blood pressure to a safe level through lifestyle changes and, if needed, medication.

## What is blood pressure?

The pumping action of your heart pushes blood into your arteries with enough pressure to keep it flowing forward. The amount of blood pumped out of your heart (cardiac output) and the resistance to blood flow in your arteries determine the amount of tension pushing against the walls of your arteries. The more your heart pumps and the smaller the arteries, the higher your blood pressure (that is, the harder your heart must work to pump the same amount of blood).

Your blood pressure normally varies during the day. It rises during activity, and decreases with rest. The medical term for high blood pressure is hypertension (*hyper* means high, and *tension* refers to the pressure inside your arteries).

The standard way to measure blood pressure is in millimeters of mercury (mm Hg). This unit of measurement refers to how high the pressure inside your arteries is able to raise a column of mercury. Each blood pressure measurement has two numbers and is written like a fraction. The top number is your systolic blood pressure, or the highest pressure within your arteries that occurs during systole, when your heart is contracting. The bottom number is your diastolic blood pressure, or the lowest pressure within your arteries that occurs during diastole, when your heart is relaxing and filling with blood.

Normal blood pressure refers to your blood pressure when you are resting comfortably. Although a typical blood pressure is considered to be 120/80 mm Hg, your blood pressure is not constant. Even a change in position from lying down to sitting or standing can change your blood pressure.

Therefore, it's necessary to take more than one reading to determine whether you have high blood pressure. About 35 percent of people who have high blood pressure on a single reading will not have an elevated value when their blood pressure is measured again. If your blood pressure is elevated during three separate measurements, it requires medical evaluation and treatment.

## What is high blood pressure?

There are gradations in severity of high blood pressure. The significance of your blood pressure and the response you and your physician should take to alter it depend on how high it is and whether it is consistently elevated, as measured when you are relaxed. Treatment recommendations also depend upon whether or not you have sustained organ damage or have other risk factors for cardiovascular disease.

Either your diastolic pressure or your systolic pressure—or both—may be elevated. Elevated diastolic pressure promotes damage to your kidneys and to blood vessels throughout your body. High systolic blood pressure is associated with a higher risk of coronary artery disease and stroke.

The National Heart, Lung, and Blood Institute, a division of the National Institutes of Health, periodically issues a report on the prevention, detection, evaluation and treatment of high blood pressure. The latest report, issued in November 1997, divides people with high blood pressure into three risk groups (A, B and C) according to blood pressure readings (high-normal, stage 1, stage 2 or stage 3; see sidebar), damage to internal organs, and risk factors for cardiovascular disease.

The report includes recommendations for treating borderline (high-normal) blood pressure, since it's likely to progress to high blood pressure if left untreated.

*Risk group A* includes you if you have high-normal blood pressure or high blood pressure without organ damage, cardiovascular disease or other risk factors. In risk group A, if your blood pressure is in the high-normal or stage 1 hypertension range, the report recommends lifestyle changes to reduce your blood pressure to a normal or optimal level. However, if you have stage 1 hypertension and if the changes don't bring your blood pressure down adequately within a year, you may need medication. Even in this lowest risk group, if you have stage 2 or stage 3 hypertension, initial treatment should include both medication and lifestyle changes.

*Risk group B* includes you—like most people with high blood pressure—if you have no organ damage or cardiovascular disease, but one or more cardiovascular risk factors (excluding diabetes). As with the previous risk group, if your blood pressure is high-normal or stage 1 hypertension, the report recommends trying lifestyle changes first. If, after 6 months, lifestyle changes haven't reduced your stage 1 hypertension, you may need medication. In this risk group initial treatment for both stages 2 and 3 high blood pressure includes both lifestyle changes and medication.

*Risk group C* includes you if you have cardiovascular disease, organ damage, diabetes or a combination of these, even if your blood pressure is high-normal. For all people in risk group C, the report recommends treatment that includes both lifestyle changes and medication.

## What causes high blood pressure?

It's normal for blood pressure to rise with increased output from your heart—as occurs with exercise, for example. But high blood pressure is abnormal when it's caused by a persistent increased resistance to blood flowing through your small arterioles (the smaller branches of your arteries). Think of the arterioles as hoses. It takes less pressure to push the same flow rate of water through a hose with a large diameter than through a narrower hose.

## Blood pressure classification

**Systolic** (top number)

120 mm Hg or lower: optimal blood pressure, with respect to cardiovascular risk

129 mm Hg or lower: normal blood pressure

130 to 139 mm Hg: high-normal blood pressure

140 to 159 mm Hg: Stage 1 hypertension

160 to 179 mm Hg: Stage 2 hypertension*

180 mm Hg or higher: Stage 3 hypertension

**Diastolic** (bottom number)

80 mm Hg or lower: optimal blood pressure, with respect to cardiovascular risk

81 to 84 mm Hg: normal blood pressure

85 to 89 mm Hg: high-normal blood pressure

90 to 99 mm Hg: Stage 1 hypertension

100 to 109 mm Hg: Stage 2 hypertension

110 mm Hg or higher: Stage 3 hypertension

*Isolated systolic hypertension is defined as a normal diastolic blood pressure lower than 90 mm Hg but an elevated systolic blood pressure of 160 mm Hg or more. About half of older adults with high blood pressure have this condition. Studies show that treating this form of high blood pressure can prevent 24,000 strokes and 50,000 severe cardiovascular problems, including heart attack, each year.

This information is based on the 1997 Report of the Joint National Committee on Prevention, Detection, Evaluation, and Treatment of High Blood Pressure.

## "White-coat" hypertension

You may find that your blood pressure is high when it's measured at your doctor's office, yet is normal if you measure it at home. This condition, called "white-coat" (or stress or office) hypertension, may affect up to 20 percent of the population.

Sometimes having someone who is not a physician take your blood pressure reading helps. And you can learn to monitor your own blood pressure at home.

In order to do that, you will need to borrow or purchase a blood pressure device. *Consumer Reports* magazine evaluates these devices periodically. Doctors don't recommend devices that take a reading from your finger or wrist. If you own a blood pressure gauge, check its accuracy at your doctor's office annually. In general, average home blood pressure readings lower than 135/85 mm Hg correspond to under 140/90 at your physician's office.

It's generally not a good idea to measure your blood pressure by an automated machine at a shopping mall. While these machines are usually accurate when they're first installed, heavy use and infrequent calibration often result in faulty readings. Furthermore, it's difficult to be as relaxed as possible in such a setting.

### Monitoring your blood pressure at home

Your doctor may suggest that you measure your blood pressure at home as part of your treatment (see page 227). To do that you need a device called a sphygmomanometer (pronounced SFIG-mo-mah-NOM-uh-tur). All blood pressure monitoring devices used on your arm have an inflatable cuff that encircles your upper arm. Check with your doctor or nurse about what cuff size is appropriate for you. When you inflate the cuff, the arteries in your arm are briefly closed.

As you gradually release the pressure with the air-flow regulator and listen over an artery with a stethoscope, you will begin to hear a pulse beat (a tapping sound). The point at which you hear the first beat indicates your systolic pressure (the top number). The point at which your pulse beat disappears indicates your diastolic pressure (the bottom number).

If your model has a mercury column, it rises and falls in response to the amount of pressure exerted on the blood pressure cuff. This device uses millimeters of mercury to measure the pressure. Other devices mechanically reproduce this method of measurement.

Spring gauge models feature a round dial activated by a spring pressure gauge that indicates the amount of pressure in the arm cuff. Each degree the needle moves in the measurement dial is equivalent to a millimeter of mercury.

Electronic digital models use built-in electronic sound and pressure sensors to read your blood pressure, which is displayed on a digital readout. Many models also have built-in pulse monitors that measure your pulse rate. You do not need a stethoscope for this type of device.

By taking your reading in different locations on a regular basis, you can give your doctor valuable information that can help tailor your treatment. Be sure your device is calibrated periodically to ensure accurate readings.

If you've just had coffee or a cigarette—or if your bladder is full—don't take your blood pressure right away. All these factors increase your blood pressure. Sit quietly for 5 minutes before taking a reading. Then follow these steps:

1. Extend your arm at heart level on a table or arm of your chair. If you are right-handed, you may find it easier to measure the pressure in your left arm, and if you are left-handed, in your right arm.

If the cause of the abnormal resistance in your arterioles is unknown—as it is in 95 percent of people with the condition—you are said to have primary, or essential, hypertension. Hypertension runs in some families, although the problem may never develop in many relatives. It affects men and women equally. It's more common among blacks than among whites. Everyone's risk increases with age.

Your risk of developing high blood pressure increases if you're a woman who takes birth control pills and smokes cigarettes. Or you may be one of those people for whom a high intake of sodium in the diet increases your blood pressure. A recent report suggests that at least part of the increased prevalence among blacks may be due to a gene that makes them more sensitive to salt.

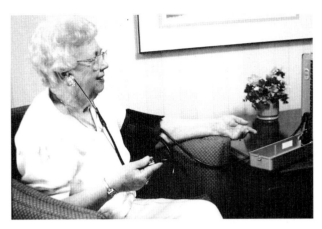

*This woman is using a blood pressure cuff with a built-in stethoscope. The mercury column measuring unit is on the table.*

**2.** Apply the cuff to your bare upper arm. It should fit snugly, with the lower edge about 1 inch above your elbow.

**3.** Where you place the stethoscope depends upon the type of unit you are using. If your unit has a built-in stethoscope, the flat disk should be placed over your pulse, 2 inches above the inside of your elbow. If you're using a stethoscope that is not attached to the blood pressure cuff, place the flat disk over your pulse at the inside of your elbow.

**4.** Repeatedly squeeze the hand bulb until the pressure gauge reads 30 mm Hg above your anticipated systolic blood pressure. Stop pumping. You should not hear any pulse sound when you listen through the stethoscope.

**5.** Deflate the cuff slowly (about 2 to 3 mm Hg per second). As the pressure falls, listen for the sound of your pulse. Note the reading on the gauge when the beating first becomes audible. This is your systolic blood pressure.

**6.** Continue deflating the cuff. Note the reading when your heartbeat ceases to be audible. This is your diastolic blood pressure.

**7.** Record your blood pressure as systolic/diastolic (for example, 140/90).

**8.** Repeat the procedure at least once to confirm the accuracy of your reading.

If your hearing is impaired, it may be a good idea to have an electronic monitoring device. Take your device to your doctor's office, fire department or public health service every 6 months or so to have the calibration checked. And occasionally check your measurement with that taken by your doctor or nurse.

Your doctor will tell you how often and at what times of the day to measure your blood pressure. Remember that blood pressure varies, so don't get too worried if one reading is unusual. Repeat the measurement in an hour.

Portable devices that continuously monitor and record your blood pressure are useful tools. They record your blood pressure during the day and night, while you're awake or sleeping. This method of recording gives you and your doctor a more realistic and accurate assessment of your true blood pressure.

## Why is high blood pressure bad for you?

Many studies clearly show the direct relationship between high blood pressure and stroke, heart disease, and kidney (renal) failure. If you have high blood pressure, you're about three times more likely to have coronary artery disease, six times more likely to have congestive heart failure, and seven times more likely to have a stroke than are people whose high blood pressure is under control. A major contributor to the decline in deaths due to stroke and heart disease over the last 50 years has been the treatment of high blood pressure.

So it's worth decreasing these risks markedly by treating your high blood pressure. If you don't treat it—or inadequately control it—high blood pressure can have detrimental effects on your heart, arteries, brain and kidneys.

High blood pressure forces your heart to work harder than normal. Blood pressure is like a weight or load that your heart muscle must lift. Like any other muscle, your heart gets larger with heavy weight-lifting. Eventually, however, your heart's pumping efficiency decreases when the muscle can no longer adapt to the excessive workload. If this occurs, your heart muscle may weaken, and you may develop congestive heart failure.

High blood pressure accelerates the development of atherosclerosis in your arteries and arterioles as you age, increasing the chances of a heart attack or stroke. A stroke is a form of brain injury caused by a blocked or ruptured blood vessel in your brain. High blood pressure can also lead to an aneurysm, or bulge, in an artery.

About 25 percent of the people who now undergo kidney dialysis have kidneys that were damaged as a result of mild, untreated high blood pressure. Frequently you can avoid or delay the need for kidney dialysis or transplantation by treating high blood pressure early and adequately.

## Evaluating your high blood pressure

If you have high blood pressure, your doctor will want to obtain a careful medical history, perform a physical examination, and do a limited number of tests in order to answer these three questions before deciding on the best method of treatment:

- Are any of your organs damaged?
- Do you have any other cardiovascular risk factors?
- Is your high blood pressure primary or a form of secondary (and possibly curable) hypertension?

To help answer these questions, your doctor may order some laboratory tests to determine whether you have cardiovascular disease and, if so, its severity. If the physical examination and laboratory findings are normal, most people with mildly elevated blood pressure don't need further tests. However, if you have any of these conditions you may need further assessment:

- Sudden onset or abrupt acceleration of high blood pressure
- Very high diastolic pressure (higher than 110 mm Hg)
- Low blood potassium level

- Evidence of kidney abnormalities
- A bruit (pronounced BREW-ee) that your doctor can hear, which is the sound of blood flowing through a narrowed vessel

Notify your doctor of any prescription or over-the-counter medications, vitamins or herbal remedies that you take. Some medications raise your blood pressure. They include cold, allergy and sinus medications, nasal sprays and diet pills. And some medications may interact dangerously with medications your doctor may prescribe for high blood pressure. These include certain heart medications, psychiatric medications, and water pills (diuretics).

Guidelines your doctor follows for treating high blood pressure are complex. They're based upon your blood pressure readings, evidence that high blood pressure has affected other organs in your body, your age, and the presence or absence of other risk factors for coronary artery disease, such as diabetes, hypercholesterolemia and tobacco use.

Although most people with hypertension eventually require medication, it's important to remember that lifestyle modifications—including weight loss, increased exercise, improved diet, reduced alcohol consumption, and the cessation of smoking—are part of the strategy for everyone with high blood pressure. Lifestyle changes can prevent the development of hypertension in some individuals whose blood pressure is in the high-normal range.

## High blood cholesterol

Your risk for developing coronary artery disease is higher than average if blood tests show that you have an elevated cholesterol level. Thus, it's reasonable to do what is necessary to keep your cholesterol in an acceptable range. In fact, the American Heart Association and the National Heart, Lung, and Blood Institute have concluded jointly that the "benefits of modifying serum cholesterol levels extend to men and women, young and old, those with high risk… and those with borderline high risk levels."

Cholesterol has recently become a household word. A great deal of advertising and many food labels focus on cholesterol. Cholesterol screening has become a nearly routine part of medical examinations and wellness programs at work sites and health fairs. However, the bits and pieces of information you may have heard from various sources may have failed to answer some basic questions such as:

- What is cholesterol?
- Why is it important?
- What constitutes an elevated cholesterol level?
- How much risk does an elevated cholesterol level pose, and when should you be concerned?
- What can you do to control your cholesterol level?

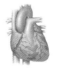

**HEALTHY HEART ♥ TIP**

*People in Asia have significantly lower levels of coronary heart disease than Americans, partly because their diets contain more soy.*

*Natural soy compounds, called isoflavones, act like human hormones that regulate cholesterol levels. To achieve optimal cholesterol-lowering benefits, you must consume a daily minimum of 25 grams of soy protein, along with a low-fat, low-cholesterol diet. Food options include soy milk, tempeh, tofu or textured soy protein, a main ingredient in many meat substitutes. Eating soy isoflavones may reduce total cholesterol levels by up to 10 percent.*

## Glossary of terms related to cholesterol

- **Apoproteins:** proteins that combine with lipids to make them dissolve in your blood.

- **Cholesterol:** a type of lipid your body uses to build cells and certain hormones. It is found only in foods derived from animal sources.

- **Fatty acids:** also called fats, they occur in several forms in the foods you eat. Different fatty acids have different effects on your lipid profile.

- **HDL cholesterol** *(high-density lipoprotein cholesterol):* a combination of about 50 percent apoproteins and 20 percent cholesterol. HDL cholesterol tends to help remove excess cholesterol from your blood.

- **LDL cholesterol** *(low-density lipoprotein cholesterol):* a combination of about 25 percent apoproteins and 45 percent cholesterol. Although LDL cholesterol provides cholesterol for necessary body functions, in excessive amounts it promotes cholesterol accumulation in artery walls.

- **Lipids:** a general term referring to fats (cholesterol and triglycerides) circulating in your bloodstream.

- **Lipid profile:** the amounts of various lipids in your bloodstream.

- **Lipoproteins:** lipids combined with apoproteins.

- **Triglycerides:** a type of lipid used by your body as a source of energy. Most triglycerides are transported through your bloodstream as a *very-low-density lipoprotein* (VLDL). Some cholesterol is also present in VLDL.

# What is cholesterol?

Cholesterol is one of several types of fats (lipids) that play important roles in your body. Because of its reputation as a risk factor for coronary artery disease, people tend to think of cholesterol only in negative terms. Nevertheless, it's an important component of cell membranes and therefore vital to the structure and function of all cells in your body. Cholesterol is also a building block in the formation of certain types of hormones.

However, cholesterol is also the predominant substance in atherosclerotic plaques, which may develop in your arteries and impede the flow of blood (see page A10). When the cholesterol level in your bloodstream becomes excessively high, the likelihood of your developing atherosclerotic plaques increases.

## What are lipoproteins, HDL cholesterol, LDL cholesterol and VLDL?

If the terms are unfamiliar to you, a discussion of cholesterol quickly starts to look like alphabet soup. Cholesterol is not the only lipid that circulates in your bloodstream. Triglycerides are another form of fat that circulates in your blood. Think of triglycerides as transportable fuel that's ultimately used for your body's energy production.

Since they are fats (lipids), neither cholesterol nor triglycerides dissolve in water. Therefore, in order to circulate through your blood—which is mainly water—cholesterol and triglycerides must be carried by protein packages called apoproteins. A lipoprotein is a combination of an apoprotein and a lipid. Each type of lipoprotein is defined by the type and proportion of lipid and apoprotein in its structure.

The main types of lipoproteins are low-density lipoprotein cholesterol (LDL) and high-density lipoprotein cholesterol (HDL). You often hear them referred to as LDL cholesterol and HDL cholesterol.

HDL cholesterol contains almost 50 percent protein and 20 percent cholesterol. LDL cholesterol contains about 25 percent protein and 45 percent cholesterol. Another type of lipoprotein, very-low-density lipoprotein (VLDL), contains mostly triglycerides and small amounts of protein and cholesterol.

## Why are LDL cholesterol and HDL cholesterol important?

The function of LDL cholesterol is to transport cholesterol to sites throughout your body. Then it's either deposited or used to repair cell membranes. Thus, LDL cholesterol promotes the accumulation of cholesterol in the walls of your arteries. Think of it as hard water promoting a build-up of lime inside the plumbing of your house. However, cholesterol deposits are a spotty, rather than even, coating on the walls of your arteries.

The task of HDL cholesterol is to carry cholesterol to your liver, where it's broken down and removed from your body. In a sense, HDL cholesterol is like a clean-up crew that sops up excess cholesterol in your system and disposes of it before it can do any damage by accumulating where you don't need it.

LDL cholesterol is mainly to blame for the risk associated with cholesterol. The opposite is true for HDL cholesterol. Since it works to eliminate excess cholesterol, the more HDL cholesterol you have, the less cholesterol will be deposited in atherosclerotic plaques. Therefore, a relatively low ratio of LDL cholesterol to HDL cholesterol is desirable for lowering your risk of developing coronary artery disease.

The role of very-low-density lipoprotein (VLDL) in determining your risk of developing coronary artery disease is not well known. A high level of VLDL seems to be an independent risk factor in women, but not in men. A high level of triglycerides corresponds to a high level of VLDL.

## Measuring cholesterol levels

Your lipids are measured by analyzing a specimen of your blood. Eating before the blood test doesn't affect your level of blood cholesterol, but it does affect your blood triglyceride level. Therefore, since one specimen will be used to measure both, you should fast before the test.

Do not eat for a minimum of 12 hours before your blood is drawn, and do not drink alcohol for a full 24 hours before the test. If you follow these guidelines, your physician will have an accurate measure of your cholesterol, triglycerides and other blood lipids. Fasting before a blood test for lipids doesn't guarantee that your results will be precisely the same two days in a row, even if you don't make any changes in your diet, exercise or medication. It's common for lipid levels to vary by about 10 percent from day to day.

Therefore, the importance of a blood lipid test is not to detect small changes or to make a large issue of a particular value that is several points too high. Rather, this test helps you know generally what your risk level is. It also helps you determine whether your body's response to changes in diet, exercise or medication is satisfactory.

## What will the results tell me?

In a way, it's inaccurate to think of your cholesterol or triglyceride level as being either strictly normal or abnormal. Although expert investigators and physicians have identified ranges of cholesterol levels that are considered too high, there's no magic number that separates risky levels from safe levels. Rather, these experts have identified levels of lipids in the blood above which the risk for developing coronary complications is high enough to warrant changes.

If your cholesterol or triglyceride levels are in the higher-risk zones, you're said to be hypercholesterolemic, hypertriglyceridemic, or simply hyperlipidemic (*hyper* means high, *lipid* means fat, and *emic* means in the blood). But, as with all risk factors, being in the high range does not guarantee that you'll develop coronary artery disease, nor does being in the low range guarantee that you'll avert it.

Lipid levels are described as the number of milligrams that are present in one tenth of a liter of blood (about 1/2 cup). The unit of measurement is expressed as milligrams (mg) per deciliter (dL), or mg/dL. Of course, this value is calculated from the measurements of lipids in a much smaller sample of your blood.

Research clearly shows that the amount of cholesterol in your bloodstream and the proportions of the different types of lipoproteins have a definite impact on your future risk for developing coronary blockages. This evidence comes from extensive studies of populations whose average cholesterol levels were compared with the prevalence of coronary artery disease and in studies that investigated whether lowering cholesterol could influence the tendency for developing coronary artery disease.

In some cases, the link between lipid levels and cardiovascular risk is striking. Because of genes inherited from their parents, some people lack certain parts of their cells that are vital to processing cholesterol and getting rid of LDL cholesterol. When they have this condition, called hypercholesterolemia, people have extremely high levels of cholesterol, especially LDL cholesterol. This makes them susceptible to developing angina pectoris or heart attacks very early in life—even in their 20s.

In other groups of people whose cholesterol levels are less markedly elevated, the link still exists, although not as strikingly. A large, careful study of heart disease and risk factors in the general population has been going on for more than 40 years in Framingham, Massachusetts. Investigators measured cholesterol in a large group of townspeople (2,282 men and 2,845 women) and then waited to determine how many of them would have coronary problems over the next 14 years.

They found a very significant trend: The higher a person's cholesterol at the outset, the greater the chance that he or she would show signs of coronary disease during the study. In fact, among people with a total cholesterol of 300 mg/dL, coronary problems developed more than twice as often as among people with a total cholesterol level of 150 mg/dL. People with cholesterol levels between these extremes had risks of coronary disease that were also in between.

Other studies demonstrate that the risk of dying from coronary artery disease increases as the cholesterol level increases. One study, called the Multiple Risk Factor Intervention Trial (its acronym, MRFIT, is pronounced Mr. Fit) studied what happened to more than 360,000 men whose cholesterol levels were measured. Six years after the test began, the results were clear: The likelihood of dying from coronary disease was nearly four times greater in people with total cholesterol levels above 300 mg/dL, compared with those whose levels were below 180 mg/dL. Numerous other studies support these conclusions.

### Lipid level goals

| Target lipid levels | The general population | People with coronary artery disease |
|---|---|---|
| Total cholesterol | Less than 200 mg/dL | Less than 200 mg/dL |
| Total triglycerides | Less than 200 mg/dL | Less than 200 mg/dL* |
| HDL cholesterol | More than 35 mg/dL | More than 35 mg/dL* |
| LDL cholesterol | Less than 130 mg/dL | Less than 100 mg/dL |

*In general, the higher your HDL and the lower your triglycerides (many physicians would like to see triglycerides under 100) the better, especially if you have coronary artery disease.*

## Measuring only total cholesterol can be misleading

Some physicians recommend having your HDL cholesterol and triglyceride levels measured initially, in addition to total cholesterol. Why? Some people have low levels of HDL cholesterol and high levels of triglycerides, but normal or even high LDL cholesterol. In these cases, a total cholesterol measurement might appear normal. You and your doctor would be unaware of the risk posed by the abnormalities that were not measured.

## Calculating your own LDL cholesterol level

LDL cholesterol levels are an important piece of information in determining your risk of cardiovascular disease. Although LDL cholesterol can be measured directly, it is more commonly calculated based on measurements of other lipids. This calculation is usually sufficiently accurate and doesn't incur the cost of an additional blood test.

Here's how your LDL cholesterol level is calculated:

• Subtract your HDL cholesterol level from your total cholesterol level.

• Then subtract one-fifth of your triglyceride level. The result is your LDL cholesterol level.

Example: If your total cholesterol level is 226, your HDL cholesterol level is 56 and your triglyceride level is 150, your LDL cholesterol level is: 226 – 56 = 170,  170 – 150/5 = 140.

*Note: If your triglyceride level exceeds 400 mg/dL, the formula for calculating LDL cholesterol may not apply.*

## Does reducing your cholesterol reduce your risk?

It's one thing to observe that people with relatively low cholesterol levels have less chance of getting coronary artery disease. But that doesn't necessarily establish that if you lower your cholesterol level you'll also lower your risk. What if your high cholesterol level was simply a signal that you are at risk of coronary disease—but not the cause? In that case, there would be very little point in doing anything to lower your cholesterol level.

In fact, much effort and expense have been expended to address that very point. The answer is now convincing: Reducing your cholesterol level is important. Several large studies done in different parts of the world in the past 5 years show that lowering serum cholesterol by using a class of drugs known as statins substantially reduces the rate of cardiac events. In some studies, overall death rates and rates of stroke also declined.

In several studies people reduced the occurrence of coronary disease by one third to one half by reducing their cholesterol levels with diet or medications. In general, if your cholesterol level is high or moderately high and you lower it by 10 percent, you will lower your risk of coronary artery disease by about 20 percent. Most of these studies also indicate that your risk of coronary disease is lower if you have higher levels of HDL cholesterol. Additional research trials also show that a reduction of coronary disease through lowered cholesterol levels translates into an actual decline in deaths due to heart disease— a very important bottom line!

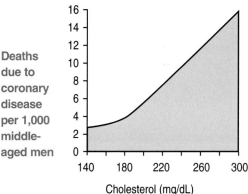

*Results from the Multiple Risk Factor Intervention Trial show the relationship between total cholesterol level and the chance of dying from coronary heart disease within 6 years. The study showed that men aged 35 to 57 years with a total cholesterol of 300 mg/dL had more than four times the chance of dying as men with a cholesterol level of less than 180 mg/dL.*

What if you already have coronary problems detected by tests, or if you have chest pain (angina pectoris) caused by a rate of blood flow in your coronary arteries that is not sufficient to meet your heart's oxygen requirements, or if you have had a heart attack? Will lowering your cholesterol make a difference? Even if you're in this group, studies show that lowering cholesterol reduces:

- The further development of coronary blockages and heart attacks
- The need to use catheters to reopen obstructed coronary arteries (percutaneous transluminal coronary angioplasty, PTCA)
- The necessity of surgery to reroute your blood supply by bypassing blocked coronary arteries (coronary artery bypass graft, CABG)
- Death rates

## Cholesterol facts

- Approximately 55 percent of American adults have total cholesterol levels higher than 200 mg/dL.
- If your total cholesterol is 300 mg/dL, your risk for developing coronary artery disease is double what it would be if your total cholesterol were 150 mg/dL.
- If your total cholesterol is 300 mg/dL, your risk of dying of coronary artery disease is four times what it would be if your total cholesterol were 190 mg/dL.
- You can usually reduce your average LDL cholesterol by 15 percent or more with diet. However, dietary measures are less likely to be effective if your triglyceride level is normal.
- Reducing your cholesterol by 10 percent reduces your future coronary risk by 20 percent.
- Increasing your HDL 1 mg/dL reduces your risk of coronary artery disease by 2 to 3 percent.
- Aggressively modifying your lifestyle (including reducing your cholesterol) has a major effect on cardiac event rates, greatly out of proportion to the small reversal of coronary artery blockage shown on your angiograms.

Even more interestingly, lowering your cholesterol may cause regression in some blockages that are already present. These changes were observed after as little as 2 years.

If you have coronary artery disease, your physician may not be satisfied if your cholesterol levels are at a point considered adequate for people without heart disease. This is due to the fact that there may be a possibility for regression of disease in people with coronary artery disease. Therefore, if you already have coronary artery disease, there's good cause for much more aggressive treatment. The goal in this case is to reduce your LDL cholesterol level to 100 mg/dL or lower.

To summarize, you will likely experience fewer coronary artery problems and live longer, on average, if you have low LDL cholesterol (and low VLDL) or high HDL cholesterol levels, even if that means using diet, exercise or medications to achieve those levels. Although everyone can benefit from lower cholesterol, you derive the greatest benefit from lowering your cholesterol if you have developed coronary artery disease or if your cholesterol levels are equal to or more than 270 mg/dL.

## What about your child's cholesterol level?

Most cholesterol research has focused on middle-aged adults. After all, this is the phase of life when the risk of coronary artery disease is higher. But lipids should also be a concern for children and older adults as well.

Although atherosclerosis typically becomes severe enough to cause problems only later in life, it begins to develop early in life. Evidence suggests that children with high cholesterol levels develop atherosclerosis earlier and have a greater chance of developing coronary artery disease as adults.

However, the evidence is not clear enough to justify recommending cholesterol testing for all children. Certainly, however, children older than age 2 who come from high-risk families should have their blood cholesterol measured. Your family is defined as one with a high risk if one parent's cholesterol level is 240 mg/dL or higher or if a parent or grandparent had evidence of coronary artery disease before age 55.

If your child's cholesterol level is elevated, dietary changes are the first course of action. Actually, all children older than age 2, regardless of their cholesterol level, should follow the same eating strategies recommended for adults. These strategies focus on reducing fat and cholesterol in your diet, maintaining a healthful weight and encouraging physical activity.

If, by 10 years of age, your child's cholesterol level remains elevated above 190 mg/dL (or above 170 mg/dL in high-risk families)—despite dietary attempts—it may be necessary to use a medication to lower your child's lipid level. Since not every medication is suitable for children, your pediatrician should prescribe an appropriate one.

| Cholesterol levels in children and adolescents from high-risk families* | | |
|---|---|---|
| **Category** | **Total cholesterol (mg/dL)** | **LDL cholesterol (mg/dL)** |
| Acceptable | Lower than 170 | Lower than 110 |
| Borderline | 170-199 | 110-129 |
| High | Higher than or equal to 200 | Higher than or equal to 130 |

*One parent has a cholesterol level of 240 mg/dL or greater, or a parent or grandparent had coronary artery disease before age 55.

## When should adults—both younger and older— have cholesterol checked?

The National Cholesterol Education Program recommends that all adults older than 20 years of age begin by having a blood test that measures total cholesterol. If your total cholesterol is more than 200 mg/dL, you should have your LDL cholesterol, HDL cholesterol and triglyceride values checked. Future regular medical checkups should then always include a cholesterol check.

If your cholesterol is high and your doctor recommends dietary changes or other treatments, you will probably have your cholesterol rechecked in about 3 months to determine the effect of treatment. Your doctor will then discuss with you what additional treatment may be advisable.

The evidence that lowering cholesterol helps to slow down the development of coronary artery disease in many people provides a strong rationale for advocating cholesterol control beyond middle age. People in their 60s, 70s, 80s and 90s who have coronary artery disease or other additional risk factors have the highest risk of problems if the disease progresses.

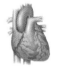

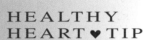

HEALTHY
HEART ♥ TIP

*Obesity is a known risk factor for heart disease. But how fat is too fat?*

*The "waist circumference method" considers only the measurement around a person's natural waist (just above the navel). A high-risk waist circumference is defined as 35 inches or more for women and 40 inches or more for men.*

## Excess Weight

You may think of being overweight as a cosmetic problem. Although appearance may be important, it's not the main drawback of obesity. Your weight is closely linked to your cardiovascular health. However, it's different from other risk factors.

Your weight interacts with several other risk factors that have a harmful effect on your health. It's a key factor in the development of high blood pressure, for example. In fact, if you're overweight, your risk for developing high blood pressure is two to six times what it would be if you maintained a healthful weight. Being overweight also promotes high cholesterol and increases your risk of diabetes. And, of course, your heart must work harder any time you want to move the extra weight you're carrying on your body.

The difference between being overweight and obese is a matter of degree. Body mass index (BMI) is a formula that considers your weight and your height in determining whether you have a healthful or unhealthful percentage of total body fat (see page 161). Federal guidelines define overweight as a BMI of 25 to 29. Obesity refers to a BMI of 30 or more. According to federal guidelines, more than 50 percent of American adults are overweight or obese—almost 30 percent are overweight and another 25 percent are obese. More than 25 percent of American children are overweight or obese. In 40 years the percentage of Americans who are obese has nearly doubled, and the percentage who are overweight has increased slightly.

While being overweight doesn't guarantee that you'll develop coronary artery disease, it significantly increases your chances. For example, a study involving more than 82,000 women found that those who gained 11 to 22 pounds (5 to 10 kilograms) during adulthood had a 70 percent increase in risk of high blood pressure compared with women who didn't gain weight after age 18. The risk was even higher for women who gained more than 22 pounds. And studies of men also have shown that being overweight increases the risk of high blood pressure.

As you put on weight, you gain mostly fatty tissue. Just like other parts of your body, this tissue relies on oxygen and nutrients in your blood to survive. As the demand for oxygen and nutrients increases, the amount of blood circulating through your body also increases. More blood traveling through your arteries means added pressure on your artery walls. Weight gain also typically increases the level of insulin in your blood—an increase associated with retention of sodium and water, which increases blood volume. Excess weight is often associated with an increase in heart rate and a reduction in the capacity of your blood vessels to transport blood.

Fortunately, just as many risk factors increase when you put on weight, they usually go down when you lose weight. Even shedding a few pounds can bring noticeable benefits. For example, the study already mentioned showed that women who lost 11 to 22 pounds lowered their risk of developing high blood pressure by more than 25 percent. Similarly, weight loss can lower your cholesterol and your risk of developing diabetes. So it's no surprise to learn that your risk of dying early (compared with the average age at death of all people in the country) progressively increases the more overweight you are.

## What's your healthful weight?

No one way is perfect for determining whether you're overweight. And you must also be realistic. If you've never in your adult life weighed what a weight table shows, the table may not be a useful, realistic goal for you. Most important, it's good to seek a realistic weight goal that reduces your risk for health problems. Three evaluations can help you determine whether your weight is healthful or whether you could benefit from losing a few pounds.

| The danger of excess weight | | | |
|---|---|---|---|
| If you are this much overweight | 5%-15% | 55%-60% | 100% |
| Your risk of early death is increased by | 1.1 times | 2.2 times | 12 times |

## Body mass index

Body mass index (BMI) is a better way to determine your health risks than simply using your bathroom scale or standard height and weight tables. To determine your body mass index, locate your height on the chart below and follow it across until you reach the weight nearest to yours. Look at the top of the table for the BMI rating. A BMI of 19 to 24 is considered healthful. A BMI of 25 to 29 signifies overweight, and a BMI of 30 or more indicates obesity. Extreme obesity is indicated by a BMI of more than 40. Your risk for developing a disease related to your weight increases if your BMI is 25 or greater.

### What's your BMI?

| | Healthy | | Overweight | | | | | Obesity | | | | |
|---|---|---|---|---|---|---|---|---|---|---|---|---|
| **BMI** | 19 | 24 | 25 | 26 | 27 | 28 | 29 | 30 | 35 | 40 | 45 | 50 |
| **Height** | | | | | | **Weight in pounds** | | | | | | |
| 4'10" | 91 | 115 | 119 | 124 | 129 | 134 | 138 | 143 | 167 | 191 | 215 | 239 |
| 4'11" | 94 | 119 | 124 | 128 | 133 | 138 | 143 | 148 | 173 | 198 | 222 | 247 |
| 5'0" | 97 | 123 | 128 | 133 | 138 | 143 | 148 | 153 | 179 | 204 | 230 | 255 |
| 5'1" | 100 | 127 | 132 | 137 | 143 | 148 | 153 | 158 | 185 | 211 | 238 | 264 |
| 5'2" | 104 | 131 | 136 | 142 | 147 | 153 | 158 | 164 | 191 | 218 | 246 | 273 |
| 5'3" | 107 | 135 | 141 | 146 | 152 | 158 | 163 | 169 | 197 | 225 | 254 | 282 |
| 5'4" | 110 | 140 | 145 | 151 | 157 | 163 | 169 | 174 | 204 | 232 | 262 | 291 |
| 5'5" | 114 | 144 | 150 | 156 | 162 | 168 | 174 | 180 | 210 | 240 | 270 | 300 |
| 5'6" | 118 | 148 | 155 | 161 | 167 | 173 | 179 | 186 | 216 | 247 | 278 | 309 |
| 5'7" | 121 | 153 | 159 | 166 | 172 | 178 | 185 | 191 | 223 | 255 | 287 | 319 |
| 5'8" | 125 | 158 | 164 | 171 | 177 | 184 | 190 | 197 | 230 | 262 | 295 | 328 |
| 5'9" | 128 | 162 | 169 | 176 | 182 | 189 | 196 | 203 | 236 | 270 | 304 | 338 |
| 5'10" | 132 | 167 | 174 | 181 | 188 | 195 | 202 | 209 | 243 | 278 | 313 | 348 |
| 5'11" | 136 | 172 | 179 | 186 | 193 | 200 | 208 | 215 | 250 | 286 | 322 | 358 |
| 6'0" | 140 | 177 | 184 | 191 | 199 | 206 | 213 | 221 | 258 | 294 | 331 | 368 |
| 6'1" | 144 | 182 | 189 | 197 | 204 | 212 | 219 | 227 | 265 | 302 | 340 | 378 |
| 6'2" | 148 | 186 | 194 | 202 | 210 | 218 | 225 | 233 | 272 | 311 | 350 | 389 |
| 6'3" | 152 | 192 | 200 | 208 | 216 | 224 | 232 | 240 | 279 | 319 | 359 | 399 |
| 6'4" | 156 | 197 | 205 | 213 | 221 | 230 | 238 | 246 | 287 | 328 | 369 | 410 |

*Modified from Clinical Guidelines on the Identification, Evaluation, and Treatment of Overweight and Obesity in Adults, National Institutes of Health (NIH), 1998.*

## Classification of overweight and obesity

| Class | BMI | Disease risk* relative to normal weight and waist circumference | |
|---|---|---|---|
| | | Men less than 40 inches<br>Women less than 35 inches | more than 40 inches<br>more than 35 inches |
| Underweight | Less than 18.5 | _____ | _____ |
| Normal | 18.5-24.9 | _____ | _____ |
| Overweight | 25-29.9 | Increased | High |
| Obesity | 30 or higher | | |
| Class I | 30-34.9 | High | Very high |
| Class II | 35-39.9 | Very high | Very high |
| Class III | 40 or higher | Extremely high | Extremely high |

*Disease risk for type 2 diabetes, hypertension and coronary artery disease.*

If you're overweight (BMI between 25 and 29.9) and have any other risk factors for heart disease, it's a good idea to lose weight. If your BMI is 30 or higher, losing weight should improve your health over the long term, regardless of your other risk factors.

## Waist circumference

This measurement indicates where most of your fat is located. If you carry most of your fat around your waist, you may be referred to as apple-shaped. If you carry most of your weight below your waist, around your hips and thighs, you may be considered pear-shaped.

Generally, when it comes to your health, it's better to have the shape of a pear than the shape of an apple. As fat accumulates around your waist, it increases your risk for coronary artery disease, as well as for high blood pressure, diabetes, stroke and certain types of cancer. This occurs because fat in your abdomen is more likely to break down and accumulate in your arteries.

To determine whether you're carrying too much weight around your abdomen, measure your waist circumference. Find the highest point on each hipbone and measure across your abdomen just above those highest points. A measurement of more than 40 inches (102 centimeters) in men and 35 inches (88 centimeters) in women signifies increased health risks, especially if you have a BMI of 25 or more.

### What's your history?

Numbers don't give you the whole picture. An evaluation of your medical history, along with that of your family, is equally important in determining whether your weight is healthful. Consider these questions:

- Do you have a family history of coronary artery disease or stroke?

- Do you have a health condition, such as high blood pressure, diabetes or high cholesterol, that would improve if you lost weight?

- Do you have a family history of illness related to weight, such as type 2 diabetes or high blood pressure?

- Have you gained considerable weight since high school? Weight gain in adulthood is associated with increased health risks.

- Do you smoke cigarettes, have more than two alcoholic drinks per day, or live with significant stress? In combination with these behaviors, excess weight can have greater health implications.

## So where do you stand?

If your BMI shows that you're not overweight, if you're not carrying too much weight around your abdomen, and if you answered no to all of the personal or family history questions, your weight is probably at a healthful level. There's probably no health advantage to changing it.

If your BMI is between 25 and 29, your waist circumference equals or exceeds healthful guidelines, or you answered yes to at least one personal and family health question, you may benefit from losing a few pounds. Discuss your weight with your doctor during your next check-up.

If your BMI is 30 or more, losing some weight will improve your health and reduce your risk for coronary artery disease.

## Diabetes

If you have diabetes, your risk of developing some types of heart disease is at least double that of the general population. Unfortunately, your symptoms of heart disease may be less apparent than they are in someone without diabetes. In fact, lacking the typical warning signs, you may be unaware that you have coronary artery disease. If you have diabetes, therefore, aggressive efforts to both prevent and diagnose coronary artery disease are very important.

Diabetes increases your risk of developing coronary artery disease in any form—angina, heart attack or sudden death. It also increases your risk of diseases of the blood vessels (vascular disease) in other parts of your body, which can lead to claudication or stroke. If you have diabetes, you're also more likely not to have the pain that usually occurs when insufficient blood and oxygen reach your heart (myocardial ischemia)—or even a heart attack. As a result, your heart may sustain significant damage before you receive any treatment.

## What is diabetes?

Diabetes is a disease in which too much sugar (glucose) accumulates in your bloodstream, rather than being carried to cells throughout your body. By itself, diabetes actually refers to only one primary sign of the disease—frequent urination. It is derived from the Greek word for siphon.

You do not get diabetes by eating too much sugar. Your body normally converts some of the food you eat into a type of sugar (glucose) that provides an energy source for your cells. Your bloodstream distributes glucose throughout your body. A hormone called insulin allows glucose to enter your cells.

If you have diabetes, either your pancreas stops making insulin or your body doesn't respond properly to the insulin it produces. In type 1 diabetes, the main problem is decreased insulin production. In type 2 diabetes, the main problem is a reduced response by your body to insulin. Both types of diabetes are associated with a higher risk of cardiovascular disease.

Type 1 diabetes often occurs in younger people (it used to be called juvenile-onset diabetes). It affects about 1.5 million Americans. It's caused when your

## What is a normal blood glucose level?

Normal blood glucose levels after an overnight fast in a person over age 1 year are 70 to 100 mg/dL (milligrams per deciliter). A deciliter is one tenth of a liter, or about one-half cup.

Levels higher than 127 mg/dL measured on two separate occasions are considered indicative of diabetes.

## Signs and symptoms of diabetes

The American Diabetes Association estimates that nearly 5 million Americans don't know that they have diabetes. Mild diabetes may produce no signs for years. People who are older than 40, or are overweight or obese, or have a family history of diabetes have the greatest chance of developing type 2 diabetes.

Signs and symptoms of type 1 diabetes usually appear rather suddenly:

- Increased thirst
- Increased volume and frequency of urination
- Weight loss despite increased appetite
- Fatigue

Signs and symptoms of type 2 diabetes usually develop more gradually and may be subtle. They include any of the above signs and symptoms (except weight loss), in addition to the following:

- Frequent or slow-to-heal infections, particularly vaginitis, skin or gum infections, or bladder infections
- Blurred vision
- Tingling or numbness in the hands or feet

pancreas produces no—or insufficient—insulin. If you have this type of diabetes, you must regulate your high blood glucose levels (hyperglycemia: *hyper* means high, *glyc* means sweet, *emia* means in the blood) with insulin injections that compensate for the insulin your body isn't producing.

More than 90 percent of the people with diabetes have type 2 diabetes—at least 9 million people. Almost 5 million people who have type 2 diabetes don't even realize it.

Most people who have type 2 diabetes are overweight. Evidently, obesity is a trigger that causes diabetes to develop in people who are genetically vulnerable. Diabetes causes both a deficiency of insulin and an inability of your body's cells to respond appropriately to insulin that is present. A high-fat diet is probably also a risk factor for diabetes.

Evidence is mounting that exercise lowers your risk of developing type 2 diabetes, even if you are overweight or have a family history of diabetes. The best treatment for type 2 diabetes is weight loss. If you are unable to lose weight, you may need to take oral medications or insulin injections.

Diabetes brings several health complications, including an increased risk for vascular disease and coronary artery disease. If everything else is equal, your risk of heart disease increases fivefold if you are a woman with diabetes—twofold, if you're a man.

## Sedentary lifestyle

Lack of exercise or a sedentary lifestyle is a risk factor for coronary artery disease, just like smoking, a poor lipid profile, high blood pressure, a family history of coronary artery disease, or diabetes. Most of the population of the United States is sedentary.

More than 60 percent of American adults do not get the recommended amount of physical activity. In fact, about a quarter of adults are totally inactive. Physical inactivity is most common among women, black and Hispanic adults, older individuals, and less affluent people. You're more likely to get regular physical activity if you have the support of your family and friends.

You are sedentary if you:

- Spend most of your day sitting
- Seldom walk more than a block
- Have leisure activities that don't require you to move from place to place
- Have an inactive job
- Don't take 20 to 30 minutes to exercise most days each week

Your body was designed to move. Sitting around is not good for it. Your heart and lungs perform their functions much more efficiently if you are physically active on a regular basis. The more you use your muscles, the more work they can perform before they become fatigued. Regular exercise is necessary if you hope to achieve optimal levels of health, performance and appearance.

If you're sedentary, your risk of having a fatal heart attack is nearly twice that of active people your age whose other risk factors are equal. Without physical activity you experience a gradual decline in your ability to perform activities that require physical effort. You lose strength, endurance and flexibility. Daily activities gradually become more difficult.

## Benefits of physical activity

If all sedentary people became moderately active, the number of persons with coronary disease would decline steeply. Remaining active helps you maintain or improve your fitness level. The best way to assure that you include adequate physical activity in your daily life is to have a personal exercise program.

Maintaining a healthful activity level benefits your heart in several ways. It gives your heart a greater capacity to pump blood and reduces your risk of dying prematurely from heart disease. It promotes weight loss. New evidence suggests that physical activity has an independent protective effect against the development of type 2 diabetes by lowering your blood sugar. Exercise may lower your total cholesterol and triglyceride levels and increase protective HDL cholesterol. It also reduces the risk of developing high blood pressure or may lower your blood pressure if you have hypertension.

All of these effects can reduce your risk of developing coronary artery disease. Furthermore, exercise also may have a direct tendency to lower your risk of developing coronary disease, apart from its effect on your other risk factors.

## Signs of deconditioning

You are not in optimal physical condition if you:

- Feel tired most of the time
- Are unable to keep up with other people your age
- Avoid physical activity because you know you will quickly become fatigued
- Experience shortness of breath or fatigue when you walk a short distance or climb a few stairs

These symptoms can also occur because of heart problems or other diseases. If there is no medical explanation for the symptoms, increasing your activity level will help you improve your physical condition.

## What exercise can do for you

The cardiovascular benefits available to you from an exercise program include the following:

- Increased ability of your heart to pump blood
- Decreased heart rate at rest and during moderate exercise
- Possibly decreased blood pressure if you have hypertension
- Possibly increased HDL cholesterol level
- Possibly reduced LDL cholesterol and total cholesterol levels
- Possibly decreased triglyceride level
- Help with weight control
- Help with stress reduction
- Help to reduce elevated levels of blood sugar (glucose), if you have type 2 diabetes

In addition, an exercise program offers other benefits:

- Increased exercise capacity, resulting in an improved ability to perform physical and mental work
- Reduced fatigue, tension, and anxiety
- Possibly improved joint function
- Potential reduction of bone mineral loss, therefore lessening the risk of osteoporosis
- Improved appearance, self-confidence and a sense of well-being
- Help to maintain bowel regularity

# Stress and your personality

The question of whether psychological stress and personality cause coronary artery disease, heart attacks, and sudden cardiac death is highly controversial. A great deal of research seems to suggest that your personality, the stressful events in your life and your body's physiological reaction to stress can increase your risk of heart disease. However, this theory is not proved. Stress is very difficult to study, because it's hard to measure psychological and physical responses to stress or to assess the social factors that may buffer the detrimental effects of stress.

Your stress may originate in many different situations, and your response to a stressor may be quite different from that of someone else. That's why researchers have difficulty identifying whether or how stress contributes to the development of heart disease.

People with heart disease commonly report that emotional peaks cause chest pain. It's also common for heart attacks to occur during emotionally difficult periods. The added stress of being emotionally upset may also disrupt the balance between your body's supply of and your heart's demand for, oxygen. The result is chest pain.

Although sometimes it seems possible that acute stress is a major factor in precipitating a heart attack, it's not clear whether ongoing stress causes the underlying coronary artery disease (atherosclerosis) that's usually associated with heart attacks. Trying to answer that question, researchers have studied the subject of stress and heart disease in terms of people's personalities, social support systems, and the body's physiological responses to stress.

Two researchers, Dr. Meyer Friedman and Dr. Ray Rosenman, developed the concept of type A personality or behavior pattern in 1964. This was the basis for a theory of a psychological or personality component to heart disease.

If you're a type A person, you're always in a hurry. You're also competitive, strive intensely for achievement, and need to be productive. In many ways, these are positive characteristics in a society that emphasizes accomplishments.

But if you have a type A personality, you may also be impatient, overcommitted to your work, and easily provoked to hostility. You may tend to have few interests outside of your work.

On the other hand, if you have a type B personality, you may be relaxed, unhurried and more easily satisfied with your pace, while still being interested in achievement. Some researchers suggest, on the basis of one large study, that people with type A personality have twice the risk of type B people for coronary artery disease.

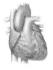

## HEALTHY HEART ♥ TIP

*First we worried about cholesterol. Now it's fat. But there are many kinds. How do they differ?*

*Saturated fatty acids raise blood cholesterol, increasing the risk of coronary artery disease. These fatty acids are usually solid or waxy at room temperature.*

*Polyunsaturated fat is usually liquid at room temperature. It helps to lower total blood cholesterol, but it also lowers the "good" HDL cholesterol. Polyunsaturated fat is susceptible to oxidation, which may enable the cells in your arteries to absorb fats and cholesterol.*

*Monounsaturated fat is liquid at room temperature. This type of fat helps lower blood cholesterol without affecting the "good" HDL cholesterol. It is more resistant to oxidation.*

*Trans fat is formed when vegetable oils are hardened (hydrogenated) into margarine or shortening. It raises blood cholesterol levels similar to saturated fatty acids.*

Research also indicates that your social situation—and how you respond to it—can affect your risk of disease. Stable social relationships seem to be associated with good health. Your potential risk may increase with a lack of social contacts or with an overload of stressful events in your life, such as divorce, death of a family member or close friend, loss or change of a job, or a move to a new home.

Dr. Robert Eliot proposed the concept that certain people are "hot reactors," which means that their bodies respond adversely to stress. If you're a hot reactor, you exhibit extreme increases in heart rate and blood pressure in response to the everyday stresses of life. According to this theory, these surges may gradually damage your coronary arteries and your heart itself. Thus, it's prudent to learn how to handle stress to limit your risk.

## What happens to your body when you're under stress?

When confronted with a difficult or threatening situation (which a psychologist specializing in stress terms a stressor), both animals and humans respond in a similar fashion: the so-called fight or flight response. Your heart rate and blood pressure increase, blood vessels in your skin constrict, muscle tension and the flow of blood to your muscles increase, your blood sugar level rises, and the tendency of your blood to clot increases. In other words, you prepare yourself for vigorous action. Your sympathetic nervous system and a discharge of the hormone epinephrine (adrenaline) from your adrenal gland trigger many of these changes.

If you have coronary artery disease, the concurrent increases in your heart rate and your blood pressure raise your heart's need for oxygen and may bring on angina. If your blood tends to clot, it may predispose you to a clot in the artery of your heart (coronary thrombus) and produce a heart attack.

If you are a hot reactor, Dr. Eliot proposed that you might have a second type of stress reaction, in addition to this alarm reaction to stress. This reaction is termed vigilance. To clarify: The reaction of a firefighter hearing an alarm exemplifies the alarm type of stress, while an air traffic controller's continuous monitoring to prevent rare but tragic problems represents the vigilant type of stress.

You, like many other people, may experience this vigilant type of stress on an ongoing basis. You may have a potentially recurring disease such as cancer—or be the parent or spouse of someone who does. You may work for a company undergoing a reorganization that may eliminate your job. Financial difficulties can be stressful, as are conflicts with spouses and children. Or you may live or work with someone who has a violent temper. Vigilance involves a chronic, low level of arousal that lacks the surge typical of alarm.

# Chapter

# 9

## Reducing your risks

There probably never will be a prescription that guarantees the health of your heart. But waiting until heart disease strikes and hoping for a guarantee of a cure is unrealistic, too.

You can take steps to prevent or delay heart disease and improve your risk factors. You can also make changes that will improve your outlook if you already have coronary artery disease. The impact of these steps goes beyond potential protection from heart disease. They can improve the way you look and feel today.

You make decisions every day that involve your lifestyle. Individual decisions that you make—whether to smoke, what to eat, how to find time for exercise, how to relax—become habits.

Remember, many of the factors that affect your heart's health interact with one another. For example, if you stop smoking, your capacity for exercise will probably improve. You'll probably find that getting regular exercise relieves stress and tension and promotes a feeling of accomplishment. Improved eating habits and exercise work together to help you lose weight, reduce your cholesterol and triglyceride levels, and improve your HDL cholesterol levels.

You can change habits that don't promote good health. Changing begins with a personal decision you make—and those decisions can become lifelong healthful habits. You'll not only improve your heart's health, but you'll feel much better overall, as well.

Don't expect to change all your habits at once. You may find that tiny changes, over years, become permanent. The size of the change is not as important as constant reinforcement. Good health habits are the work of a lifetime.

Don't switch to alternatives such as a pipe or cigar. Chewing tobacco is the most dangerous of all.

## How to stop smoking

Most smokers—85 percent, in fact—have either tried to quit or would like to quit. However, 75 to 90 percent return to smoking after any single attempt. Fear of failure may make you reluctant to even try to stop smoking. However, it may help to remember that the average person tries to stop smoking four or more times before achieving sustained abstinence. Think of a relapse not as a failure, but as an opportunity to learn how to avoid future relapses. Few people succeed in quitting without making changes or seeking outside help.

## Change your attitude

A serious attempt to stop smoking often depends on recognizing that the negatives of smoking outweigh the positives. You will find it helpful to develop a very negative image of cigarettes.

Although you may look at tobacco products as friends that will help you through any situation and will always be there for you, consider the terrible cost. Think of these products as the insidious killers that they are. Examine the positive aspects of quitting, instead of all that you're giving up. If you have children, setting an example for them can be a strong motivator.

It may help you stop smoking if you consider how smoking interferes with your other lifetime goals. The social stigma of smoking has encouraged many people to quit. Only 28 percent of Americans currently smoke. You needn't look far to see that smoking makes you less welcome in many environments and social circles.

Part of a successful abstinence program is changing your patterns and thoughts associated with smoking. Start by getting rid of tobacco products and ashtrays in your house. Make it inconvenient to respond to your urge to smoke.

Analyze when you smoke and what triggers you to smoke. Then identify behaviors that you can use to replace smoking. For example, if you have the urge to smoke during telephone conversations, find something other than smoking to replace that behavior. Something as simple as doodling on a notepad near the phone may help.

## Getting ready to stop

When you are ready to stop completely, set a firm stop date. Let your family and friends know how they can help and support you with words and by their actions. Stay away from situations in which other people smoke, especially in the early weeks and months after you quit. If you generally smoke while having an alcoholic beverage, you may need to stop drinking for a while. Alcohol lowers your inhibitions and resolve, and frequently promotes a relapse.

Select a method of stopping that has the highest likelihood of success. There's no single best way to stop smoking. The best way is one that you believe will work for you. Ask your health care professional to help you evaluate your options.

Several techniques are effective in helping people stop smoking. Stopping "cold turkey" is one frequently used. However, a decision to stop is usually not as effective if it's made spontaneously. Rather, the most successful stopping strategy is the result of planning. This may include:

- Selecting a specific date or event as the time you'll stop smoking
- Telling others of your intent to stop on a certain date, to increase your commitment
- Having a celebration or ceremony on the day you quit

Most researchers, doctors and ex-smokers agree that the more concrete and explicit your decision and act of quitting, the greater the likelihood of your success.

There are many different ways to quit, including nicotine replacement therapy (gum, patches or inhalers), self-help programs, group programs, and other medications.

## Nicotine replacement products

Part of the difficulty of trying to refrain from a habit of using tobacco products has to do with the addictive nature of nicotine. That's one reason you may need additional assistance in overcoming its effect on you. Nicotine withdrawal begins within hours of your last smoke. Withdrawal symptoms can include craving, irritability, anxiety, headache, depression, restlessness and difficulty concentrating. Although it's usually best to stop smoking abruptly, it may be more manageable to withdraw nicotine more gradually.

You can accomplish this with the use of nicotine gum, nicotine patches, and nicotine inhalers or nasal sprays. These all ease withdrawal symptoms by releasing low levels of nicotine into your bloodstream.

Nicotine replacement products are more effective when used as part of a smoking cessation program. Your doctor can prescribe the nicotine nasal spray or inhaler for you with specific instructions for its use. You can buy nicotine gum and patches over the counter without a prescription.

*Nicotine gum* can help you withdraw from nicotine, if you use it correctly. Chew it only until you feel a tingling sensation in your mouth (about 10 seconds), then park it between your cheek and gums. Periodically chew and park it for about 30 minutes. How much gum you use will vary, according to how much you would have smoked. Use enough pieces to reduce the urge to smoke to a manageable level. Taper off using the gum until you stop using it altogether in 3 to 6 months.

*Nicotine patches* also can help you stop smoking by reducing withdrawal symptoms. The main advantage patches offer over nicotine gum is the ease with which you can use them. The nicotine is slowly released through your skin and enters your bloodstream. As you decrease the patch dose, the nicotine levels decrease. Your ability to abstain from tobacco use will depend on the behavioral adjustments you have made.

*Nicotine nasal spray* delivers nicotine to the lining of your nose in the form of a fine mist. Your body absorbs nicotine through this. From there it enters your bloodstream. To use it properly, tilt your head back slightly and don't inhale as you press the spray. One dose is a spray in each nostril. Most people start with one dose per hour. Side effects include nasal irritation, sneezing, and a runny nose. These generally subside after you've used the spray for a few days. The typical length of therapy is 6 to 12 weeks, tapering down to fewer doses per day at the end of the period.

*A nicotine inhaler* delivers nicotine in a vapor form to the lining of your mouth, where it's absorbed. Note that the nicotine isn't actually inhaled. The nicotine inhaler is a plastic holder into which cartridges with a sponge containing nicotine vapor are placed. You puff on the inhaler to draw the nicotine vapor into your mouth. In order to extract the amount of nicotine you need to relieve withdrawal symptoms, you need to puff frequently. Each cartridge lasts about 1 to 2 hours. Initially you'll probably need at least six per day. The usual length of therapy is 6 to 12 weeks, and you can taper down at the end of the period by using fewer cartridges per day.

The antidepressant bupropion (Zyban, Wellbutrin) also can help reduce symptoms of nicotine withdrawal and help you stop smoking. The FDA has approved these prescription medications for smoking cessation. The dose used for smoking cessation is less than when they are used as antidepressant. Start with one pill per day for 3 days, then one pill twice daily. The length of therapy will vary, but is usually 6 to 12 weeks. Side effects include a dry mouth and insomnia. Don't take these medications if you've had a seizure, serious head trauma, stroke or other illness predisposing you to seizures. Because they are not nicotine products, you can use it in conjunction with nicotine replacement products.

## General strategies for successfully stopping smoking

1. Stay away from opportunities to smoke. Do not go where you are likely to be tempted.
2. Analyze when you smoke and what triggers your smoking, and then identify activities that can replace smoking.
3. Develop a negative image of smoking. It's smelly, dirty, and disgusting. It turns your fingers and teeth yellow, makes your breath and clothes smell, costs you money and offends your friends.
4. Remind yourself of all the benefits you have gained from not smoking.
5. View relapses as learning experiences.
6. Read and use helpful materials and programs from the American Cancer Society, the American Lung Association and the American Heart Association.

## Basic responses to fears you may have about quitting

*I have failed before, and I will probably fail again.*
Fewer than 25 percent of smokers are able to quit on the first try. Most take four or more tries. Stopping smoking is like learning anything new: It takes several tries.

*I will have unbearable cravings.*
Most cravings last less than 5 minutes. Plan what you can do until the urge goes away.

*I will get irritable and frustrated.*
While you are quitting, make fewer demands on yourself. Give yourself a break.

*I will be unable to concentrate.*
Consider quitting smoking during your vacation, when your need to concentrate is not as great.

*I cannot stand feeling so restless.*
Take walks or other time-out periods. Handle objects. Use your hands for other things.

*I need the stimulant effect of smoking.*
Increase your activity and begin an exercise program. Work toward a more regular pattern of exercise.

*I will gain weight.*
While many ex-smokers gain weight, not all do. The average weight gain after stopping smoking is 5 to 8 pounds. It may help to plan snacks that are low in fat and start an exercise program when you quit.

*I will not be able to sleep.*
For good sleep hygiene, don't read or watch television in bed. Go to bed only when you are tired. Do not nap during the day. Exercise earlier during the day and avoid caffeine at night. If you do not fall asleep in 30 minutes after you go to bed, get up for a while.

### Can you handle smoking just one?

Frequently, the problem with quitting is not the moment of stopping, but the process of never smoking again. Many recent ex-smokers fool themselves into believing they can handle just one. Most can't. It's best if you don't even try. Experts now recognize that prevention of relapse is the key to success. The mainstay is your commitment to stay smoke-free each day. However, strategies to prevent relapse are designed to give your commitment a better chance.

Setting measurable goals that are well defined, recording your behavior to monitor your progress, having frequent contact with health care providers, and arranging for social support and positive reinforcement will help you succeed. Many people use rewards to encourage their progress. It's also important to maintain daily vigilance over a long time to avoid relapse.

Regardless of the specific assistance you may need to stop smoking and maintain abstinence, a nicotine dependence treatment center may enhance your effort. In these settings, counseling, prescriptions, instructions and follow-up can focus on your specific needs.

Quitting smoking is probably the single best thing you can do to reduce your risk of heart disease. Modifying other risk factors certainly will help, but nothing can help more than getting rid of tobacco products. The combination of smoking and other risk factors greatly amplifies your risk of developing coronary artery disease.

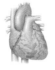

### HEALTHY HEART ♥ TIP

*Quit smoking today—especially if you're under 50 years old. In this younger age group, smoking produces a greater relative risk for heart disease than it does for people over 50. In addition, women who smoke and use oral contraceptives greatly increase their risk of coronary heart disease, compared with women who neither smoke nor use oral contraceptives.*

## Eating for a healthy heart

Although researchers don't yet have all the answers, they do know that nutrition plays a key role in many risk factors for coronary artery disease. Risk factors influenced by nutrition include high cholesterol (hyperlipidemia), high blood pressure (hypertension), excess weight, and diabetes.

For the past three decades, medical experts have focused on dietary components that increase risk for heart disease. Now there's a growing awareness that some components in foods can decrease risk as well. The first part of this section reviews food components that may affect your risk for coronary artery disease. Then you'll find practical guidelines for heart-healthy eating.

### Hyperlipidemia: getting the fats straight

If you assume that cholesterol from food is the greatest dietary contributor to elevated total blood cholesterol levels, guess again. While you shouldn't ignore the amount of cholesterol you consume, the most important culprit in raising your blood cholesterol level is saturated fat. Lowering your intake of saturated fat is the most important dietary step you can take to protect your heart from heart disease. Here's a primer on the fat in your diet.

## Saturated fat

Your body makes "bad" LDL cholesterol from the saturated fat you eat. Therefore, decreasing your saturated fat intake is key to improving your lipid profile. Most saturated fat comes from foods of animal origin—especially meats, milk and milk products. Plant sources include the tropical oils: coconut, palm kernel oil, palm oil and cocoa butter. Unlike other plant oils, the tropical oils are composed predominantly of saturated fatty acids. They're common ingredients in commercial cakes, cookies and other snack foods.

## Monounsaturated fat

Monounsaturated fat has good qualities. In recommended amounts it helps to lower total blood cholesterol and resists oxidation, the process that enables cells in your arteries to absorb fats and cholesterol. Over time, oxidation speeds the build-up of plaque in your arteries and increases your risk of heart attack and stroke. Olive, peanut and canola oils are sources of monounsaturated fat.

## Polyunsaturated fat

Like monounsaturated fats, polyunsaturated fatty acids (PUFAs) help to lower your blood cholesterol level and are an acceptable substitute for saturated fat in your diet. However, unlike monounsaturated fats, PUFAs are susceptible to oxidation. Since no population has consumed a diet high in this type of fat over a long period of time, the health effects of consuming large amounts of polyunsaturated fats are unknown. Therefore, medical researchers suggest that you avoid large quantities of PUFAs.

## Trans fats

Recent studies suggest that another type of fat, trans fatty acids (trans fats), may raise your total cholesterol and "bad" LDL cholesterol levels, and lower the "good" HDL cholesterol levels. Trans fats are produced when polyunsaturated fats, such as those found in vegetable oils, undergo the chemical process of hydrogenation. The greater the degree of hydrogenation, the more saturated the fat becomes. Major sources of trans fats include margarine and vegetable shortening—and products made from them, including cookies, desserts, crackers and other prepared foods. The trans fat content of the typical American diet is a significant contributor to coronary artery disease.

## Cholesterol

Even though saturated fat is the main dietary culprit in high blood cholesterol levels, that doesn't mean you can ignore your cholesterol intake. The cholesterol you eat does raise the level of cholesterol in your blood, although not as much as saturated fat raises it. Because your body can make all the cholesterol it needs, you don't need to consume additional cholesterol in your diet. Cholesterol is present only in foods from animals: meat, poultry, seafood, eggs, dairy products, and animal fats such as butter and lard. You can lower your intake of both saturated fat and cholesterol by cutting back on animal products and substituting foods that are lower in fat for their counterparts that contain more fat.

## Butter versus margarine

Most of the fat in butter is saturated. Most of the fat in margarine begins as polyunsaturated fat.

When margarine is hydrogenated, some of its polyunsaturated fatty acids are converted to saturated fats or trans fats. This process makes the fat more solid. Therefore, stick margarine is more saturated than tub margarine.

The American Heart Association considers a hydrogenated product acceptable if it contains less than 2 grams of saturated fat per tablespoon and if the ingredient listed first is a liquid vegetable oil. However, the amount of fatty spread you use is just as important as the type you choose.

## Triglycerides

Triglycerides, like cholesterol, are a type of fat. After you eat, your body digests the fat in food and releases triglycerides into your blood. Your liver also changes excess calories from carbohydrate, fat and protein into triglycerides. Alcohol also increases your blood triglyceride level. Recent research suggests that elevated triglycerides may contribute to coronary artery disease. A blood triglyceride level below 200 milligrams per deciliter (mg/dL) is considered normal, between 200 and 400 mg/dL is considered borderline and above 400 mg/dL is high. If your triglyceride level is high, it's a good idea to exercise regularly, maintain a healthy weight, and limit your intake of sugar, alcohol and dietary fat.

## Taking it step by step

The National Cholesterol Education Program's Step I and Step II diets may be your first line of defense in reducing your risk of coronary artery disease.

### Reducing cholesterol and fat one step at a time

| Nutrient | Typical American intake | Step I recommendations | Step II recommendations |
|---|---|---|---|
| Cholesterol | Men: 333 mg<br>Women: 213 mg | Less than 300 mg | Less than 200 mg |
| Fat | 33 percent of total calories | 30 percent or less of total calories* | |
| Saturated | 11 percent of total calories | 8 to 10 percent of total calories | 7 percent or less of total calories |
| Monounsaturated | 13 percent of total calories | Up to 15 percent of total calories* | |
| Polyunsaturated | 7 percent of total calories | Up to 10 percent of total calories* | |
| Carbohydrate | 51 percent of total calories | At least 55 percent of total calories* | |
| Protein | 16 percent of total calories | About 15 percent of total calories* | |
| Calories | Men: 2,500<br>Women: 1,600 | Just enough to achieve and maintain a healthy weight | |

*Apply to both Step I and Step II recommendations.

Use these guidelines to evaluate and adjust your intake of saturated fat and cholesterol and set a calorie level that promotes your desired weight. If you have high blood cholesterol, your doctor probably will recommend the Step I diet. You can use the Step II diet to further lower your cholesterol. If your cholesterol level is more than 240 mg/dL initially, or if you have coronary artery disease, your doctor will probably recommend starting with the Step II diet. Ask your doctor to refer you to a registered dietitian, who will translate these nutrient guidelines into practical and tasty food selections.

The Step I diet can lower "bad" LDL cholesterol about 7 to 9 percent. The Step II diet can lower LDL cholesterol about 10 to 20 percent. A very low fat diet, such as the Ornish diet (see page 190), may reduce your cholesterol 20 to 25 percent. However, individuals respond differently to dietary changes, and some people require medication to lower cholesterol levels sufficiently.

## Excess weight

Although health experts don't totally understand how and why people become overweight, they do know that it involves an interaction of genes and environment. Clearly, being seriously overweight has major implications for your health. Experts know that obesity raises triglyceride levels, raises total cholesterol and LDL cholesterol, lowers "good" HDL cholesterol, raises blood pressure, and can induce diabetes. Even a modest reduction in weight—5 to 10 percent—can reduce these health risks.

### Were you born to be fat?

Being overweight arises from the interaction of several factors:

- Genetics. Children of parents who are overweight tend to be overweight, too. A family history of obesity increases your chances of becoming obese by about 25 to 30 percent.

- Sex. Muscles use more energy than fat tissue uses. Women have a higher percentage of body fat than men have. Men burn between 10 and 20 percent more calories during rest than women do, because men have more muscle.

- Age. As you get older, you need fewer calories. The amount of muscle in your body tends to decrease, and fat accounts for a greater percentage of your weight. This lower muscle mass leads to a decrease in metabolism. In addition, physical activity tends to decrease with age.

- Physical inactivity. Usually, overweight adults are less physically active than people of average weight. It's not clear whether this is a cause or consequence of excess weight.

- Diet high in fat. Ounce for ounce, fat provides more than twice as many calories as carbohydrate or protein. This calorie difference may contribute to weight gain.

- Society and environment. Efficient transportation, household conveniences, and the easy availability of foods discourage physical activity and promote increased caloric intake.

- Cigarette smoking. Because nicotine raises your metabolic rate, men and women who smoke tend to weigh 6 to 10 pounds less than nonsmokers. When you stop smoking, you burn fewer calories—and many people eat more. However, the advantages your heart and lungs gain by stopping far outweigh the risk associated with moderate weight gain.

- Medical problems. Experts can trace less than 2 percent of all obesity cases to metabolic disorders such as low thyroid function or hormonal imbalances.

## Understanding weight control

Have you ever wondered how food gives you energy? Food contains various nutrients—some of which provide energy, while others help your body use the energy. Carbohydrate, protein, fat and alcohol all provide energy. Every day your body requires a certain amount of energy from carbohydrate, protein and fat to function properly. Calories measure both the energy in food and the energy your body needs.

## Energy comes in different forms

Carbohydrates, protein and fat found in foods—and alcohol found in some beverages—provide calories. Fat provides more than twice the calories per weight of carbohydrates or protein. That's why reducing fat intake is an effective way to trim calories. All fats—saturated, mono-unsaturated, polyunsaturated and trans—provide the same amount of calories.

| Nutrient | Calories per gram* |
|----------|--------------------|
| Carbohydrate | 4 |
| Protein | 4 |
| Fat | 9 |
| Alcohol | 7 |

*A gram is about the weight of a small paper clip.*

## Calculating your daily calorie requirement

The following formulas show the approximate number of calories you need to maintain your weight:

*If you are sedentary:*
  Current weight (in pounds) x 12
*If you are moderately physically active:*
  Current weight (in pounds) x 14
*If you are extremely active:*
  Current weight (in pounds) x 16 or 18

**Example:**
Pat is sedentary and weighs 165 pounds.
  165 x 12 = 1,980
Maintaining Pat's current weight requires about 1,980 calories a day.

When you use more calories than you eat—through physical activity and exercise, for example—you lose weight.

Foods high in fat are also high in calories, because fat is the most concentrated source of energy. Compared to carbohydrates and protein, which weigh in at 4 calories per gram, fat adds calories fast—a whopping 9 calories per gram. It's easier to eat more calories from fatty foods than foods high in carbohydrates. Foods that are rich in complex carbohydrates tend to be bulkier, so you're more likely to feel full after eating them than after eating foods high in fat. A diet that promotes heart health consists of foods that provide the right balance of carbohydrate, protein, fat and other nutrients in amounts that help you achieve and maintain a desirable weight.

## Principles of weight control

Your weight is determined by your energy balance. If you eat more calories than you burn, you gain weight. If you burn more calories than you eat, you lose weight. If you burn the same amount of calories you eat, your weight stays the same. The number of calories you need each day depends on several factors, including whether you are at a desirable weight, overweight or underweight. Your level of physical activity is also a factor.

It takes about 3,500 excess calories to gain a pound. On the other hand, if your body uses at least 3,500 calories more than you take in, you lose a pound. Losing weight requires a steady energy deficit. You can create this deficit in one of two ways: eat fewer calories or increase the amount of calories your body uses through physical activity. Health experts find that the most effective way to lose weight is to combine both.

A slow, steady approach is safest and is most likely to be permanent. The general rule of thumb is to lose about 1 to 2 pounds a week. To do this, you need to create a deficit of at least 3,500 calories—or a deficit of 500 calories a day on each of the 7 days. For example, you can create that deficit by eating 250 calories fewer than your body typically needs to maintain its weight and by expending 250 additional calories through physical activity, such as brisk walking.

It's not a good idea to consume fewer than 1,200 calories a day without your doctor's advice, because it's difficult to get all the nutrients you need with limited quantities of food. In addition, weight loss may occur too rapidly in people who eat fewer than 1,200 calories. Also, rapid weight loss doesn't allow for the time it takes to adapt to a new lifestyle. Therefore, it often leads to rapid regain of the weight.

It takes time to break old habits and make new ones. You're much more likely to stick with new eating patterns over the long term if you make changes gradually. Slow and steady weight loss allows the changes you've made to become habits. Set yourself up for success by taking the time to do it right the first time.

## Hypertension and diet

Because sodium can affect your blood pressure, it's important to control your sodium intake (see page 178). Sodium is an essential mineral. Its main role is to help maintain the appropriate balance of fluids in your body. It also helps transmit messages through your nerves that influence the actions of your muscles.

You need less than 500 milligrams of sodium each day. However, most Americans consume about 4000 milligrams of sodium a day. Your kidneys, which regulate the amount of sodium in your body, typically can compensate for high or low sodium intake. But if your heart, kidneys, liver or lungs are diseased, your body may be unable to regulate its sodium level. Furthermore, high levels of dietary sodium can cause some people's blood pressure to rise. Unfortunately, there's no easy way to tell if you're sensitive to sodium other than to limit your intake of sodium and see if your blood pressure goes down.

## What's a reasonable and safe level of sodium consumption?

The National High Blood Pressure Education Program recommends that all Americans limit daily sodium intake to 2400 milligrams a day. Many health professionals and organizations, including high blood pressure specialists at Mayo Clinic, support this recommendation. Here's why:

### What if you took "phen-fen"?

The United States Food and Drug Administration (FDA) approved fenfluramine, dexfenfluramine, and phentermine—all appetite suppressants—for management of obesity. The FDA action covered only the use of the drugs individually and for a short period of time. Use of a combination of phentermine and fenfluramine (often referred to as phen-fen) became popular after early reports suggested it was effective and had few side effects. However, the FDA never approved the use of these drugs in combination.

After 24 women taking the combination of phentermine and fenfluramine reported unusual thickening and leakage in their heart valves in 1997—and following further investigation—the two drugs were withdrawn from the market. Phentermine was not withdrawn, as there were no reported cases of valvular heart disease (disease of the heart valves) associated with this medication when used alone.

If you took fenfluramine, phentermine or dexfenfluramine—or any combination of these drugs—you should be examined by your physician. If you have any symptoms that suggest cardiac valvular disease—or if your doctor detects a heart murmur—you should have an echocardiogram (an ultrasound examination of your heart).

The good news is that more recent large studies indicate that the vast majority of people who have taken these drugs will not develop any significant heart valve problems. This should be greatly reassuring to the many people who have taken these drugs in the past.

- If you have high blood pressure and you're sensitive to sodium, limiting sodium intake can lower your blood pressure. Combined with other lifestyle changes, such as eating a healthful diet and increasing your physical activity, this may be enough to ward off the need for medication.

- If you're taking blood pressure medication, limiting sodium can improve the effectiveness of the drug.

- If you're at risk for developing high blood pressure, you may avert it by limiting sodium and making other lifestyle changes.

- Even if you're healthy, it's safe and reasonable to limit sodium as part of a healthful diet. This may reduce your risk for coronary artery disease as you get older, when high blood pressure is more common and your sensitivity to sodium often increases.

Large studies show that, on average, when people lower their sodium consumption, their blood pressure decreases—and there are fewer deaths from heart attack and stroke. This suggests that the average person may benefit from reducing sodium in the diet.

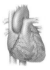

## HEALTHY HEART ♥ TIP

*Salt is widely blamed for raising blood pressure. But everyone responds to salt differently.*

*If you're sodium-sensitive, salt may raise your blood pressure, whereas cutting back may lower it. Most of your daily salt intake comes from prepared or processed foods—and not the salt shaker in your hand. Read food labels to determine how much sodium is contained in items you're about to buy. Avoid salt at the table and when you cook. If you're taking blood-pressure-lowering medications, cutting back on sodium helps them do their job.*

## Lowering your sodium intake

Table salt is the most obvious source of sodium (it contains 40 percent sodium and 60 percent chloride). Just one teaspoon of salt contains about 2400 milligrams of sodium. The salt you add in cooking or at the table may be only the tip of the iceberg in your total sodium consumption. Even many natural foods—such as milk, meat and vegetables—contain some sodium. But sodium that is added to foods in processing is, by far, the greatest contributor (at least two thirds) to the total amount of sodium in your diet.

Food manufacturers are responding to consumers' demands for foods with lower sodium levels. They offer reduced-sodium counterparts to an array of foods that typically are high in sodium, such as soups, frozen dinners, canned vegetables, luncheon meats, salad dressings, cheeses, chips and crackers. Read the nutrition facts labels to find the sodium content (shown in milligrams). While you're checking for sodium content, check for fat as well, because some foods with reduced sodium levels are still high in fat.

Use fresh foods in place of processed foods, so that you can control the amount of sodium that's added. Fresh or frozen vegetables are a much better choice over canned vegetables, because sodium is often added in the canning process.

Dairy products are a natural source of sodium. Three 8-ounce glasses of milk (whole, reduced-fat, low-fat or skim) a day contain 375 milligrams of sodium, which is not an excessive amount. However, if you drink more than 3 glasses and also eat cheese, ice cream or frozen yogurt, the amount of sodium quickly adds up.

When you're cooking, go for fresh flavors, instead of masking the natural flavor with salt. Use blends of herbs and spices for added flavor. Don't add salt at the table. Finally, have patience—it may take 6 to 8 weeks to learn to appreciate less salty flavors. You'll begin to taste a variety of other flavors after you reduce the salt in your diet.

## The DASH diet

For years, doctors' main dietary approach to high blood pressure was a recommendation to reduce sodium intake. Now researchers have discovered that a diet rich in fruits and vegetables, adequate in dairy products, and low in fat can lower blood pressure—possibly enough to reduce or eliminate your need for medication.

The DASH diet evolved from a 1997 Dietary Approaches to Stop Hypertension study (hence, the acronym). This study suggests that other dietary factors, in addition to sodium, influence blood pressure in a positive way. During this study, participants followed one of three diets for 8 weeks:

- A diet that matched the average American diet
- A similar diet with higher amounts of fruits and vegetables, or
- A combination diet that reduced saturated fat and emphasized fruits, vegetables and low-fat dairy products

The study established that while both the diet enriched with fruits and vegetables and the combination diet (reduced saturated fat and abundant fruits, vegetables and low-fat dairy products) lowered blood pressure, the combination diet was more effective. In that group, the decrease in blood pressure was the greatest for those whose blood pressure was above 140/90. That group saw an average drop of 11.4 points in the systolic pressure (the top number) and 5.5 points in the diastolic pressure (the bottom number). That is about the same effect that some medications have on blood pressure.

A word of caution: Don't stop or alter your medication without first consulting your doctor.

All three diets limited sodium to about 3000 milligrams daily, more than the recommended 2400 but less than a typical American's consumption. A second study (DASH2) is evaluating whether lowering sodium further can produce even greater blood pressure reductions.

The DASH diet is also a diet that promotes heart health. It increases your consumption of grains, fruits, vegetables and low-fat dairy products, and encourages you to reduce your intake of animal products, including meat. But the DASH diet alone can't produce an ideal blood pressure. It's still important to exercise, lose excess weight, stop smoking, and limit your alcohol consumption. However, of all the lifestyle factors related to blood pressure, weight loss is the most effective in lowering blood pressure for most people.

## Precautions about salt substitutes

If you've been advised to reduce your sodium intake, you may wonder about using a salt substitute. Before you try one, check with your doctor.

Here's why:

- Some salt substitutes or "lite" salts contain a mixture of sodium chloride (salt) and other compounds. To achieve that familiar salty taste, you may end up using more of a salt substitute. As a result, you may not reduce your sodium intake at all.

- Potassium chloride is a common ingredient in salt substitutes. Too much potassium can be harmful for people who are taking certain medications for their high blood pressure or for heart failure. It can also be harmful for people with kidney problems.

Some diuretics such as amiloride (Midamor), spironolactone (Aldactone) and triamterene (Dyrenium), and medications (such as Moduretic, Aldactazide, Dyazide or Maxzide) that combine hydrochlorothiazide with one of the above generic drugs, cause your kidneys to retain potassium. If you take one of these medications, you may need to limit the amount of potassium you eat.

## The DASH diet

| Food group | Daily servings* |
|---|---|
| Grains and grain products | 7 to 8 |
| Vegetables | 4 to 5 |
| Fruits | 4 to 5 |
| Low-fat or fat-free dairy foods | 2 to 3 |
| Meats, poultry and fish | 2 or fewer |
| Nuts, seeds and dried beans | 4 to 5 per week |
| Fats and oils | 2 to 3 |

*For serving sizes, see the discussion of the Food Guide Pyramid on page 291.*

## Diabetes and your diet

Excessive blood sugar can damage many of your organs and tissues, leading to atherosclerosis, coronary artery disease, kidney disease and other conditions. A full discussion of diabetes is beyond the scope of this book. However, when it comes to coronary artery disease, the most important thing to remember about diabetes is that good blood sugar control may help delay cardiovascular complications.

Exercise, weight control and good regulation of dietary factors—including fats, sweets and alcohol—promote good blood lipid and glucose management. If you have type 2 diabetes, you're probably overweight and could benefit from weight loss.

## Dietary components under investigation

Researchers don't know everything they'd like to about how nutrition affects your heart. Ongoing research yields new information on a continuous basis.

### Fiber

Experts believe that certain components of foods may decrease your risk for coronary artery disease. One such component is dietary fiber. When eaten as part of a diet that is low in fat and saturated fat, fiber can help lower your blood cholesterol.

## Carbohydrates

Carbohydrate is one of the nutrients in food that provide energy. In fact, it should be your body's main fuel source. Most carbohydrates come from plants. Typical sources include grains, vegetables, fruits and legumes (such as peas and beans). Dairy products are the only significant animal source of carbohydrates.

Three types of carbohydrates

| Type | Calories per gram | Simple or complex | Source |
|---|---|---|---|
| Sugars | 4 | Simple | Table sugar, milk, fruit, some vegetables, processed foods, desserts |
| Starches | 4 | Complex | Grains, breads, cereals, pasta, vegetables |
| Fiber | 0 | Complex | Whole grains, whole-grain breads, cereals and pasta, vegetables, legumes, fruits |

Large population studies link diets high in complex carbohydrates (see page 180) and fiber with lower death rates from coronary artery disease and some other chronic diseases.

Dietary fiber is a term used for several parts of plants that your body can't digest. Most dietary fiber passes through your body unchanged. As it passes through your body, however, fiber affects the way your body digests food and absorbs nutrients.

There has been much speculation about the role of fiber in preventing or treating a variety of diseases, including coronary artery disease, diabetes and cancer. While fiber is not a magical cure, it is an important part of your diet.

The two main categories of fiber are soluble and insoluble. Each has its own characteristics and is part of a healthful diet. Soluble fiber may help lower blood cholesterol and blood sugar levels and reduce your risk of heart attack. It's not definitively proved, but researchers believe that consuming insoluble fiber may also reduce your risk of heart disease. Fiber also aids in normal bowel function, helping you avoid hemorrhoids and diverticulosis (multiple pouches that project outward from the wall of the colon).

Foods high in soluble fiber include oat bran, oatmeal, beans, peas, rice bran, barley, citrus fruits, strawberries and apple pulp. You can find insoluble fiber in whole-wheat breads, wheat cereals, rye, rice, barley, most other grains, cabbage, beets, carrots, brussels sprouts, turnips, cauliflower and apple skin. In short, it's important to eat a wide range of foods high in fiber.

## Soy

In cultures where soy is the main source of protein, rates of cardiovascular disease and some kinds of cancers are low. Research into the role of soy continues, and results appear promising.

Increasing evidence shows that isoflavones—plant estrogens found in soy—may have some effects on your body that closely resemble the effects of the human estrogen hormone. Research suggests that eating about an ounce (25 grams) of soy protein a day can reduce three important numbers in your lipid profile by about 10 percent: total cholesterol, "bad" LDL cholesterol, and triglycerides. Eating soy also may help improve your "good" HDL cholesterol.

Researchers aren't yet sure how soy may lower cholesterol and triglycerides. But it's not difficult to substitute soy foods for animal products that are high in saturated fat and cholesterol. Researchers have also suggested that proteins in soy may change the levels of certain hormones in your body, which in turn may cause your liver to make less cholesterol.

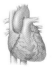

**HEALTHY HEART ♥ TIP**

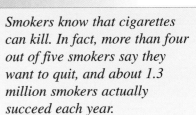

*Smokers know that cigarettes can kill. In fact, more than four out of five smokers say they want to quit, and about 1.3 million smokers actually succeed each year.*

*With good smoking cessation programs, 20 to 40 percent of participants can quit smoking and stay off cigarettes for at least one year. Stop-smoking programs appear to be especially helpful for heavier, more addicted smokers, such as those who smoke more than 25 cigarettes a day. Combining interventions, such as physician advice and follow-up with nicotine gum and behavior modification, may increase success rates.*

### Fish and fish oils—and omega-3 fatty acids

About two decades ago, researchers discovered something surprising about people living in Greenland. They had a low rate of heart attacks, despite eating a diet laden with fat that included about a pound of fatty fish and whale meat each day. Since then, scientists have found that consumption of fish in moderate amounts is associated with less coronary heart disease and sudden death. The key seems to be a unique type of fat.

Some fish—particularly fatty types prevalent in cold water—such as salmon, mackerel and herring—contain high amounts. Omega-3 fatty acids are also present in smaller amounts in green leafy vegetables, soybeans, nuts and canola oil.

### The benefits of omega-3 fatty acids

Research indicates that omega-3 fatty acids in your diet may:

- Lower your blood triglyceride level. Persistently high triglyceride levels may add to the risk for coronary artery disease. If your triglyceride level is extremely high and doesn't respond to prescribed medication, your doctor may suggest that you use fish oil supplements, in addition to your medication. This is the only use of fish oil capsules the American Heart Association supports.
- Reduce the risk of dangerous blood clotting. Omega-3 fatty acids act as a natural anticoagulant by altering the ability of platelets in your blood to clump together. The platelets become less sticky, so clot formation is less likely.
- Lower blood pressure. Several studies have examined the effects of omega-3 fatty acids on blood pressure. One study compared people on a diet based on fish with those on a vegetarian diet. The group eating fish had a lower incidence of borderline or high blood pressure.
- Decrease the risk of abnormal heart rhythms and sudden death.

### How much fish?

Dietitians generally recommend at least two meals of fish every week for possible heart benefits. Fish oil capsules shouldn't be a substitute for fish in your diet. In high doses they pose potential risks, especially if you're regularly taking aspirin or blood thinners, such as warfarin.

### The fish hook

No one's certain whether the apparent benefits of eating fish stem from omega-3 fatty acids alone, the fatty acids combined with other nutrients in fish, or because as you eat more fish you probably eat less animal and saturated fat. But the bottom line is that eating fish can't hurt and may very well help.

## Alcohol: is it good for you?

There's still a lot that researchers don't know about whether alcohol's health benefits outweigh its risks. It's not an easy judgment, because several factors influence results.

*A toast to your health*

Dozens of studies show that moderate alcohol consumption lowers the risk of heart attack for people in their middle ages by roughly 30 to 50 percent. This result seems to hold up, even when you consider other factors that may play a role, such as age and tobacco use. Apparently, the greatest protective effect of alcohol is for men over age 50, especially smokers and former smokers. Alcohol appears to raise levels of "good" HDL cholesterol and may help prevent blood clots, reducing the likelihood of a heart attack, stroke or other disorders.

Some studies suggest that light alcohol consumption may offer other health benefits, including a longer life, significant reduction in your risk for the most common type of stroke (ischemic stroke), a reduction in blockages in your leg arteries and a lowering of your risk for macular degeneration related to aging, the leading cause of blindness in people over age 65.

There's no unanimity on whether wine is more beneficial than beer or liquor. Some studies suggest that wine's benefits are superior, because of beneficial compounds in wine (resveratrol, for example). Other studies document the same cardiovascular benefits for all three. No matter which you prefer, ask your physician for guidelines. If you drink alcohol, do it with meals. Food slows alcohol absorption, and people who drink at meals tend to do so in moderation.

*Beware of the health risks*

When you consider the potential benefits of moderate alcohol consumption, don't forget the potential risks. Studies often reveal conflicting information about alcohol, and many results are still preliminary. Misuse or abuse of alcohol leads to accidents, emotional problems, and alcoholism.

Heavy or binge drinking increases your risk for accidents and falls. Over time, heavy drinking raises your risk for liver, kidney, lung and heart disease, stroke, osteoporosis, high blood pressure, and obesity, as well as certain cancers, including those that affect your throat, stomach, colon and, perhaps, breast.

Even in small amounts, alcohol can have negative effects on your health. As it slows your brain activity, it affects your alertness, coordination and reaction time. It can interfere with your sleep and sexual function, and it can bring on high blood pressure. Alcohol can interact with many common prescriptions and over-the-counter medications. It can weaken the effects of certain beta-blocker medications. If you combine it with tranquilizers, sleeping pills, antihistamines or pain relievers, such as aspirin, it can be dangerous. If you combine alcohol with aspirin, you face an increased risk of stomach bleeding.

*Moderation is vital*

Until researchers know more about how alcohol affects your health, your best bet is to drink in moderation, if at all. Don't feel pressured to drink. And don't drink every day. Few, if any, medical experts advise nondrinkers to start drinking.

## What is moderate drinking?

For men, moderation means no more than two drinks per day. Because women and older people are more sensitive to alcohol's effects and process it more slowly, moderation means one drink for women or anyone over 65 years of age.

A drink is defined as:

- A 4- to 5-ounce glass of wine
- A 12-ounce can of beer
- A 1½-ounce shot of 80-proof liquor

Some people should refrain from drinking for health reasons, such as those with high blood pressure, high blood triglyceride levels, liver disease, ulcers, severe stomach acid reflux and sleep apnea. You should also abstain if you are trying to conceive, are pregnant or are breastfeeding. Discuss any questions with your doctor.

## Caffeine: does it affect your heart?

Caffeine may be the world's most controversial stimulant. It wakes you up, gives you energy, increases your alertness and quickens your reaction time. Scientists have studied the potential health risks of caffeine for several years. Evidence that coffee—the most common source of caffeine in the American diet—causes serious health problems is unclear. For every study that implicates coffee as a possible health risk, there seems to be another that finds no link.

If you have coronary artery disease—or are at risk for it—most experts recommend that you limit yourself to two cups or less per day of decaffeinated coffee or beverages that contain caffeine (coffee, tea, cola). If you have a heart arrhythmia, high blood pressure, or both, your doctor may recommend that you avoid caffeine entirely. There's strong evidence that caffeine affects heart function by increasing the force of your heart's contractions and altering the regularity of its beats. Caffeine also temporarily elevates blood pressure. However, regular use seems to bring a tolerance to the effects on blood pressure.

Research into coffee's effects on health continues. Over the years, coffee has been linked to slightly elevated cholesterol levels and an increased risk for coronary artery disease and heart attack. But a 1996 study of more than 121,000 female nurses found that after researchers adjusted for cigarette smoking among coffee drinkers, coffee consumption—even at high levels—didn't increase heart attack risk.

There is some evidence that compounds in coffee may increase cholesterol levels. But the compounds are found only in boiled coffee—not in filtered or instant. Take this into account if you drink unfiltered coffee (percolated, boiled, espresso).

## Caffeine content of various types of coffee

Here's a handy comparison of caffeine content for various types of coffee. Note that amounts can vary, depending on several factors—how strong it is, for example.

| Type of coffee, 6-ounce cup | Milligrams of caffeine per serving |
|---|---|
| Brewed, drip method | 115 |
| Brewed, percolator method | 80 |
| Instant, 1 rounded teaspoon | 65 |
| Decaffeinated | 2 |
| Espresso (1½ to 2 ounces) | 100 |

## Can vitamins help you avoid coronary artery disease?

Although medical specialists have recognized the value of some vitamins for many years, there are still many unknowns. Researchers are investigating the effects on heart health of many vitamins.

### Niacin

Sometimes doctors prescribe large doses of niacin (vitamin B-3) to help patients improve the levels of fats in their blood. Niacin can lower "bad" LDL cholesterol and triglycerides and raise "good" HDL cholesterol. Studies show that niacin can slow—and even reverse—the progression of the enlargement of plaque in your arteries when used with other drugs that help lower cholesterol and a diet designed to improve heart health and exercise. However, in doses typically needed for these effects (usually more than 1000 milligrams), niacin is being used as a medication, not a vitamin. At doses higher than 2000 milligrams, niacin has potentially serious side effects that can include liver damage, high blood sugar and irregular heartbeats. As little as 50 milligrams can cause flushing, headaches, cramps and nausea. Take increased supplemental niacin only upon your doctor's advice.

### What about antioxidants?

Antioxidants may help prevent cholesterol from damaging the lining of your arteries. Antioxidants include vitamins C and E and the carotenoids, such as beta-carotene. Antioxidants come mainly from fruits and vegetables.

Antioxidant vitamins can slow the oxidation process—hence the name. Oxidation is a chemical process that causes changes in fatty acids and "bad" LDL cholesterol in your blood. These changes enable cells in your arteries to more easily absorb fatty acids and LDL cholesterol, a process that can cause plaque enlargement and block your arteries. Antioxidants may reduce the risk of coronary artery disease by slowing oxidation.

The strongest evidence for using naturally occurring antioxidants to protect yourself against coronary artery disease is for vitamin E. Evidence is weakest for vitamin C, and information on the role of beta-carotene is limited and contradictory. Beta-carotene from fruits and vegetables appears to have a beneficial effect; however, several studies that are well designed found that beta-carotene in the form of a supplement offers no protection against heart disease. In two studies, beta-carotene supplements appeared to increase the risk for lung cancer in smokers. Researchers need to do more research to establish the safety and benefits of antioxidants.

Studies on vitamin E use doses that are so high that you can't get it all from food—around 400 international units (IU) or more a day. At these levels, vitamin E has pharmacological effects and is considered a drug. By comparison, the Recommended Dietary Allowance (RDA) for vitamin E is only 15 IU for men and 12 IU for women. Potential side effects include gastrointestinal complaints, as well as bleeding, if you're taking medications to thin your blood. Even though news about vitamin E is promising, consult your doctor before taking any supplements.

### How folic acid, vitamin B-6, and vitamin B-12 affect homocysteine

Homocysteine is a natural by-product of your body's use of protein. Many studies have established a relationship between high homocysteine levels in your blood and increased risk of coronary artery disease.

Your diet strongly influences your homocysteine levels—especially your consumption of folic acid and vitamins B-6 and B-12, which help break down homocysteine in your body. Although both folic acid and vitamin B-6 supplementation

---

**Where to find antioxidants in your food**

**Vitamin C:** green and red peppers, collard greens, broccoli, spinach, tomatoes, potatoes, strawberries, oranges, grapefruit and other citrus fruits.

**Vitamin E:** vegetable oils and products made with them, wheat germ, nuts.

**Carotenoids:** deep yellow, dark green and red vegetables and fruits.

lower homocysteine levels, folic acid does so more effectively. Vitamin B-12 lowers homocysteine only if you're deficient in that vitamin.

While this is encouraging, no studies have yet shown that vitamin treatment to lower homocysteine levels results in decreased risk for coronary artery disease. Nevertheless, if you're at high risk, you should probably follow an overall diet that ensures adequate intake of folic acid and vitamins B-6 and B-12.

You can get an adequate amount of these vitamins from ample servings of a variety of vegetables, fruits and legumes and small amounts of poultry, fish and beef. Many breakfast cereals are fortified with these vitamins as well.

## Food versus supplement

The use of dietary supplements—especially vitamins, minerals and herbs—has become quite controversial. Millions of Americans take dietary supplements for various reasons, including health promotion and disease prevention. Unfortunately, there is no clear scientific proof of any benefits from most supplements. And because they aren't considered drugs, the government doesn't require testing for effectiveness, content levels, or safety.

Some dietary supplements show promise for promoting heart health, but the jury is still out on most of them. Here's a look at a few of the most popular supplements.

## Garlic

Garlic may ward off more than vampires, according to an increasing body of research on this pungent herb's disease-fighting properties. The most convincing research thus far suggests that garlic may alter some factors that contribute to increased risk for coronary artery disease.

Researchers from Pennsylvania State University found that garlic reduces the production of triglycerides and cholesterol in the livers and blood of rats. High levels of triglycerides and cholesterol increase the risk for coronary heart disease. Researchers are currently performing similar studies on humans.

Garlic also thins your blood and makes clotting less likely. Researchers have discovered that sulfur compounds in onions, similar to those in garlic, make platelets slippery and less likely to stick together and form clots that can block blood flow and lead to heart attack and stroke. Garlic may help prevent and even reverse the enlargement of plaque in the walls of your arteries. One study found less stiffening of the heart's main artery among older adults taking standardized garlic powder for at least 2 years.

The claims made for garlic don't go unchallenged, however. While there's reasonable certainty of garlic's ability to lower cholesterol and reduce clotting, there's still not enough proof of some of the other potential benefits.

### *What form and how much?*

The best way to increase your garlic consumption is not yet clear. Questions remain about a safe and effective dose and what form of garlic you should consume. Eating garlic as a food may reduce its effectiveness, because apparently your stomach

---

**Good sources of folic acid and vitamins B-6 and B-12**

**Folic acid:** green leafy vegetables, citrus fruit and fruit juices, legumes (such as lentils, dried peas and beans).

**Vitamin B-6 (also called pyridoxine):** whole (but not enriched) grains, cereals and bread, spinach, green beans and bananas.

**Vitamin B-12 (also called cobalamin):** occurs naturally only in animal sources (meat, fish, eggs and milk).

---

breaks down allicin, the sulfur-containing compound responsible for much of garlic's health benefits. Fresh garlic may lose its effectiveness quickly after you cut or crush it. And cooking may either decrease or increase the potency of various compounds in garlic. Taking very large amounts of garlic may cause anemia and irritation of your intestinal tract. Many people consider garlic's odor offensive.

One solution is to use odorless, enteric-coated garlic tablets. The coating allows the tablet to pass through your stomach intact so that the garlic can be absorbed by your small intestine. Some researchers use aged garlic extract, which contains possibly more effective sulfur compounds than those found in fresh garlic. However, two studies showed no benefits from garlic extract.

Foods have been tried and tested over centuries, and are probably the best and safest way to get your fill of garlic for now. The U.S. Food and Drug Administration (FDA) doesn't regulate supplements, so it's difficult to know if what you're getting is pure. Despite the questions that remain about the health benefits of garlic, there's nothing wrong with enjoying this versatile herb in your foods. As is the case with vitamin E, no official medical organization has endorsed the use of these preparations for preventing heart disease, and the decision to use this substance is an individual and personal one.

## Cholestin

Cholestin is a new dietary supplement that appears to lower blood cholesterol levels. But the American Heart Association agrees that it's too soon to recommend using it.

Cholestin is made from rice fermented in red yeast. In China, red yeast has been used for centuries to enhance the color and flavor of food. It has also been used medicinally by Chinese people to improve circulation. Among the components of red yeast rice are several naturally occurring compounds, called statins, that act to lower cholesterol levels. Several of the drugs approved by the FDA to lower cholesterol contain statins.

A small number of short-term studies in humans suggest that Cholestin lowers cholesterol. One study in the United States involved 88 people with LDL cholesterol levels that were above average. After 12 weeks, LDL cholesterol levels decreased 22 percent in those taking the Cholestin. Their HDL cholesterol levels were unchanged. Although Cholestin may prove to be a useful tool for lowering cholesterol, more study is needed to determine if the supplement is safe and effective over the long term. For now, the FDA considers it to be an unapproved drug.

## Dietary supplements: the bottom line

Remember that humans eat whole foods, not supplements. Your body may best use nutrients in the concentrations and combinations present in whole foods. The more you vary your diet, the more likely you'll be to get the benefits of nutrients you need.

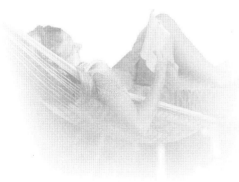

If you're thinking of taking a supplement, talk it over first with your doctor. Some supplements are proved to be unsafe, and others may affect the actions of medications you're taking.

## Functional foods for the future

There is increasing interest in an emerging field of nutrition: functional foods. These are foods or food ingredients that are modified to provide a health benefit beyond the traditional nutrients they contain. Often, the boost comes from phytochemicals, substances that occur naturally in plants. Some may reduce your risk of cardiovascular disease and some cancers. Studies now under way are testing the potential health benefits and possible risks of many functional foods.

Functional foods captured national attention recently, when two appeared in dairy cases in supermarkets across the United States. Take Control and Benecol are trade names for spreads designed to replace margarine or butter in your diet.

Phytochemicals incorporated into these spreads are derivatives of plant sterols called stanols, or plant sterols themselves—natural components of vegetable fats and oils. Plant sterols and their derivatives have demonstrated a cholesterol-lowering effect by blocking cholesterol from being absorbed in the digestive tract.

It's important to remember that these margarines are intended to replace some of your daily intake of fat, rather than add to it. It's better to eat less fat and saturated fat than to add this margarine on top of your typical fat intake.

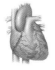

### HEALTHY HEART ♥ TIP

*You've reduced your fat intake to 30 percent of your diet. What should you replace those calories with?*

*Increase your carbohydrate intake to 60 percent or more of your total calories by emphasizing complex carbohydrates such as vegetables, fruits and whole grains. The complex carbohydrates—as opposed to the simple carbohydrates found in sugars—help you add more fiber to your diet. Foods high in complex carbohydrates are usually low in calories and have a wide variety of vitamins, minerals, and phytochemicals.*

Plant sterols aren't the only plant substances being used in functional foods. Currently, the other major components are the soluble fibers found in oats and in a plant seed called psyllium (SILL-ee-um). Psyllium is a primary ingredient in many laxatives. Soon, you may find a number of new food products enhanced with oat and psyllium fibers on your supermarket shelves. These functional foods will include dried pasta, frozen entrees, breads, cereals, baked potato crisps, and cookies.

There probably will be many more functional foods designed to help lower cholesterol. But if you're going to benefit, these foods must be part of a diet low in saturated fat and cholesterol. In addition, you should get regular physical activity.

## Is there an optimal diet to promote heart health?

While many diets claim to be the latest and greatest, it's important to remember that what's best for you may not be best for everyone else. There's a wonderful, colorful and tasteful variety of foods from which to choose, and you can tailor your selections to fit your preferences.

Several eating patterns, or diets, appear to be very effective in reducing the risk of heart disease. They include the Mediterranean diet, the Asian diet, and the Ornish diet (a vegetarian diet that's very low in fat). All of these diets share two common features: They are lower in saturated fat and cholesterol than the typical American diet and they are higher in plant foods. However, this is where the similarity ends.

## Mediterranean diet

Until recently, several areas in the Mediterranean region enjoyed the lowest recorded rates of chronic disease and the highest life expectancy. Studies have linked this good health to the diet of people who live in this region.

In 1999, the final report of an important study of the Mediterranean diet was published, and the news was good. In the Lyon Diet Heart Study, researchers tested whether a Mediterranean diet would reduce the occurrence of a second heart attack and sudden death more than a typical diet low in saturated fats and cholesterol. It did—by about 70 percent!

In addition to emphasizing monounsaturated fats, a Mediterranean diet is rich in alpha-linolenic fatty acids. Alpha-linolenic acid, a type of omega-3 polyunsaturated fatty acid, is found mainly in soybean and canola oils and in fish. The study linked this type of polyunsaturated fat to the reduced death rate.

## Asian diet

The diet and health statistics of some Asian countries and peoples are well documented, while those from others are not readily accessible. But there is enough reliable information available to show a general pattern. Asian people who eat their traditional diets have low rates of chronic diseases.

Researchers suspect that the healthfulness of the typical Asian diet is linked to its emphasis on plant-based foods, including rice and other grains, noodles, fruits, vegetables, beans, various soy foods, other legumes, nuts, seeds, vegetable and nut oils, herbs and spices, and plant-based beverages, including tea, wine and beer. This diet can provide all the known essential vitamins and minerals, fiber, and other plant substances that scientists believe promote health.

### Characteristics of traditional Mediterranean and Asian diets

| Characteristic | Mediterranean | Asian |
|---|---|---|
| Emphasizes an abundance of food from plant sources | X | X |
| Is low in saturated fat | X | X |
| Is low in total fat | * | X |
| Uses olive oil as the principal fat | X | |
| Includes fish in moderate amounts on a weekly basis | X | X |
| Includes poultry and eggs in low to moderate amounts on a weekly basis | X | X |
| Includes red meat in low amounts on a monthly basis | X | X |
| Includes low to moderate amounts of cheese and yogurt (low-fat and nonfat versions preferred) on a daily basis | X | ** |
| Includes wine in moderation and with meals | X | X |
| Includes tea and beer and other alcoholic beverages in moderation | X | X |

*The Mediterranean diet has total fat ranging from less than 25 percent to more than 35 percent of total calories.*

**The typical Asian diet excludes dairy foods, except in India, where yogurt and cheese are consumed, and some parts of China.*

*Note that regular physical activity is also part of both lifestyles.*

## Ornish diet

Also called the "Reversal Diet," the Ornish diet is a vegetarian diet that is very low in fat. It has minimal amounts of saturated fat, with 10 percent of its calories from total fat. It includes no meat, no added fat, and only nonfat dairy products. It emphasizes whole grains, vegetables, fruits and beans. This diet is part of a comprehensive treatment program for people who already have coronary artery disease. Many people find that the program, founded by Dr. Dean Ornish, requires substantial lifestyle changes. The regimen requires regular moderate exercise, stress management, group support and psychological counseling, and smoking cessation for smokers. Research shows that, over the long term, this diet—along with other lifestyle changes—can bring about substantial regression of even severe coronary artery disease without the use of drugs to lower lipid levels. Even after just one year, participants experienced a mild reduction in atherosclerotic plaque.

One study compared a group of patients who followed the Ornish diet and lifestyle program with a group who followed a diet similar to the Step II diet (see page 174). As a whole, coronary artery disease progressed in those who followed the less vigorous diet and lifestyle plan. They experienced more than twice as many cardiac events over the five years of the study, including heart attacks, strokes, unstable angina, heart failure, sudden death, and other events. Although a vegetarian diet limiting fat to 10 percent may not be practical for some people, this diet and these recommended lifestyle changes offer a choice that can reduce risk for coronary artery disease.

## 'How-to' for heart-healthy eating

A diet that is good for your heart is not unlike plain, healthy eating! Because heart disease is the number 1 killer in the United States, all Americans by about the age of 2 should follow the same dietary principles as people who are at risk for heart disease.

Scientists now know much more about how diet influences the risk for and management of heart disease. Researchers have known for years that a diet high in saturated fat, total fat, and cholesterol increases your risk for coronary artery disease. Now they also know—thanks to a great amount of interest and research in nutrition over the past decade—that some components in foods help you reduce your risk. You can find these components in grains, vegetables and fruits. By eating more of them, you can more easily curb your intake of meats, dairy products and other foods that contain high levels of saturated fat and cholesterol.

## Unified Dietary Guidelines

By adopting a healthful diet, you can lower your risk for many of the nation's most powerful killers: heart disease, stroke, cancer and diabetes. Under the Unified Dietary Guidelines, a typical day's healthy diet includes:

- Less than 10 percent of total calories from saturated fat
- About 30 percent of calories from all types of fat
- At least 55 percent of total calories from complex carbohydrates

- No more than 300 milligrams of cholesterol

- A maximum of 6000 milligrams of salt per day (2400 milligrams of sodium)

- Enough calories to maintain a healthy body weight

These are good guidelines for all Americans older than 2 years of age. They closely follow the United States Department of Agriculture's food guide pyramid and ensure that the diet contains enough vitamins, minerals, fiber and other essential nutrients.

1. Eat a variety of foods.

2. Choose most of what you eat from plant sources.

3. Eat five or more servings of fruits and vegetables each day.

4. Eat six or more servings of bread, pasta and cereal grains each day.

5. Eat foods that are high in fat sparingly, especially those from animal sources.

6. Keep your intake of simple sugars to a minimum.

## The U.S.D.A. food guide pyramid

The U.S.D.A. food guide pyramid is a tool that helps you implement the dietary guidelines. It calls for eating a variety of foods every day to get the nutrients you need and the right amount of calories to help you maintain or improve your weight.

### Alternative food pyramids

The U.S.D.A. food guide pyramid is based on the typical American diet. By popular demand, health researchers have developed food pyramids for several alternative eating patterns, to help you implement these healthy variations. The illustrations on the following pages show the Mediterranean diet pyramid, Asian diet pyramid and vegetarian diet pyramid, as devised jointly by the Oldways Preservation & Exchange Trust, the Harvard School of Public Health and other institutions. These pyramids are scientifically based on research into the traditional and alternative diets described earlier. Regardless of which pyramid you choose to follow, the message is the same: Eat more plant-based foods!

**U.S.D.A. food guide pyramid**

Fats, oils and sweets — *Use sparingly*

Milk, yogurt and cheese group — Meat, poultry, fish, dry beans, eggs and nuts — *2-3 Servings*

*3-5 Servings* — Vegetable group — Fruit group — *2-4 Servings*

Bread, cereal, rice and pasta group — *6-11 Servings*

All of the pyramids follow the basic principles described in the dietary guidelines. Use these principles when you eat, shop and plan meals, as well as when you eat out. In reviewing all of the pyramids, start from the base and move up. You'll also find on these pages specific suggestions for grocery shopping, reading labels and cooking. With a few simple substitutions, you and your family can eat more healthfully and enjoyably.

## Mediterranean diet pyramid

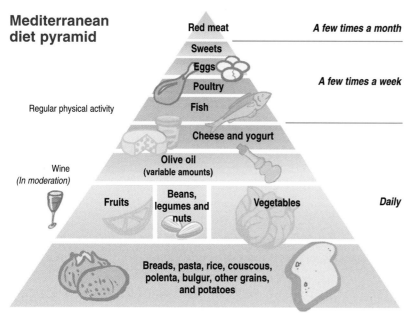

### Goodness grains

Eat 6 or more servings of grain products every day—preferably whole-grain breads, cereals, rice and pasta.

A serving is 1 slice of bread, 1 ounce of ready-to-eat cereal, 1/2 cup of cooked cereal, rice or pasta.

If you eat less fat and fewer high-fat meats and dairy products, it's likely you're eating more of something else to fill the void (unless you're trying to lose weight). That something is probably carbohydrate. The grain group, found at the base

## Asian diet pyramid

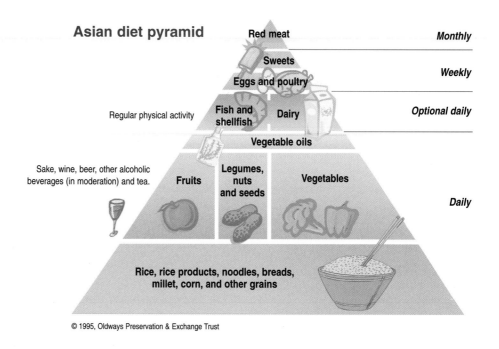

of the pyramid, is rich in carbo-hydrates. Yet, contrary to popular belief, most are low in fat and calories. You do need to be careful about what you add to these foods. Croissants, many dessert breads and some crackers are high in fat, so you should limit the amount of these that you eat.

Select whole-grain breads and cereals over refined products. Whole grains retain the bran and germ. Because they have bran, you will automatically increase the amount of fiber you eat.

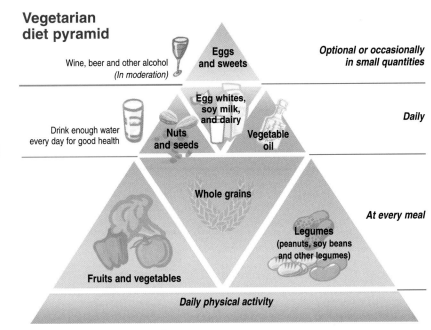

**Vegetarian diet pyramid**

Wine, beer and other alcohol (In moderation)

Eggs and sweets — *Optional or occasionally in small quantities*

Drink enough water every day for good health

Nuts and seeds

Egg whites, soy milk, and dairy

Vegetable oil — *Daily*

Whole grains

Fruits and vegetables

Legumes (peanuts, soy beans and other legumes) — *At every meal*

*Daily physical activity*

© 1997, Oldways Preservation & Exchange Trust

## Choosing grains

| Best choices (whole grains that are low-fat)* | Whole grain breads, cereals and pastas, English muffins, bagels and bread sticks, brown rice, crackers,* plainpopcorn, pretzels |
| --- | --- |
| Go easy on (contain moderate amounts of total fat) | Egg noodles, refined grains (such as white bread, pasta and white rice) |
| Limit or avoid (highest in total fat) | High-fat snack crackers and chips, biscuits, croissants |

*\* Check the label for fat, fiber and sodium contents. Low-fat is defined as less than or equal to 3 grams of fat per serving. Foods that are a good source of fiber have 2.5 or more grams per serving. Low-sodium foods have 140 milligrams or less per serving.*

### Anatomy of a grain

**Endosperm**—makes up the majority of the seed and is where you find most of the protein, carbohydrate and small amounts of vitamins and minerals.

**Germ**—the part from which a new plant sprouts, and where you find B vitamins, trace minerals and some protein.

**Bran**—the outer layer of the grain seed, which is full of B vitamins, trace minerals and fiber.

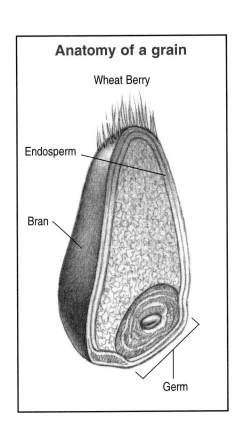

**Anatomy of a grain**

Wheat Berry

Endosperm

Bran

Germ

If you eat a typical American diet, you consume only about half of the fiber you should. Aim for between 20 and 35 grams of fiber a day from food, not from supplements (see page 180.) Fiber supplements don't provide the other nutrients found in grains, vegetables and fruits that your body needs. The new Nutrition Facts labeling makes it easier to figure out which foods are good sources of fiber, because manufacturers are required to show the total amount of dietary fiber per serving.

Increase your fiber intake gradually, so that your body can adjust to the bulk. If you eat too much fiber before your body is accustomed to it, you may experience bloating and gas. Be sure to drink plenty of fluids—about 8 glasses of water a day. Because fiber absorbs up to 15 times its weight in water, inadequate fluid intake—if you're on a diet high in fiber—can lead to constipation and may cause intestinal blockage.

### Vital vegetables!

Eat 3 to 5 servings of vegetables every day. A serving is 1 cup of leafy vegetables, 1/2 cup of other vegetables (cooked or raw), 3/4 cup (6 ounces) of vegetable juice.

### Choosing vegetables

| | |
| --- | --- |
| Best choices | Fresh, plain frozen, canned* or dried vegetables |
| Go easy on | Olives* |
| Limit or avoid | Vegetables with cream or heavy sauces, butter or dips |

*These are higher in sodium. Buy canned vegetables with no added salt if you must limit your sodium intake.*

Studies show that vegetables are more important than just acting as replacements for foods that are high in fat, saturated fat and cholesterol. Phytochemicals, substances found in plants, may help prevent cardiovascular disease and some cancers. Some known phytochemicals include antioxidants (see page 185), plant sterols (see page 188), isoflavones (see page 197) and allicin (see page 187). Researchers are identifying many more phytochemicals and their roles in maintaining health and fighting disease. Others are yet to be discovered.

Vegetables are sources of folic acid and vitamin B-6, two vitamins that decrease homocysteine levels in your blood (see page 185). Because high homocysteine levels are linked to increased risk for heart and vascular disease, scientists believe that folic acid and vitamin B-6 may protect your heart. Good vegetable sources of these B vitamins appear on page 186.

Vegetables contain no cholesterol and are naturally low in fat, sodium and calories. They also are high in fiber. You can improve your diet easily without cutting back on the volume of food you eat by eating more vegetables in place of foods that have more fat and calories. You'll find there is a wonderful array of flavors in vegetables. Try a new one each week, find your favorites, and treat yourself often.

Fresh vegetables are best, but frozen vegetables are great, too. Most canned vegetables are high in sodium, because sodium is used as a preservative in the canning process. If you use canned vegetables, look for labels that indicate that no salt is added.

Don't smother vegetables in fats (butter, margarine, oils), high-fat salad dressings or rich creams. Steam vegetables or cook them in a microwave oven with a small amount of water. This helps preserve the vegetables' natural flavors, and you won't need butter or sauces. Experiment with different spices, herbs and flavored vinegars to add zest to vegetables.

You can also enjoy eating many vegetables raw. Keep celery, carrots, cauli-flower, broccoli, cherry tomatoes, bell peppers and other raw vegetables ready to eat in the refrigerator, and reach for them when you have the urge to snack. Select commercial dips that are low in fat—or nonfat. You can also make your own with low-fat or nonfat yogurt or cottage cheese mixed with various herbs and seasonings.

### Fit fruits!

Eat 2 to 4 servings of fruit every day. A serving is 1 medium-sized piece of fresh fruit, 1/2 cup chopped or canned fruit, 3/4 cup (6 ounces) of fruit juice.

Like vegetables, fruits are great sources of soluble fiber (see page 181), vitamins, minerals and phytochemicals (see page 194). They are low in calories and virtually free of fat (except for avocado), so they help you control your weight and reduce your risk for developing diabetes and high blood pressure. Fruits and vegetables are an integral part of the DASH diet (see page 179), which can significantly reduce blood pressure in people with borderline or high blood pressure—in some cases enough to reduce or eliminate the need for medication.

Fruits make tasty snacks. If you get the urge to munch on something between meals—or if you have a sweet tooth that just won't quit—keep a bowl of fresh fruit nearby. Citrus fruits are an excellent source of vitamin C, an antioxidant that may help protect your heart (see page 185). Citrus fruits are also high in folic acid. One word of caution: Some people with high triglyceride levels may not be able to eat all the fruit they want because of its natural sugar content.

### Low-fat milk, yogurt and cheese, please!

Eat 2 to 3 servings of low-fat or nonfat milk, yogurt or cheese every day. A serving is 1 cup of milk or yogurt, $1^1/_2$ ounces of natural cheese, 2 ounces of processed cheese.

Dairy products do not have to be a significant source of fat and cholesterol in your diet. You can still get the benefits of milk products by choosing low-fat or nonfat varieties. Many people have the mistaken notion that skim milk products are not as nutritious as those made from whole milk. Actually, except for the lower amount of fat, calories and cholesterol in skim milk, there is little difference between the two. Try skim milk, low-fat or nonfat yogurt and reduced-fat cheeses.

Milk and dairy foods are an important part of your diet. They are an excellent source of calcium. Calcium is especially important for children, because it promotes

| Choosing fruits | |
| --- | --- |
| Best choices | Fresh, frozen, canned or dried fruits |
| Go easy on | Avocado (high in fat—primarily monounsaturated) |
| Limit or avoid | Coconut, fruits in cream or heavy sauces |

| Choosing dairy products | |
| --- | --- |
| Best choices | Nonfat (skim, fat-free, zero-fat or no-fat), low-fat, light or "little fat" (1/2 to 1 percent) milk; nonfat (fat-free) yogurt; low-fat cheese*; low-fat (1 to 2 percent) cottage cheese*; buttermilk made from skim, or 1 percent fat milk; nonfat or low-fat soy milk or soy yogurt |
| Go easy on | Reduced-fat (2 percent) milk, ice milk, creamed cottage cheese (4 percent fat), part-skim-milk cheeses (mozzarella, ricotta, farmer cheese,* reduced-fat yogurt, buttermilk |
| Limit or avoid | Whole milk, cheese* or yogurt made from whole milk, ice cream |

*Check labels for fat and sodium contents. Low-fat is defined as less than or equal to 3 grams of fat per serving. Low-sodium foods have 140 milligrams or less per serving.*

bone growth. And it's also important for both women and some men because, as they grow older, the risk for osteoporosis (a degenerative bone disease) increases. Milk is fortified with vitamin D, which helps your body use calcium.

Some dairy products are higher than others in fat, cholesterol and calories. These are whole milk and reduced-fat dairy products. By choosing skim milk instead of whole milk, for instance, you can save 8 grams of fat, 35 milligrams of cholesterol and 65 calories per serving (see Boning up on milk math). Instead of eating a slice of regular American cheese, you can cut the fat in half and reduce the calories by three fourths by choosing reduced-fat American cheese.

### Boning up on milk math

|  | Fat (grams) | Saturated fat (grams) | Cholesterol (milligrams) | Calories |
|---|---|---|---|---|
| Whole milk (3.5 percent fat) | 8 | 5 | 34 | 150 |
| Reduced-fat milk (2 percent fat) | 5 | 3 | 18 | 120 |
| Low-fat milk (1 percent fat) | 3 | 2 | 10 | 100 |
| Nonfat (skim) milk | 0 | 0 | 4 | 85 |

Beware! Imitation milk products, such as nondairy creamers, can be high in fat and saturated fat. Read the label, because calories and saturated fat can add up fast with such products. Stay far away from milk substitutes that contain coconut oil, palm oil or palm kernel oil, since these are very high in saturated fat.

Consider trying soy milk and soy yogurt as a complement to or substitute for dairy products. Soy milk is the liquid from soaked, ground and strained soybeans. Because of their isoflavones (see page 197), these products can be a healthy addition to your diet. Use soy milk in cereal or in recipes that call for milk, such as creams or sauces, or drink it as a flavored beverage by mixing it with fruit in a blender. You can also use it to make lower-fat custards or add to pancake or waffle mixes.

### Meats and their mighty substitutes!

Eat 2 to 3 servings of lean meats, poultry, fish, dried beans, eggs or nuts every day. A serving is 2 to 3 ounces of cooked lean meat, skinless poultry or fish (no larger than the size of a deck of cards). Note that 1/2 cup of cooked dried beans, 1 egg, 2 tablespoons of peanut butter, or 1/3 cup of nuts counts as 1 ounce of meat.

### Choosing meat, poultry, fish and beans

| Best choices | Lean meats ("select" or "choice" grade), fish, poultry (without the skin), egg whites or egg substitutes, tuna or salmon* (packed in water), peanut butter, nuts* dried beans, lentils |
|---|---|
| Go easy on | Low-fat cold cuts,* low-fat hot dogs,* fish (canned in oil)*, oysters, shrimp, egg yolks |
| Limit or avoid | Organ meat, fatty and heavily marbled meats, spare ribs, cold cuts, hot dogs, sausage, bacon, fried meats |

*Check the label for fat and sodium contents. Low-fat is defined as less than or equal to 3 grams of fat per serving. Low-sodium foods have 140 milligrams or less per serving.*

This food group sounds like a mouthful—meat, poultry, fish, dried beans, eggs, nuts. What's really the point here? Simply put, this is the food group from which you get most of your dietary protein. Your body needs protein to build and maintain body tissues, to produce hormones, enzymes, antibodies, and various fluids and body secretions and to help maintain normal body fluid pressure. Studies show that you can meet your body's protein needs by eating a varied diet that emphasizes vegetables, grains and legumes (dried beans, peas, lentils). You don't need much, if any, animal protein. Most Americans eat too much protein.

Meat, poultry and fish are also important sources of B vitamins (including B-12, which is only found naturally in animal foods), iron and zinc. But because some of these foods are high in fat, saturated fat and cholesterol, eat them in moderation.

You may want to make three changes, when you choose from this group.

1. Try more meatless meals. Plan meals around meat substitutes, such as legumes. Legumes are low in fat and contain no cholesterol, but are high in protein and fiber. Choose from black beans, butter beans, kidney beans, lima beans, navy beans, pinto beans, baked beans, black-eyed peas (cowpeas), chickpeas (garbanzo beans), lentils, split peas, soybeans and soy products (see below). In addition to being an excellent source of high-quality protein, soybeans contain isoflavones, naturally occurring plant estrogens that behave similarly to human estrogen and may have benefits for your heart. Combine legumes with whole grains for a high-fiber, high-protein, low-fat, low-cholesterol meal. Try bean tacos, meatless chili and corn bread, rice and beans, and hummus and low-fat crackers.

## Using your bean!

Try adding several of these soy products to your daily diet.

| | |
|---|---|
| Soybeans | Soybeans contain more plant estrogen than prepared soy foods. To soften the dried beans, soak them overnight, then cook them for $2\frac{1}{2}$ hours. Add beans to your favorite chili or baked bean recipe, stir-fry or pasta sauce. Fresh (frozen) soybeans may be steamed or lightly sautéed in water. |
| Tempeh and miso | Both are made from fermented soybeans. Tempeh is available in a thin cake, while miso is a paste. Find recipe ideas on the packaging. Next to soybeans, these are the highest in plant estrogens. |
| Soy milk | Use soy milk on cereal or in recipes that call for milk—or enjoy it, flavored, as a snack. |
| Soy flour | Substitute for up to 20 percent of the total flour in baked goods. Replace eggs in baking recipes by substituting 1 tablespoon of soy flour and 2 tablespoons of water for each egg. |
| Tofu | A curd that's made from soybeans in a process similar to that used for making cheese. Because it has a bland taste and spongy texture, it's a good flavor chameleon, absorbing flavors of other foods around it. Use it in stir-fry dishes or scramble it like an egg. When it's frozen, you can crumble it into recipes that call for ground meat. |
| Textured soy protein (TSP) | Available in the frozen food section, TSP looks like browned meat and can be used in foods such as tacos, chili and meatloaf. Also in the frozen food section: soy burgers. |

*Note: Soy sauce doesn't contain healthful amounts of soy and is very high in sodium.*

Eggs can also stand in for meat. But even though eggs are rich in protein and relatively low in calories, don't forget that they're also high in cholesterol (found in the yolks). Limit your egg yolk consumption to three or four a week. When you make scrambled eggs, discard half the egg yolks. Substitute two egg whites for each whole egg in most baked products. You may also choose a commercial egg substitute, which has no cholesterol, for cooking or for making scrambled eggs, omelets or quiches.

2. Next, reduce the amount of meat you eat to the recommended serving size. The American Heart Association recommends no more than 6 ounces of lean meat, fish or poultry daily. One way to adjust to this change is to shift your meal planning from making meat the centerpiece to making meat the

## Lower-fat meat choices

These meats are good choices, when you're limiting fat and cholesterol in your diet. All figures below are for a 3-ounce serving with all visible fat removed. No fat was added in preparing the meats. (Figures are rounded.)

| Name of cut | Calories | Fat (grams) | Cholesterol (mg) |
| --- | --- | --- | --- |
| **Beef** (lean only, choice grade) | | | |
| Top round steak, broiled | 165 | 6 | 70 |
| Eye of round, roasted | 160 | 6 | 60 |
| Tip round, roasted | 165 | 7 | 70 |
| Sirloin, broiled | 180 | 8 | 75 |
| Tenderloin, broiled | 180 | 8 | 70 |
| Bottom round, braised | 190 | 8 | 80 |
| Chuck arm pot roast, braised | 200 | 9 | 90 |
| **Pork** (lean only) | | | |
| Tenderloin, roasted | 140 | 4 | 80 |
| Ham, boneless, water added, extra lean (about 5 percent fat) | 110 | 4 | 40 |
| Center loin chop, broiled | 200 | 9 | 80 |
| **Poultry** (roasted) | | | |
| Turkey, light meat, without skin | 130 | 2 | 60 |
| Chicken breast, without skin | 140 | 3 | 70 |
| Chicken drumstick, without skin | 150 | 5 | 80 |
| Chicken breast, meat and skin | 170 | 7 | 70 |
| Chicken drumstick, meat and skin | 180 | 9 | 80 |
| **Fish, shellfish** (baked or broiled) | | | |
| Cod | 90 | 1 | 50 |
| Lobster, boiled | 100 | 1 | 100 |
| Shrimp (steamed or boiled) | 110 | 2 | 160 |
| Tuna, light, canned in water | 90 | 2 | 30 |
| Halibut | 120 | 2 | 30 |
| Salmon, Atlantic/coho | 150 | 7 | 50 |

*Note: Venison (deer, elk, mouse caribou, antelope) and lamb are also good choices. Avoid marbled steak cuts such as filet mignon, T-bone, and New York strip.*

accompaniment. Prepare more casseroles or mixtures with meat as one of the ingredients. Reducing the amount of meat you eat will become easier if you increase your consumption of grains, vegetables and fruits.

3. Finally, switch to leaner cuts of the meats you eat. For instance, instead of ground beef, switch to well-trimmed round steak, or try the chicken breast rather than the leg or thigh. Generally, fish, chicken (remove the skin before eating) and well-trimmed pork are somewhat lower in fat than beef. But you don't need to give up on beef. Some cuts are nearly as low in fat as dark-meat chicken.

Red meats. U.S. Department of Agriculture (USDA) meat grades tell you about the amount of fat in beef. USDA Prime beef has the highest proportion of fat, USDA Choice beef has less fat than Prime, and USDA Select grade has an even lower amount. Even if you closely trim a piece of meat, particles of fat that are interspersed in the meat (called marbling) contribute to the fat content. The amount of marbling is one of the factors considered in grading beef. The same amount of Prime beef may have nearly twice as much fat as Select beef. The amount of cholesterol, on the other hand, is fairly equal among the various grades, because cholesterol is found in the muscle portion of the meat, rather than in the fat.

Poultry. Unless you eat the giblets—the liver, heart and gizzard, which have a high amount of cholesterol—you're fairly safe with chicken and turkey, as long as you don't prepare them with added fat. Poultry is low in fat. Since most of the fat is in the skin, if you remove the skin before you eat it you cut the fat by about half. The lowest amounts of total fat and saturated fat are in the skinless white meat. Ground turkey can be a lower-fat alternative to ground beef, if the skin is not ground with the meat. Ask the butcher or read the label before you buy it.

Fish. Fish is one of the lowest-fat meats you can choose. Even the fish with the highest fat content compare favorably with the leanest cuts of red meat and poultry. Seafood contains little saturated fat, too. As noted earlier in this chapter, fish also contains omega-3 polyunsaturated fatty acids, which are associated with lower triglyceride levels, lower blood pressure, a reduced risk of blood clotting and a decreased risk for abnormal heart rhythms and sudden death. For these reasons, you should include various types of fish on your menu at least twice a week.

In the past, experts believed that some types of shellfish have very high cholesterol and as a result didn't recommend them as part of a heart-healthy diet. However, new measuring techniques show that their cholesterol content is similar to that of lean beef and poultry. Of the shellfish—clams, crab, lobster, oysters, scallops and shrimp—shrimp contains the most cholesterol, but is very low in fat. A 1996 study suggests that the elevation in blood total cholesterol levels associated with a diet rich in shrimp may be due to an increase in good HDL cholesterol.

### Fats, oils and sweets

Use them with care. Fats, oils and sweets are located at the small tip of the Food Guide Pyramid to indicate that you should eat these foods sparingly. You don't need to eliminate them entirely to make your diet healthful. But keep in mind that these foods are high in calories, yet contribute few essential nutrients.

| Choosing fats | | |
|---|---|---|
| Best choices (in small amounts) | Monounsaturated oils (olive, canola or peanut oil); polyunsaturated oils (safflower, corn, sunflower, soybean, sesame or cottonseed); salad dressings made with unsaturated oils; tub margarine with the first ingredient listed as liquid oil | |
| Go easy on | Mayonnaise, creamy salad dressings, reduced-fat sour cream or cream cheese, stick margarine | |
| Limit or avoid | Saturated fats (butter, lard, bacon, fat, gravy and cream sauces, cream, half-and-half, sour cream, cream cheese, shortening, cocoa butter, coconut oil, palm oil, palm kernel oil, most nondairy creamers | |

Check labels for fat and sodium contents. Low-fat is defined as less than or equal to 3 grams of fat per serving. Low-sodium foods have 140 milligrams or less per serving.

Fats and oils. The fats you add to foods basically fit into one of the main categories of fats: monounsaturated, polyunsaturated and saturated. When you add fat to a food—for any reason—remember to use small amounts. Your best choice is one that is high in monounsaturated fat, such as olive oil, canola oil or peanut oil. Polyunsaturated fats are acceptable too, and include safflower, sunflower, corn and soybean. Limit your use of saturated fats—such as butter, lard and tropical oils (coconut, palm and palm kernel oils)—because they increase your cholesterol levels.

Salad bars can be a good place to get a variety of healthful, fresh vegetables and fruits. But don't go overboard with salad dressing. One tablespoon of regular salad dressing contains 6 to 9 grams of fat—equivalent to about two pats of butter or margarine. Salad dressings are also high in sodium. To reduce fat and calories, choose one of the lower-fat or fat-free salad dressings that also have reduced sodium.

Margarine is less saturated than butter and contains no cholesterol. The softer (more liquid) the margarine, the more unsaturated it is. Tub margarines are softer than stick margarines, and liquid margarines are softer than tub margarines. But the important thing to remember is that your choice of a fatty spread is less important than the total amount you consume.

No matter what its chemical structure, fat is fat. All three types provide 9 calories per gram. Whether it's olive oil, margarine, or butter, a tablespoon contains about 14 grams of fat and 125 calories. Too much fat of any kind can contribute to extra weight (body fat), which can increase your risk for diabetes, hypertension and early death, among other conditions.

Desserts and sweets. Choose them wisely, use them sparingly.

Don't attempt to give up desserts and sweets entirely. But be smart about your selections and portion sizes. Traditional desserts and sweets are a major source of calories (and often of fats, too), yet they contribute very few other beneficial nutrients to your overall diet. The first worthwhile change you might make is to

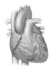

**HEALTHY HEART♥TIP**

*You want your kids to make heart-healthy food choices. The best way to get them on the right track is to set an example.*

*Children acquire eating habits in the same way they assimilate other vital behaviors—by emulation. To make sure they're doing what you want them to do, take an inventory of your own eating habits. Even by choosing healthful snacks— carrot sticks or a crisp apple instead of full-fat ice cream or cinnamon buns—you encourage your children to do the same.*

avoid keeping desserts and sweets that are high in fat and calories at home routinely. Getting rid of the temptation before it can cause a problem is both easy and effective.

Another technique that some people find helpful is to plan ahead. Think about upcoming situations in which you will be tempted to splurge—a reception, a family birthday, a special anniversary, your retirement party. Then, do some extra exercise that week, eat a little less that day, and enjoy the pleasure of eating the dessert. Consult the sidebar for suggestions on acceptable desserts that you can have sparingly.

| Desserts and sweets | |
| --- | --- |
| Best choices | Angel food cake, vanilla wafers, fig bar cookies, sherbet |
| Go easy on | Cakes, cookies, muffins and other bakery products made with polyunsaturated fats |
| Limit or avoid | Rich baked goods, such as pies, cakes, cookies, donuts, commercial sweet rolls, pastries and muffins |

If you have high triglycerides, you should be very careful about eating desserts and sweets, because increased amounts of sugar and calories in your diet can further elevate your triglyceride level. If your triglyceride level is high, you can usually reduce it by:

- Losing weight and then maintaining a healthy weight
- Cutting back significantly on sugar and foods that contain sugar. The sugar in beverages—sweetened soft drinks, coffee or tea, for example—can add up quickly. It's even important to keep your intake of fruit and fruit juice at a reasonable level, because they contain sugar naturally
- Drinking less alcohol
- Increasing your level of physical activity (see page 207)

Low-fat and reduced-fat foods. Just because some of the fat is gone doesn't mean the calories are gone, too. When you check the label, you'll often find that a reduced-fat snack you're eating still has a significant amount of calories—sometimes even as much as the food they're replacing. Pay attention to the label, especially the serving size and total calorie content, so that you don't wind up with more calories than you intended.

### Alcohol

Drink in moderation, if at all.

Earlier in this chapter you learned that moderate alcohol consumption may help lower your risk for coronary artery disease (see page 182). The benefits accompany only light drinking, defined as no more than 1 drink per day for women and 2 for men. But don't forget that alcohol itself, as well as alcohol mixers, contains calories. A 2.5-ounce martini has about 155 calories, while a 2-ounce Manhattan has 130 calories. A 12-ounce beer has about 150 calories, and a 4-ounce glass of white or red wine has about 80 to 85 calories. Even wine coolers tip the scale at more than 200 calories for a 12-ounce serving. To conserve calories, you can try light beer (100 calories) or nonalcoholic beer (60 calories). Or, make your own wine spritzer by adding club soda to half a glass of wine.

## Quick shopping tips

- Plan a week's worth of menus and prepare a shopping list of ingredients you'll need.
- Buy only the items on your list.
- Don't shop when you're hungry.
- Shop when you have time to read food labels.
- When possible, select fresh foods rather than mixes or ready-to-eat foods. This enables you to control the ingredients that are added.
- Shop the perimeter of the store. Many grocery stores place some of the most healthful foods on the convenient perimeter aisles.
- Be an informed shopper.

## Shopping guide

The grocery store is the site of many decisions you make about eating healthfully. If you plan ahead, you can select ingredients and prepared foods that fit into a heart-healthy lifestyle. Without planning, it's easy to slip back to your old way of eating or to stock up on impulse buys.

The Quick shopping tips guide (left) helps you make wise choices in the grocery store. It also makes meal preparation easier.

### Making food labels and the Food Guide Pyramid work for you

New federal regulations developed in the 1990s mean that most foods in the grocery store have food labels with specified nutrition information. The easy-to-read format of the "Nutrition Facts" panel helps you find more quickly the information you need to make healthful choices. Serving sizes are standardized to reflect not only the amounts people actually eat, but also to make nutritional comparisons of similar products easier. Listings contain crucial information on the amount of nutrients of major health concern (per serving)—saturated fat, cholesterol, dietary fiber and others. You can use the Percent Daily Value references to see how a food fits into your overall daily diet. For example, if a serving contains 12 grams of fat, the label shows you that this amount represents 18 percent of the daily limit for fat.

The Percent Daily Value information on food labels is based on a daily diet of 2,000 calories. While this was chosen as an average level, it's not appropriate for everyone. To determine the level appropriate for you, consult the table below.

## How much do you need each day?

| | Many women, older adults | Most children, teen girls, active women, most men | Teen boys, active men |
|---|---|---|---|
| Calorie level | About 1,600 | About 2,200 | About 2,800 |
| Grain group servings | 6 | 9 | 11 |
| Vegetable group servings | 3 | 4 | 5 |
| Fruit group servings | 2 | 3 | 4 |
| Milk group servings | 2 or 3* | 2 or 3* | 2 or 3* |
| Meat group servings | 2 (5 ounces total) | 2 (6 ounces total) | 3 (7 ounces total) |
| Total fat (grams) | 53 | 73 | 93 |

*Women who are pregnant or breastfeeding, teenagers, and young adults to age 24 need 3 servings.*

When you shop, the most important thing to remember is to choose plenty of plant foods and go easy on animal foods. This helps put the Food Guide Pyramid to work for you. It helps you cut fat intake quickly, since many animal foods contain more fat than plant foods. Initially, keeping track of the fat grams listed on the labels of the foods you eat will help you determine which foods fit best into your overall diet. Eventually, you won't need to count fat grams every day, but doing a "fat checkup" once in a while will help keep you on the right track.

### 'Low-fat,' 'reduced fat' and 'light' foods

In terms of fat, foods with these claims on their labels are better choices than their counterparts with the regular amount of fat. If your weight is normal, they're probably acceptable. However, if you need to lose weight, they may not be appropriate for you, because these foods often contain nearly as many calories as their counterparts with the regular amount of fat.

But don't get caught up in one-word descriptors and advertising hype designed to catch your eye. The most meaningful parts of a food label are the figures shown for calories, fat, saturated fat, cholesterol and sodium—and the ingredient list. Manufacturers are required to list all of the ingredients used in the product by weight, from the most to the least. Once you know your daily limits of calories, fat, cholesterol and sodium, you'll be in a much better position to compare products and to choose those that fit your desire to eat more healthfully.

### 'Low' nutrient content claims

The term "low" can be used for one or more of these components: fat, saturated fat, cholesterol, sodium and calories. The term "very low" can only be used for sodium. The descriptors are defined as follows:

- Low-fat: 3 grams or less per serving
- Low saturated fat: 1 gram or less per serving
- Low sodium: 140 milligrams or less per serving
- Very low sodium: 35 milligrams or less per serving
- Low cholesterol: 20 milligrams or less and 2 grams or less of saturated fat per serving
- Low calorie: 40 calories or less per serving

Synonyms for "low" include "little," "few," "low source of" and "contains a small amount of."

## Cooking

A few simple changes in your food preparation methods will also help you improve your heart's health. One of the most important changes you can make in the kitchen is to learn to cook with little or no oils or other fats. These tips can help:

1. Check cookbooks, magazines and newspapers for low-fat recipes that provide a nutritional analysis.

2. Invest in nonstick cookware, so you can fry or brown foods without added fat. Or use a 1-second spray of vegetable oil cooking spray, which adds only about a gram of fat and few calories.

3. Stock and use fat-free flavor enhancers such as onions, herbs and spices, colorful fresh peppers, fresh garlic, ginger root, Dijon mustard, fresh lemons and limes, flavored vinegars, sherry or other wines, soy sauce, bouillon granules, and plain nonfat yogurt.

4. Microwave or steam vegetables. Then dress them up with flavored vinegars, herbs, spices, or powders that have a buttery flavor. (If sodium is a concern, choose flavor enhancers that are also low in sodium.)

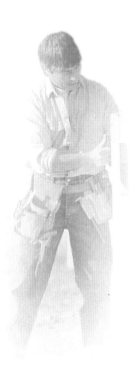

5. Poach fish or skinless poultry in broth, vegetable juice, flavored vinegars or wine. Add herbs or spices, too. A covered roasting pan is an inexpensive alternative to a fish poacher.

6. Cut the amount of meat in casseroles and stews by a third to a half and add more vegetables, whole grain rice or pasta.

7. Substitute low-fat sour cream, processed cheeses or cream cheese for their higher-fat counterparts that recipes may suggest.

## Eating out

You probably don't think of eating out as shopping—but it really is. Some considerations help you shop for appropriate restaurants. Once you're there, other strategies can help you make healthful selections.

Although you have less control over how food is prepared and what ingredients are used when you eat out, you can control your selections of where, what and how much you eat. Opt for restaurants that offer:

- Choices in types of foods. Greater variety means greater possibility for low-fat selections and more fruits, vegetables and grains.

- Choice in cooking methods. Ask for items that are prepared without added fat. This can save 100 to 300 calories and 10 to 30 grams of fat per entrée.

- Choice in portion size. Smaller portions can mean fewer calories and less fat. You also can ask up front to have half of your entree wrapped to go, so there's less on your plate. Tomorrow's lunch is prepared!

Cut back on fat. Even small amounts of fat may add unwanted calories. Specify low-fat cooking methods, such as baking, broiling, boiling, roasting, grilling, steaming and poaching. Order sauces on the side. Control portion sizes of foods that contain fat—especially meats and fatty sauces.

Limit your alcohol intake to one or two drinks per day. Alcoholic beverages add significant calories but no nutrients. Excessive amounts of alcohol are harmful. However, there's evidence that moderate alcohol consumption is associated with a lower risk for coronary artery disease in some people. Moderation is defined as no more than two drinks per day for men and 1 drink per day for women.

## The bottom line

Improving your diet can be as easy as adding more grains, vegetables and fruits and cutting back on animal products, such as meat (especially red meat) and dairy products that are high in fat. Add more meals styled after Mediterranean, Asian or vegetarian diets to your weekly pattern. Try a new food every week: a grain, a vegetable or fruit, or a new food product made from soy. Try new preparation methods. And don't forget about enhancing the flavors of your foods with herbs and spices.

The next time you're in a bookstore, look for a new, healthful cookbook. There are many creative, tasty and healthful recipes that can help you shift your eating habits—and those of your family—toward a more plant-based diet. *The Mayo Clinic*

*Williams-Sonoma Cookbook,* published in 1998, for example, offers simple solutions for eating well. It contains 140 recipes that feature a wealth of grains, vegetables, fruits, seafood, poultry and lean meats, as well as tips for planning meals, shopping and cooking.

### A healthful attitude about eating

Don't be rigid with your diet every minute of your life. An indulgence every now and then in your plan to eat more healthfully is not a tragedy, and it should not turn into an excuse for giving up. If you overindulge once in a while, you can balance things out over the long term. What is important is that you eat right most of the time. Then it becomes a habit, and good habits can be as difficult to break as bad ones. Once you notice how good you feel and how enjoyable healthful eating can be, eating right will be a habit you won't want to break.

## How to improve your cholesterol level

Three main avenues can help you achieve and maintain cholesterol levels that minimize your risk of future coronary artery disease: diet, exercise and medication. The first two are nearly universally advisable. Even small changes may be very important in improving your personal coronary risk—and from a public health standpoint. Furthermore, you can achieve small changes at a very low economic cost. If your lipid profile is not very abnormal, you can still reduce your risk.

On the average, moderate dietary measures can reduce your cholesterol level by about 10 percent. Some people respond even more impressively. If your cholesterol is strongly influenced by genetics, changes in diet and exercise may not be enough to improve your blood cholesterol levels.

### How can I lower my cholesterol with dietary changes?

Dietary changes are an important aspect of cholesterol management. See pages 173 to 175 for more complete information on dietary changes you can make to reduce your total blood cholesterol. The key concepts in making dietary changes to lower cholesterol are to reduce your total fat (especially saturated fat) and cholesterol intake and to lose weight, especially if your triglyceride level is elevated. Serious dietary changes can lower LDL cholesterol levels 25 percent or more.

New research shows that a subgroup of individuals with high levels of "bad" LDL cholesterol will experience a very marked drop in LDL cholesterol levels with a low-fat diet. The decrease in LDL cholesterol levels in most clinical trials using moderate dietary programs (less than 30 percent of calories from fat) has generally been less than 10 percent. However, highly motivated

HEALTHY
HEART ♥ TIP

*Many researchers believe that vitamin E can slow the development of atherosclerosis. It also inhibits lipoprotein oxidation, which can lead to a build-up of arterial plaque. Some evidence suggests that vitamin C may be beneficial because it also inhibits oxidation.*

patients who adhere to diets that are very low in fat can experience excellent results with a 50 percent reduction.

Another subgroup may experience a rise in "good" HDL cholesterol level. Interestingly, individuals who are at the greatest risk for heart attack and stroke due to two major genetic variants of hyperlipidemia may benefit the most from the cholesterol-lowering effects of a low-fat diet.

## The effect of exercise on cholesterol

Regular aerobic exercise often offers the benefit of reducing blood triglyceride levels and increasing the proportion of your total cholesterol that is made up of HDL cholesterol. Total LDL cholesterol improves slightly or usually stays the same with exercise. However, you can often improve the ratio of LDL cholesterol to HDL cholesterol.

The appeal of increased activity and dietary changes is that, in addition to improving lipid levels, they can also contribute to lowering other cardiovascular risks such as obesity and high blood pressure. Changing your exercise habits and diet usually doesn't require an all-or-nothing approach. Anyone with the knowledge of what to do and the desire to do it can make healthful changes that can rapidly become second nature.

## What about medications that reduce cholesterol?

Although it was clearly established by the 1980s that high cholesterol levels were major risk factors for coronary artery disease, cholesterol-reducing drugs available at that time had only a modest effect on lowering cholesterol levels. In addition, they were often associated with side effects that made it difficult for patients to take the drugs.

In the past 10 years, however, the treatment of elevated cholesterol levels has been revolutionized by the introduction of a group of drugs known as the statins. The fact that these drugs are effective—and have few side effects—has widened the group of patients who will benefit from treatment, according to treatment objectives published by the National Cholesterol Education Program expert panel (see page 157).

If periodic rechecks of lipid levels show little response to changes in diet and exercise, your doctor may recommend medications to lower your lipid levels. Some medications have their greatest effect on "bad" LDL cholesterol, others on triglycerides and others on "good" HDL cholesterol. Despite the benefits they potentially offer, medications are reserved for people for whom diet and activity alone are not sufficiently successful or for people with more severe hyperlipidemia.

There are several reasons to be conservative in the use of medications. All entail an expense. There is always the potential for side effects, and occasionally they can be severe. Taking medications is at least a little disruptive of your daily routine. Nevertheless, if other measures have failed, you may need to take medication.

The decision to use a medication is a decision best made jointly by you and your physician. These factors enter into the decision:

- The severity of the cholesterol or triglyceride abnormalities
- Evidence of existing coronary artery disease
- The presence of other risk factors that you can't modify (such as a family history of heart attacks at a young age)
- Ineffectiveness of dietary and exercise changes

As a rule, the use of medications is advisable if you have two risk factors or if there is already evidence of coronary disease and dietary measures have not succeeded in moving your lipid profile out of the higher-risk range.

One aspect of evaluating and treating high cholesterol and triglyceride levels is to determine whether they may be caused by another problem that needs treatment. High blood lipids can be caused by low thyroid function, diabetes, kidney disease and liver disease.

The variety of drugs that can help lower serum cholesterol and triglycerides includes niacin, fibrates, and bile acid sequestrants (see page 363). One recent study showed that gemfibrozil (Lopid) was moderately effective in raising the HDL cholesterol level and in reducing heart attacks and cardiac deaths in people with normal total cholesterol levels. Some may be effective, but none are as powerful as the statins for lowering LDL cholesterol and total cholesterol levels. Physicians often prescribe niacin, fibrates, and bile acid sequestrants together with the statins or in particular situations in which the goal is primarily to lower elevated triglyceride levels or to raise HDL cholesterol. Fibric acid preparations include clofibrate, gemfibrozil and fenofibrate. Bile acid sequestrants include cholestyramine and colestipol.

## Becoming more active

If you begin to exert yourself a little more than usual—and do it regularly—your body is designed to respond by improving its capacity for exercise. By gradually increasing the amount of exercise you perform, you can noticeably improve your fitness level in 8 to 12 weeks.

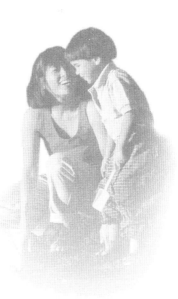

If you want to become fit, it's not necessary to engage in extremely strenuous exercise. A moderate amount of daily physical activity can improve your fitness level. You'll probably stay with a moderate level of activity more faithfully than you will with overly strenuous exercise. You'll benefit, whether your activity is in longer sessions of moderately intense activity (such as 30 minutes of brisk walking) or in shorter sessions (perhaps as short as 10 minutes, three or more times a day). And you benefit just as much if your week's activity is broken down into three sessions during the week.

Although current guidelines recommend 30 minutes of daily activity, this doesn't have to be formal exercise. Activities such as yard work qualify. You gain additional health benefits from greater amounts of activity. Build up gradually and avoid excessive amounts that can lead to injury.

## Examples of aerobic activities

Walking
Jogging
Cycling
Swimming
Rowing
Cross-country skiing
Stair-climbing
Dancing

Aerobic exercises increase your cardiovascular fitness. Aerobic activities are those in which the demand for oxygen and nourishment by your exercising muscles does not surpass the ability of your lungs and circulatory system to supply it. It consists of continuous, rhythmic contracting of your large muscle groups.

Aerobic exercise increases the rate and depth of your breathing. Your body becomes warmer, and if you exercise long enough and vigorously enough, you will perspire. However, aerobic exercises are not so intense that the need of your muscle cells for oxygen exceeds their supply. This deficiency may occur with such activities as isometric exercise or weight-lifting—activities that may increase muscle tone and bulk but are not clearly beneficial from a cardiovascular standpoint.

## Before you start

For most people, the health advantages of regular exercise far outweigh any risks. However, if you have any chronic health conditions or several major risk factors for heart disease (such as smoking, high blood pressure, high blood cholesterol, diabetes), some special precautions may apply.

It's a good idea to check with your doctor before you begin an exercise program if you:

- Have heart or lung disease, diabetes, arthritis, or kidney disease

- Are age 40 or older

- Are very overweight

- Have parents or siblings who had evidence of coronary artery disease before age 55

- Are unsure of your health status

Your doctor may recommend that you take an exercise stress test to help determine whether exercise is likely to cause an insufficient supply of blood and oxygen to reach your heart or to provoke heart rhythm abnormalities. Discuss with your doctor any limitations that he or she would suggest because of your existing health conditions.

Discuss with your doctor your plans to start a program of physical activity. If you've previously been sedentary, plan to start with short (5- to 10-minute) sessions of physical activity and gradually build up to your desired level of activity.

## A fitness plan for your heart

You don't need to develop a formal fitness plan or sign up for organized activity (unless that's the only way you'll commit to regular conditioning). Just remember that a cardiovascular fitness program has three parts: warm-up, conditioning aerobic exercise, and cool-down. The exercise should be frequent enough, intense enough, of sufficient duration, and of the appropriate type to gradually improve your condition.

In general, try to expend about 1000 to 2000 calories a week with exercise. Walking 10 to 20 miles per week accomplishes that goal for the average person.

Unless you're trying to lose weight, there's no evidence that you'll reduce your cardiovascular risk further by exercising to burn off more than 2000 calories per week.

A warm-up phase develops and maintains muscle and joint flexibility and prepares your body for the conditioning phase of the program. The essential parts of the warm-up are stretching and endurance exercises of low intensity, which gradually increase your heart rate, body temperature and the flow of blood to your muscles.

## Three important warm-up exercises

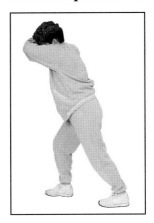 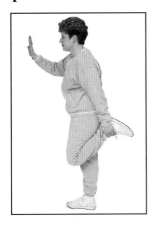 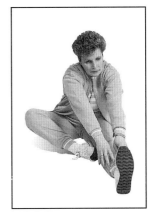

*Left: Calf stretch.*
*Starting position: Stand an arm's-length away from a wall and rest your forearms on the wall with your forehead on the back of your hands. Point your toes straight ahead. Bend your right knee and bring it toward the wall. Keep your left leg straight with your heel on the floor. Movement: Slowly move your hips forward, keeping your back straight until you feel a stretch in your left calf. Hold this position for 30 seconds and then repeat with your other leg.*

You may include muscle strengthening and toning exercises to improve your total fitness level. The warm-up phase should last 5 to 10 minutes.

The aerobic conditioning phase of your program may include any aerobic activity that requires continuous rhythmic muscle contraction of your legs and perhaps your arms. Walking, biking, swimming, jogging, cross-country skiing, rowing, rope-skipping, dancing and racket sports are good examples of aerobic exercises. Choose something that you enjoy and will want to continue.

Adjust the frequency, intensity, time and type (FITT) of your exercise program to enable you to expend the desired amount of energy to achieve your fitness goals. For example, you might walk 4 miles five times one week, and 5 miles four times another week. You may spend an hour walking 4 miles one day, but jog 4 miles in 40 minutes on another day.

## How often should you exercise?

To develop and maintain a good level of cardiovascular fitness, it's best to exercise at least three times a week on nonconsecutive days. Again, the emphasis is not on a formal exercise program, but on physical activity. If you're exercising to lose weight and improve fitness, you can increase the frequency to more days or increase the duration of your exercise to burn more calories.

*Middle: Thigh stretch. Starting position: Stand and place your right hand on a wall or a solid piece of furniture to help you balance. Reach behind you and grasp your left foot or ankle from the outside with your left hand. Movement: Slowly pull your left foot toward your buttock until you feel muscles stretch in the front of your thigh. Hold this position for 30 seconds. Then repeat it with your right leg (and right hand). If you cannot reach your foot or ankle, grasp the hem of your pants.*

*Right: Hamstring stretch. Starting position: Sit on the floor with your left leg extended straight forward and your toes pointing toward the ceiling. Bend your right knee and place the sole of your right foot on your inner left thigh. Movement: Bend forward at the waist and slowly move both hands down your left leg until you feel a stretch in the back of your left thigh. Hold the position for 30 seconds. Repeat, using your right leg.*

## Counting your pulse

Taking your pulse can help you determine whether the intensity of your exercise program is appropriate. To take your pulse, do the following.

1. Stop your exercise.

2. Place two fingers between the bone and the tendon over your radial artery on the thumb side of your wrist and exert gentle pressure. If your fingers are positioned properly, you will feel the pulsing of your artery.

3. Do not press so hard on your blood vessel that the flow of blood is blocked.

4. Count your pulse for 10 seconds and then multiply by 6 to determine your pulse rate per minute.

## The talk test

A very easy way to regulate the intensity of your exercise is to carry on a conversation with a companion. If you are too winded to talk, you are probably pushing too hard and should slow your exercise pace.

## Judging the intensity of your exercise

The intensity level of your exercise should be strenuous enough that you feel you're working, but it need not be exhausting. Exercise physiologists describe exercise intensity in terms of percentage of maximal exercise capacity. They recommend an intensity of 50 to 80 percent of your maximal exercise capacity. You can determine the intensity of your exercise by counting your pulse or using The talk test (lower left).

Many people exercising on their own use their pulse rates to determine whether their exercise is intense enough. Ask your doctor to suggest an appropriate target heart rate for you during exercise. The harder you exercise, the higher your heart rate or pulse rate climbs.

Your maximal heart rate decreases with age and is affected by cardiovascular disease and some cardiovascular medications. However, regular exercise doesn't influence your maximal heart rate. If your heart rate is very irregular, you may not be able to use the heart rate method to monitor your exercise intensity.

Another way to gauge the intensity of your exercise is to use the Borg Perceived Exertion Scale (see page 211). It rates the intensity of exercise on a scale from 6 to 20: 6 indicates a minimal level of exertion (such as sitting comfortably in a chair) and 20 corresponds to a maximal effort (such as jogging up a very steep hill). Doctors usually recommend ratings between 11 and 15 on the scale. A rating of 13 usually corresponds to 70 percent of maximal exercise capacity and is considered a good intensity for most people. If you use the scale, don't become preoccupied with any one factor, such as leg discomfort or labored breathing. Instead, try to concentrate on your overall feeling of exertion.

Unless you are or wish to become an athlete, there's no real advantage to exercising at a high intensity. You don't get major health benefits beyond moderate exercise, and you increase your risk of muscle or joint soreness or injury. A moderate exercise program shouldn't cause discomfort. If any of the following symptoms develop, stop exercising and call your doctor:

- Chest discomfort or pressure (or arm, jaw, neck or back discomfort)
- Severe shortness of breath
- A burst of very rapid or slow heart rate
- An irregular heart rate
- Excessive fatigue
- Marked joint or muscle pain
- Dizziness or fainting

## How long should you exercise?

Ideally, the duration of your exercise should be about 30 minutes, and the type of exercise, mentioned earlier, should be aerobic. However, periods of exercise less than 30 minutes are still beneficial.

If you haven't exercised for a long time, start conservatively with 5 minutes or less. Gradually increase the duration as you become accustomed to exercising.

If your goal includes weight loss, increase the duration of your exercise sessions. If you find that you enjoy exercising at a lower intensity level, you can increase the duration and still get the fitness benefits.

The last phase of your exercise program is the cool-down right after the conditioning exercise. The cool-down lets your heart rate return to pre-exercise levels gradually, prevents blood from pooling in your legs (which may cause dizziness), and stretches the muscles you've used in the conditioning activity. Walk slowly, or do some other low-intensity exercise for 3 to 5 minutes. Then do a few stretching exercises to help relax your muscles, improve or maintain flexibility, and help prevent soreness. The cool-down period usually should last 5 to 10 minutes.

## Stay motivated

No single form of aerobic exercise is best. Choose an activity that fits your personality and lifestyle. Do you like to exercise alone or in groups? If you prefer solitude, walking may be your first choice. Or perhaps you'd like to walk with a friend or family member.

If group activities appeal to you and motivate you, enroll in an aerobic dance class or water aerobics class. Do you like to be outdoors, or would you prefer to stay indoors? To combat boredom, watch television or listen to tapes while you use indoor exercise equipment. To keep things interesting, change your activity periodically. Consider using an exercise log to record your progress.

If it seems tough to find time to exercise, remember it only takes 30 minutes 3 days a week to improve your fitness level greatly. Although a moderate amount of physical activity every day will make you feel even better, daily exercise is especially important if you want to lose weight.

Think of ways to fit exercise into your regular routine. Could you walk for half an hour during your child's music lesson? How about taking your bike—instead of the car—to the store, when you need a loaf of bread? Perhaps you can swim and shower at a nearby pool over a shortened lunch hour, and save the time you normally spend showering in the morning.

| Borg Perceived Exertion Scale | |
|---|---|
| 6 | |
| 7 | Very, very light |
| 8 | |
| 9 | Very light |
| 10 | |
| 11 | Fairly light |
| 12 | |
| 13 | Somewhat hard |
| 14 | |
| 15 | Hard |
| 16 | |
| 17 | Very hard |
| 18 | |
| 19 | Very, very hard |
| 20 | |

### More reasons to exercise

Your body requires a certain amount of energy to continue functions you need to sustain life—breathing, circulating your blood and operating your vital organs. These needs, called the resting metabolic rate, account for 65 to 70 percent of the calories you burn in a day.

Exercise is an important variable in determining how many calories you burn. Exercise itself, because it requires your body to work harder than resting, requires more fuel (or calories). Even after you stop exercising, your body continues to burn calories at a modestly increased rate for a few hours. The effect of regular exercise over the long term is that your proportion of body fat decreases while the proportion of lean tissue (muscle, bone) increases. The more lean muscle you have, the higher your resting metabolic rate will be.

## Average number of calories burned in 10 minutes*

| Activity | Weight | | |
|---|---|---|---|
| | 120-130 pounds | 160-170 pounds | 190-200 pounds |
| Aerobic dance | 60-105 | 75-140 | 90-165 |
| Bicycling | | | |
|   Outdoors | 40-145 | 50-195 | 60-230 |
|   Stationary | 25-145 | 30-195 | 40-230 |
| Calisthenics | 40-105 | 50-140 | 60-165 |
| Dancing | 30-80 | 40-105 | 45-120 |
| Gardening | 30-80 | 40-105 | 45-120 |
| Golf (carry or pull bag) | 30-80 | 40-105 | 45-120 |
| Jogging | | | |
|   5 mph (12 minutes/mile) | 90 | 115 | 135 |
|   6 mph (10 minutes/mile) | 105 | 140 | 170 |
| Skiing | | | |
|   Cross-country | 60-145 | 75-195 | 90-230 |
|   Downhill | 40-90 | 50-115 | 60-135 |
| Swimming | 50-125 | 65-165 | 75-200 |
| Tennis | 50-95 | 65-130 | 75-150 |
| Walking | | | |
|   2 mph (30 minutes/mile) | 30 | 40 | 45 |
|   3 mph (20 minutes/mile) | 40 | 50 | 60 |
|   4 mph (15 minutes/mile) | 55 | 70 | 85 |

*10 minutes of continuous activity.*

Use your leverage as a member of your community to encourage opportunities for physical activity in your area. Lobby community leaders for safe, accessible trails for walking, biking and in-line skating, and sidewalks with curb cuts. Encourage your school district to open their facilities for community recreation and mall owners to provide extended hours for safe walking in any weather. Talk with your employer about ways your work place can be more supportive of employees who want to incorporate moderate physical activity into their daily lives.

If you're determined, careful with managing your time and just slightly creative, you can find the time to get regular exercise. Make it part of your daily routine. Remember—you're worth it! Don't think of it as a luxury, but as a necessary component of good health—like brushing your teeth and fastening your seat belt.

## Handling stress

It's one thing to understand that your personal style of approaching problems, conflicts and stressful events in your life can cause your body to react in a way that increases your risk of heart disease. But it's also important to know what to do about it.

Although you'll encounter numerous things in life that you can't control, you can control how you manage stress. A series of stressful life events does not condemn you to a heart attack or other serious illness, although it may increase your risk. Many health care professionals believe that you can raise or lower your risk by your own behavior and lifestyle.

Stress comes from many sources: your physical environment, unexpected events, and your own thoughts and actions. Remember, you can change your own behavior and attitudes. Frequently, people try to change the behavior of a spouse, children, boss, or people with whom they work, if they view those individuals' behavior as causing their own stress. Usually those efforts are futile.

To manage your stress, you must first recognize your symptoms of stress. These may include muscle tension, headache, insomnia, irritability, changes in eating habits, apathy, mental or physical fatigue, and frequent illness. Once you see that you're under stress, it's possible to identify the factors that produced the symptoms and develop ways to overcome them.

It's not easy to admit that you need to modify your behavior. For some, it takes the terrifying ordeal of a heart attack to motivate them to reevaluate their personal priorities and to work on changing thinking and communicating. But you don't need to wait until that happens.

## Adapting your behavior

Making simple changes in your lifestyle can help reduce your stress. Try walking at a more relaxed pace, driving more slowly, and providing ample time to complete your work. Use relaxation techniques such as biofeedback, brisk walking, or programs of regular physical activity.

In advising people on how to modify the so-called hot reactor response, experts emphasize using positive self-talk. The messages and images that you generate in your mind and send to yourself during periods of stress can greatly affect your physiological responses. For example, instead of getting upset and frustrated when you must wait for an appointment, tell yourself that waiting for some appointments in inevitable. Then plan for other ways to deal with the situation, such as reading a magazine, asking to reschedule, or calling work to say you may be late.

By changing your own thoughts and actions, you may interact with others more effectively—in fact, you may even elicit new responses from them. For example, you may complain that your spouse doesn't do anything but watch television in the evening. Instead of complaining, find a quiet room in which to read, do other work that interests you, go out for evening walks with a neighbor, sign up for an adult education course, or go to a movie with a friend. You'll not only enjoy yourself, but may find before long that your spouse turns off the television to join you.

View stress management techniques as options, not as strict rules about how you should act in certain situations. You can manage your stress level as you see fit, rather than being dragged into an increasing number of commitments by an overdeveloped sense of obligation or fear of hurting the feelings of others. Finally, you cannot expect stress management to give you a relaxed, carefree life. Unexpected problems—even catastrophes—will still happen.

While most people can view stress management as a challenge, you may be one of those who need to take more serious steps to cope with your stress. If psychological or physical symptoms persist, see your doctor as a first step in assessing the situation and devising a plan for gaining control of the stress in your life. Low self-esteem or depression can undermine your motivation

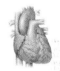

**HEALTHY HEART ♥ TIP**

*Some people just can't find the right exercise program—especially when they don't have time for the recommended 20 to 40 minutes of aerobic activity three times a week.*

*Although the gain may not be as great, recent evidence indicates that you'll benefit even if you can manage only 10 minutes of activity at a time. Regular exercise, even for a brief interval, leads to better cardiovascular health.*

to make healthful, positive changes. You may need the assistance of a psychiatrist or therapist for depression or other emotional difficulties. Many communities also offer formal stress management programs, ranging from workshops for executives to public lectures and classes. Most stress management programs include an introduction to relaxation training and techniques for solving problems.

## Techniques for managing your stress

One psychologist put it this way: It's not what happens to you that causes your stress, but rather how you react to what happens to you. These techniques can help you manage your stress more effectively:

*Maintain good social relationships*

Let your family, spouse and friends know that you love and appreciate them. Knowing that will make them more ready to help you when times get rough.

Keep in touch with a circle of friends. Many religious groups and social agencies offer marriage enrichment sessions, parenting classes, and self-improvement workshops that can help you make new friends and strengthen ongoing relationships.

*Eliminate irrational thinking*

Much of your stress may come from irrational beliefs, according to therapist Albert Ellis. Many of these irrational beliefs are absolutes and include the words "should," "always" and "never." For example, you may tell yourself, "I should never make a mistake," or "Everyone should like me," or "I should never become angry."

Modifying these expectations for yourself and others into something more realistic can be a powerful stress-reducer. Use positive self-talk to tone down your critical or negative feelings. For example, instead of "I should never make a mistake," tell yourself, "I'll try to be more careful next time." Instead of "Not everyone likes my ideas," say to yourself "Many people do seem to respect my opinions." These approaches create less intense negative feelings than more absolute statements.

*Improve your communication skill*

The technique of active listening is very helpful in dealing with difficult, angry people. It helps reduce their stress—and yours. It also keeps you from getting involved in arguments or becoming the target of their frustration. One active listening technique that may be helpful at times is to repeat or paraphrase what the other person said.

For example, suppose a friend complains to you about unfair demands placed on him or her by an employer. Using active listening techniques, you may say, "It sounds as if things are quite difficult for you at work," or "As you describe it, work seems to be very demanding." In this way you provide support without offering advice or offending the angry person.

Use assertive, effective communication. Assertiveness training can teach you how to get what you want through effective communication. You can learn to express your needs and desires without being ignored or offending others. Assertiveness training can be helpful for you if you are either someone with an overly aggressive, hostile personality who generates arguments in conversation, or if you are a passive person who frequently feels taken advantage of by others.

Assertiveness is based on the idea that everyone has basic rights—to express an opinion, to have some privacy, to make a mistake, for example. Passive people often give up their rights and then feel hurt and angry about it. Aggressive people don't respect the rights of others and assert their own rights. Assertive communication, on the other hand, involves freely expressing your ideas, avoiding sarcasm, and not criticizing those with whom you disagree.

Suppose that your spouse refuses to accompany you to an important, but potentially boring, social function that's related to your job. If you're acting passively, you may say, "Well, if you really don't want to go, I suppose I can go by myself." Meanwhile you may be thinking, "Just wait until you want me to go somewhere with you." If you're being aggressive, you may say, "You're really inconsiderate. You'd better go to this with me if you expect me to do the same for you." A more effective, assertive approach may be to say, "This is a very important meeting for me. I'd very much like you to be there with me."

Whether or not you seek additional training in communication skills, take a few moments to listen to others without offering your own ideas immediately. Avoid making conversations a win-or-lose contest, and state your opinions or feelings without criticizing others or their opposing ideas at the same time.

Practice positive thinking and positive self-talk. Avoid confusing daily problems with real crises. Do try to look for the silver lining in the clouds, and try not to make mountains out of molehills.

### Get organized

Keep a written schedule of special events, so that you're not faced with conflicts or last-minute rushes to get to your child's ball game. Keep your bills orderly in a desktop file or filing cabinet. Use drawer and closet organizers to eliminate that frustrating 5 minutes when you can't find your keys. Take a few minutes to plan your approach and rehearse before you go into important meetings or make important phone calls.

It takes time and effort to organize. You may have to learn some new habits and give up some old notions about spontaneity. The time you spend organizing yourself will pay off several times over during the ensuing months and years. It'll give you more free time to do the things you enjoy.

### Get sufficient rest

Avoid depending on stimulants such as excessive caffeine, alcohol and nicotine to regulate your moods. You can catch up on sleep you lost during the week—to some degree—by getting a little extra rest on the weekends. Don't feel guilty about taking an occasional nap or sleeping late when you can do so.

Try to break late-night television habits, and avoid food and beverages right before bedtime. If you have a serious problem sleeping, look into a nearby sleep disorder center at a hospital or large clinic.

### Have a life away from family and work

Find a hobby or activity that gives you satisfaction, outside of your work or family spheres. Consider gardening, collecting, crafts, or artistic activities. Avoid letting your hobby grow into another job or business—unless you really have the time and interest for it. Reserve a little private space for yourself where you can work undisturbed.

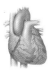

Volunteering provides an opportunity for you to have social interaction and develop new friendships (with people away from your work environment, if you work away from the home). It also enables you to make a worthwhile contribution to your community. Similarly, adult education enables you to meet new people—while learning at the same time.

While many of these suggestions may seem to apply primarily to married people who work outside the home or raise an active family, you may face different kinds of stress if you're single or older and no longer employed. Your stress may focus on loneliness, isolation, boredom and feelings of being unproductive. If you're in this category, consider the suggestions above for volunteering or adult education—or consider getting a pet. Pets can be extremely valuable as companions, and caring for a pet can also be rewarding.

*Get moving!*

Henry David Thoreau found that chopping wood not only helped cure him of loneliness in his self-imposed isolation at Walden Pond, but also helped him get over mental blocks when he was writing. Exercise can:

- Improve your blood pressure
- Lower your triglycerides and raise your HDL cholesterol
- Improve your glucose tolerance and prevent or reverse type 2 diabetes
- Help you lose weight
- Make you more physically fit
- Help reduce your anxiety
- Reduce mild depression
- Raise your self-esteem

Exercise is also the appropriate action for the physiological "fight-or-flight" stress response.

*Do away with negative thoughts and interpersonal conflict*

Numerous strategies can help you stop wasting time on nonproductive negative thinking and conflict with those around you.

For example, if you're in a prolonged argument with someone, take a time out. Then sit down together and each make a list on paper of the points on which you agree, those on which you disagree, and those that are irrelevant. As you shift from talking to writing—and from arguing to a cooperative effort—you can reduce your stress and reach a compromise solution to the problem.

Or if you've hit the wall in a thought process privately or cannot express yourself clearly, take a break. Move around. Do something. Sometimes it's more helpful to discuss problems while doing the dishes or taking a walk, rather than just sitting around a table.

*Use meditation or relaxation techniques*

In order for relaxation techniques to be helpful, it's important to make them a habit. Practice them regularly when you are already somewhat relaxed. Yoga, tai chi, and other Eastern exercises that use defined postures and repetitive movements can help you relax, if you'll take the time to learn and practice these techniques. Simple, favorite and repetitive prayers can also be a form of meditation.

## Do alternative medicines offer any valid help?

Alternative forms of medical therapy are becoming increasingly popular. These include therapy forms generally not prescribed or used in traditional, Western medical practices under the guidance of licensed physicians.

People use numerous alternative medical approaches to treat cardiovascular disease. Some people believe that these therapies are superior to standard medical therapy. Others are willing to try them, feeling that they pose little risk, even if they're not helpful. Perhaps you, like others, find some of the alternative medical practices more natural and holistic, with their emphasis on the interaction of mind, body and spirit.

*Chelation therapy* has been used to treat atherosclerosis since the 1950s. Atherosclerosis causes the blood vessels of your heart to become clogged with a build-up of complex fatty deposits that form plaques on the walls of your blood vessels. As blood vessel remodeling takes place, calcium is laid down at the vessel wall and bonds as a means of natural healing by the body.

Chelation therapy consists of multiple intravenous injections of a chemical, edetic acid (EDTA), for as many as 30 to 50 treatments. EDTA binds to various minerals—including calcium—in your bloodstream, and they're excreted in your urine. You must then replace these minerals with an oral medication. The primary theory behind chelation is that removing calcium from the build-up in your arteries reduces that build-up and softens your arteries. Proponents use chelation therapy in an effort to avoid more invasive procedures, such as coronary artery bypass surgery and angioplasty. However, in addition to being expensive, there's no published scientific proof that chelation therapy offers any benefit for atherosclerosis. Therefore, it's not a recommended treatment and there are reports of serious side effects.

*Herbal therapy,* in which plants or their extracts are used as medicine, has been used for medical treatment for centuries. In fact, many drugs commonly used today originated as herbal therapy. For example, drugs of the digitalis family come from plants in the foxglove family and are used to strengthen the heart and treat rhythm disturbances. These drugs are extremely toxic at high doses. Another common drug, aspirin, originally came from willow bark. Modern versions of these drugs—unlike herbal therapies—are synthetic and avoid using the plant directly. Active ingredients are chemically manufactured, with careful attention to strength, purity and dosage. If you use an herbal therapy—such as hawthorne (which some studies suggest may help improve heart function), rosemary, ginkgo, or ginseng—you need to understand several facts:

- There is little scientific evidence of the usefulness, side effects or dosages required for most of these preparations.

- Much of the information about their use has been orally passed down over the years.

- The active ingredients are often not well standardized and may vary greatly in products you purchase.

- You can experience side effects and undesirable interactions with your other medications.

Some herbal remedies may be useful, but their usefulness is best established by scientific studies. Although some studies are currently examining herbal remedies, lack of funding makes it difficult to do large, standardized studies that could establish their value. This occurs because the lack of available patent opportunities with herbal remedies means that drug manufacturers don't have the financial incentive to prove the usefulness and side effects of these substances. Drug companies are, however, studying plants from the rain forest for potential medical benefits. If you're considering using an herbal remedy, discuss it with your physician first, to avoid undesirable side effects and interactions with your other medications.

Because the production of alternative remedies is largely free from regulation by the U.S. Food and Drug Administration (including the costly testing required by the FDA), there is currently a tremendous financial incentive to sell these products. Burgeoning marketing efforts are intense and are directed at consumers, pharmacists and physicians. Information is often misleading, incomplete, and riddled with errors. You may hear about these remedies from friends who use them or you may read about them in publications that look official. The best advice is to proceed with great caution, and be sure your physician knows about any nonprescription drugs, herbals or alternative therapies you use.

## On the horizon

Research into causes, prevention and treatment of coronary artery disease is following several other avenues as well. However, it's still too early to draw any conclusions.

*Inflammation,* a term used to define a localized response of your body to an injury, may play a role in coronary artery disease. An inflammatory response to an insect bite, for example, causes redness, pain and swelling at the site of the bite. This is a complex response, which involves the movement of special blood cells to the area of injury. Similarly, when smoking causes injury to the wall of your artery, your body sends special cells to the site of the injury and your immune system is activated. Evidence of the immune response can be detected some distance away from the injury.

Some researchers suggest that infectious agents may trigger an inflammatory response as coronary artery disease develops. They note the increased activity of the immune system in patients with coronary artery disease, a level that is greater yet in patients with unstable angina or heart attack. It's possible that the degree of increased immune system activity may help predict cardiac events. Although there is a flurry of activity to pursue various hypotheses in this area, there is no evidence at this time that would justify recommending specific treatments.

*A genetic approach* to coronary artery disease recognizes that this disease may be caused by a combination of genetic factors and environment. In other words, if you have high cholesterol, it may be partly due to heredity and partly a result of your diet and other lifestyle factors. Researchers now recognize that an increasing number of diseases affecting the cardiovascular system are a result of defects in one or more genes.

These and other cardiovascular diseases may be candidates for gene therapy. This procedure introduces genetic material into human cells. These efforts involve, for example, inserting new genes into vascular cells to prevent a vein from again becoming narrowed or using genes to grow new blood vessels in areas of the heart where the blood supply is insufficient. These studies are in the very early stages, and the side effects and potential value of such treatments still need to be determined.

## A word to the wise

There is no substitute for a healthful lifestyle in preventing or stabilizing coronary artery disease. Research suggests that your best bet is to follow a vegetarian diet that's low in fats, coupled with an active exercise program. Some research also suggests that a diet more typical of people living in areas near the Mediterranean may protect your heart. These diets include many vegetables, fish and olive oil. If you, like many other people, feel that you can't adhere to a strict diet, your best bet is to at least try to eat less fat and leaner and smaller portions of red meat. Obesity, which is widespread in the United States and other Western countries, has recently been shown to be an independent risk factor for coronary artery disease.

Exercise offers the potential benefits of helping you lower your blood pressure and cholesterol levels. It also improves glucose control, helps reduce stress and increases relaxation. It's a good idea to establish a regular exercise program of at least one half-hour of aerobic exercise (such as walking or biking) a minimum of three times a week. In addition, you may find it helpful to improve your relaxation skills by using meditation, yoga, or tai chi.

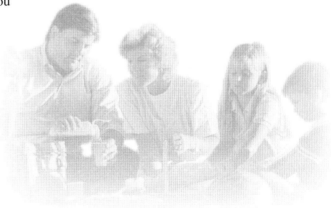

# Part 4

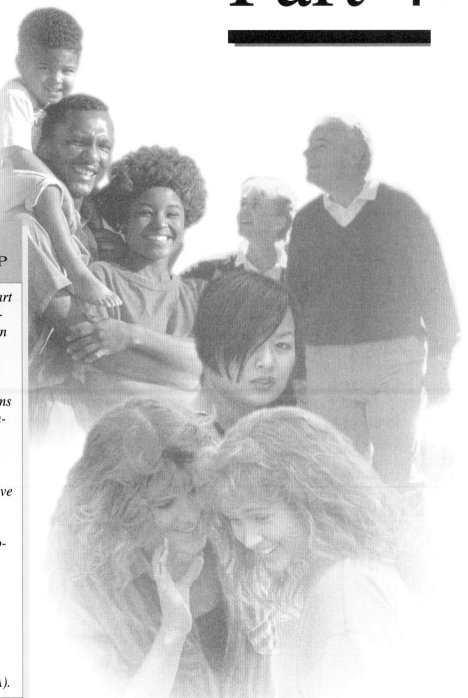

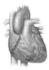

HEALTHY
HEART ♥ TIP

*If you're concerned about heart disease, rest assured that doctors have several tests that can help them assess your health. The choice of which tests will depend on your risk factors, heart history, current symptoms and the physician's interpretation of these details.*

*Tests usually start with the simplest and least invasive, then go from there. Noninvasive tests might include a resting electrocardiogram (ECG), signal-averaged electrocardiogram (SAECG), chest X-ray, Holter monitor (ambulatory electrocardiogram), echocardiogram, exercise stress test, computed tomography (CT) scan, magnetic resonance imaging (MRI) or magnetic resonance angiography (MRA).*

# Diagnosing heart disease

In many ways, your doctor is like a detective. Information gathered from you and about you provides clues to your condition. Your doctor solves the puzzle of your problem and makes a diagnosis by putting these clues together and drawing upon his or her medical training to interpret them. Medical tests provide the information your doctor needs to do this.

There are many different tests for heart disease. You're probably already familiar with some of the most basic tests. A physical examination and medical interview are part of the medical detective work for any condition. Another test you may have heard of is an ECG—an electrocardiogram, which involves recording the electrical activity of your heart.

Other tests, however, may sound more complicated and involve technology that you're not acquainted with. Not knowing about them can make these tests seem more intimidating than they need to be. Fortunately, most tests—even those with high-tech names—aren't difficult to understand. A little detective work of your own about heart disease tests will boost your confidence and comfort levels.

## Chapter

# Chapter

# 10 Medical evaluation: what to expect

The kinds of tests you'll need depend on your symptoms, your medical history and your risk factors, among others. Just as treatment is tailored to an individual, so are the processes that help your doctor make a diagnosis.

Before discussing tests specifically, it's helpful to understand the diagnostic process in general, when tests may be called for and what their limitations may be.

The medical interview and physical examination are the first steps in determining whether you have any medical problems. Tests performed later are more specific and can define your condition more precisely. Often, they're more complicated and more expensive.

Instead of screening everyone with these tests right away, doctors begin with a medical interview to find out your family history, other health risk factors, and what kinds of symptoms you're experiencing. Of particular interest are symptoms that suggest heart disease.

The physical examination often follows the interview. Listening, palpating (feeling), and observing specific areas of the body give your doctor more clues about your condition. If the medical interview and physical examination do not indicate any problems, your doctor may recommend that you undergo only a few screening tests. The results of these tests will help your doctor decide whether you need any further tests and what treatment you might need.

Screening tests are usually simple procedures that can single out people who might have medical problems. However, because many people who undergo screening tests don't necessarily have any medical problems, screening tests must be safe, convenient, and cost-effective.

## How often should you see your doctor?*

- Twice in your 20s (every 5 years)
- Three times in your 30s (every 3 to 4 years)
- Four times in your 40s (every 2 to 3 years)
- Five times in your 50s (every 2 years)
- Every year if you're 60 or older

*If you're apparently healthy.

Cardiologists would like to know the exact condition of the coronary arteries of each of their patients, but of course they cannot have everyone go to a hospital and undergo angiography and other tests that may be expensive and complicated and entail risk (see page 260). Although they might find some people who have blocked coronary arteries, they'd find many people have normal arteries. It's neither logical nor cost-effective to subject everyone with normal arteries to such a complicated procedure.

After taking the medical history and performing a physical examination, the doctor can be reasonably sure whether blockage of coronary arteries is causing the chest pain. However, to have coronary angiography, the person must go into the hospital for this invasive procedure.

Your doctor's other option is to order an exercise stress test (see page 241). If it shows no signs of inadequate coronary blood flow, your doctor can be reasonably confident that you don't have a significant coronary problem. However, he or she can't be certain, because in some situations the exercise test may not be conclusive, even when there is a significant blockage. Whether or not additional testing, including angiography, needs to be performed cannot be simply answered. Your doctor's recommendation will be based on an assessment of the potential for significant blockages.

If the results of an exercise stress test are abnormal, there is a reasonable chance that you have coronary artery disease. Coronary angiography may be necessary to settle the issue and to help determine appropriate treatment. Doctors reserve the more complicated tests for people who have a higher chance of having heart disease or for those in whom the results of screening tests don't give a clear-cut or logical answer.

Although very sophisticated tests are available to help diagnose heart disease, no test is perfect. There is always a chance that a test will give incorrect information, no matter how carefully it's done or analyzed.

## Heart disease tests

Blood tests

Electrocardiography

Chest X-ray

Nuclear scanning

Echocardiography

Catheterization and angiography

Electrophysiology studies

Noninvasive tests of your blood vessels

Advanced imaging techniques to visualize your heart.

## Is more testing necessary?

Your physical exam, medical history and prior test results help your doctor determine whether more tests are needed and which may be helpful. Here are some common testing situations:

| Situation | Action Taken |
| --- | --- |
| Exam, medical history, early test results, and doctor's impression suggest there's a problem | No further tests are required and treatment is begun. Or more advanced testing is needed to make a specific diagnosis and select treatment |
| Doctor's impression and early test results suggest that no problem exists | No further testing, no treatment |
| Doctor's impression and test results are unclear | Advanced tests are needed to make specific diagnosis |

Occasionally, a test may indicate that there is no problem when there really is one. This is called a false-negative result. Sometimes a test may indicate that there's a problem when there really is not. This is called a false-positive result.

When evaluating your condition, your physician must consider whether the test is accurate and whether the test result fits with other information about you.

Why would a doctor ever use tests that are not completely accurate? To begin with, no test is 100 percent accurate, and all tests are open to interpretation. And remember, doctors usually try to gain as much information as possible from tests that have the least risk, expense, and inconvenience. The screening tests are used to identify whether you may need more extensive (and definitive) testing.

In addition, even tests with incomplete details can give important information. For example, a chest X-ray cannot directly show the coronary arteries, valves, and other complex structures of the heart, but it can show the size and shape of the heart, which may be very useful information to the doctor. Chest X-rays are generally quick, safe, and fairly inexpensive. Using the information from the chest X-ray, your doctor may be satisfied that all is well, or may decide that more precise tests are needed to determine the problem exactly.

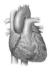

HEALTHY
HEART ♥ TIP

*If you have a healthy heart, one of the most compassionate things you can do is to sign a donor card. That way your family will know that, in case of a mortal accident, you wanted to help someone else by donating your heart.*

*You'll be a suitable donor if you're a young to middle-aged person who's been declared brain dead (based on standard criteria) with a heart that still functions properly. Doctors screen donors to make sure they don't have hepatitis B or C or any human immunodeficiency (AIDS-producing) viruses. Seriously ill patients at nearby transplant centers will be given priority.*

## Taking your medical history

Providing an accurate medical history is the best way you can begin helping your physician choose the most valuable diagnostic tools for you.

The medical history is a report to the doctor of your "medical biography," or a history of all the significant medical events in your life. The questions asked about your medical history will be more extensive during your first visit with a doctor than on subsequent visits. You'll also be asked more questions during a general exam than during one for a specific problem.

The medical interview is often conducted by your doctor. However, a nurse or physician assistant may also ask you questions. Sometimes the information is collected with a questionnaire. Regardless of the format, it's helpful if you think about and organize this information before coming to the doctor. And when you are at the doctor's office, don't be shy about bringing up concerns. If you feel that something is worth mentioning, say it.

The medical history that you provide helps the doctor decide where and how to focus the subsequent evaluation. The medical history will likely consist of the following parts:

- Chief complaint
- Medical history
- Family medical history

- Social history
- A review of your organ systems

## Chief complaint

The chief complaint is simply what brought you to the doctor's office. In describing it, be as complete and concise as possible, covering all aspects of the symptoms. Where is the problem? How does it feel? How often does it happen? How long does it last? What provokes the problem? What makes it better? What other things happen when you have this problem?

During the first visit, it's especially important to relate information in a logical order and to use specific dates and duration of events. It's always a good idea to bring notes with you to help get your story across accurately.

## Medical history

Your medical history is a review of your health throughout your life. This information not only helps sort out possible causes for the present problem but also may indicate whether your doctor will need to rule out possible treatments. For example, your chief complaint may be chest pain that turns out to be angina related to coronary artery disease. However, if you also have asthma, you may not be able to use certain medications to treat angina. The reason is that some of these medications can make your asthma worse.

Be specific when you relate your medical history. Tell your doctor about all prior illnesses, hospitalizations, accidents, operations, and allergies. In addition, discuss symptoms that concern you, medications you are taking, and questions you have. Again, jotting down a brief list of the things you want to cover is helpful.

If you're giving your medical history to a specialist after you've been examined by other doctors, it's important to make sure the specialist has copies of earlier evaluations, X-rays, or other tests you've had. In many cases, it's a good idea to have these sent ahead of the appointment so that the specialist can review them before the actual medical interview. A special note to those who have had a test called an arteriogram, which is an angiogram of the coronary arteries: It's a good idea to bring with you the actual film from the test rather than just the report.

## Family medical history

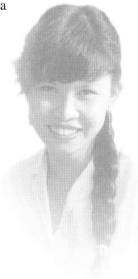

Your family medical history is valuable in making a diagnosis. It's a clue to your doctor about possible hereditary aspects of disease and also helps identify risk factors. For example, if a close family member had a heart attack at a young age, you may have a higher risk of coronary artery disease.

Make a list of any chronic diseases affecting your parents, grandparents, brothers, sisters, and children, and be sure to bring it with you.

### Social history

Your social history includes information about your lifestyle or living habits that may affect your risk of heart disease. These habits include smoking and alcohol use or job-related factors, such as toxic exposures. Not all lifestyle habits negatively affect your risk. Recreational activities, such as those involving regular exercise, may reduce your risk of heart disease. Your doctor will need to know about these, too.

### Reviewing your organ systems

Your doctor will review potential symptoms related to each of your organ systems during the medical interview. This review is a checklist for you and the doctor to go through to make sure that nothing is overlooked. For example, someone who complains of chest pain may neglect to mention that he or she experiences tiredness in the calves of the legs when walking a short distance. This information is important to the doctor because both chest pain and discomfort or tiredness in the calves can be related to blockage in the coronary and leg arteries. Gathering critical information such as this makes the organ review an important addition to your medical interview.

## The physical examination

The physical examination is a crucial component of your medical evaluation. The main parts of a cardiovascular physical examination include:

- Taking your blood pressure
- Measuring heart rate and rhythm
- Checking all pulses
- Inspecting the veins of your neck
- Checking for swelling
- Listening to breath, heart and blood vessel sounds

### Taking your blood pressure

You've probably had your blood pressure checked many times. Measuring blood pressure is a safe, simple, and standard way to detect a medical condition that is one of the key risk factors for heart disease. This test also can give your doctor clues about the pumping ability of your heart and the resistance offered by your arteries.

In general, the harder your heart pumps and the narrower your arteries, the higher your blood pressure is. To understand more fully, think of the effort it would take to push water through a hose with a $1/2$-inch diameter. Then, compare this to the effort needed to push the same amount of water through a hose with a 1-inch diameter. The pressure will be higher in the hose with the smaller diameter.

Your blood pressure should be measured when you are resting quietly. Changes in blood pressure may be detected when you are lying down, sitting, and standing. A drop in blood pressure when you stand up could explain some types of light-headedness associated with body position.

Your doctor may also measure your blood pressure in both arms. The reason? A difference between the arm pressures may indicate a partial blockage in the aorta or either of the arteries going to your arms. Blood pressure downstream from a blockage is lower than the pressure upstream from a blockage.

Something important to note is that nervousness and anxiety can increase blood pressure. The anxiety that some people have during medical examinations can lead to a phenomenon known as "white-coat" hypertension. People who have "white-coat" hypertension really may have normal blood pressure throughout most of the day. But when they have it checked by a doctor, it's high.

For this reason and others, doctors don't rely on just one measurement of blood pressure to diagnose high blood pressure. Some variation in your blood pressure measurements is normal. For an accurate diagnosis of high blood pressure, your blood pressure needs to be measured on three separate occasions.

## Understanding your blood pressure reading

Sphygmomanometer (SFIG-mo-ma-NOM-uh-ter) is the tongue-twisting name given to the device used to check your blood pressure. It consists of a cuff, which goes around your arm, and a gauge that looks a thermometer. The gauge contains mercury. This is why blood pressure readings contain the abbreviation "Hg," which is mercury's scientific symbol.

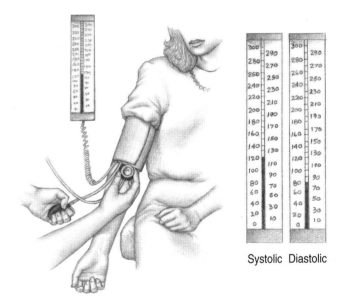

Systolic Diastolic

*Measuring your blood pressure with a sphygmomanometer. After the cuff is pumped up, air is slowly released to reduce the pressure constricting the arm. The doctor or nurse notes the pressure on the mercury-column gauge at which the heartbeat can first be heard. This is the systolic pressure, the top number in your blood pressure reading (**above, left**). The pressure at which the sounds disappear is the diastolic pressure, the bottom number in your blood pressure reading (**above, right**).*

Having your blood pressure checked is a painless, routine procedure. What you mostly feel is a slight pressure on your arm when the cuff is inflated, something that's necessary to measure your blood pressure. The top number in a blood pressure reading, which normally averages about 120 millimeters (mm) of mercury (Hg), is called the systolic blood pressure. It is the point at which the person taking the measurement hears the pulse in your arm as the pressure is deflated in the cuff. This number represents the pressure in the arteries of your arm at the time your heart is squeezing blood out into the circulation.

The bottom number in the blood pressure reading (which normally averages about 70 mm Hg) is called the diastolic blood pressure. It is the point at which the heart sounds disappear as the pressure continues to be deflated in the cuff. This number represents the pressure in the arteries of your arm at the time your heart relaxes between beats.

## Measuring heart rate and rhythm

Doctors can quickly assess your heart rate and rhythm by feeling (palpating) the pulse at your wrist, the carotid arteries in your neck, or the femoral arteries in the groin. Doctors can also tell whether your pulse is regular, has skipped or extra beats, or is irregular—something that happens if you have a condition called atrial fibrillation.

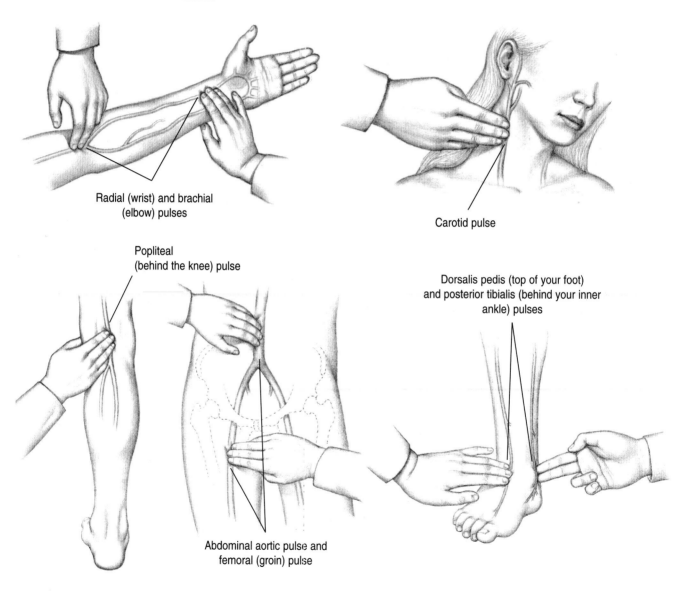

Radial (wrist) and brachial (elbow) pulses

Carotid pulse

Popliteal (behind the knee) pulse

Dorsalis pedis (top of your foot) and posterior tibialis (behind your inner ankle) pulses

Abdominal aortic pulse and femoral (groin) pulse

*There are many different places on your body where your pulse normally can be felt easily. Absence of a pulse at any of these points may signal a blockage in the artery upstream.*

Health professionals usually count your pulse for 15 seconds and multiply that number by 4 (4 x 15 seconds = 1 minute) to calculate your heart rate in beats per minute. In a thorough examination, you will have your pulses palpated at a wide range of areas on your body: both your wrists; the pulses at the inner part of both elbows (brachial pulse); the carotid pulses in your neck; the aortic pulse in the abdomen; the femoral pulses in the groin; the popliteal pulse behind each knee; the dorsalis pedis pulse on the top of each foot; and the posterior tibialis pulse (on the inside of each leg, behind your inner ankle). An absent or reduced pulse at any of these sites may indicate a blockage upstream from it.

## Inspecting the veins of your neck

Doctors examine pulses in your veins, called "venous pulses," by looking rather than by listening or palpation. They carefully look at your neck when you are lying down with your head partially raised or when you are sitting up. As your heart beats, they observe the slight expansion made by the main vein in your neck—the jugular vein. The jugular vein is a reliable indicator of the pressure on the right side of your heart. When the pressure on the right side of your heart is high, the blood flowing from the jugular vein into the heart backs up a bit, causing the top of the expansion to be at a higher point on your neck. Doctors can estimate the approximate pressure in the right side of the heart and also get an idea of how much extra fluid there is in your cardiovascular system by observing your jugular vein.

## Checking for swelling

Doctors routinely look for excess fluid by examining parts of your body that are prone to swelling. If you spend most of your time upright during the day, swelling can occur in the ankles and legs. The medical term for swelling is "edema" (eh-DEE-muh).

To gauge fluid retention, the doctor presses on the skin (for example, over the ankle) and watches how far it can be pushed in—something doctors call indentation. If the spot pushed in remains indented, this is called pitting. Pitting edema can occur in the ankles and the area over your shin, thighs, the lower back and abdomen, or your hands, depending on the severity of your fluid retention.

Edema can also occur if you have a blockage in a vein carrying blood back from one of your arms or legs. If you have kidney failure or if the main vein that carries blood from your head (called the superior vena cava) is obstructed, you may have edema in the face, causing it to look puffy and rounded.

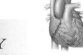

**HEALTHY HEART ♥ TIP**

*Few diners would choose to eat bland food, but that's sometimes what you get when cutting back on fat and salt.*

*Instead of reaching for the butter dish or the salt shaker, try these other methods to enhance flavor:*

- *Stock up on plenty of herbs and spices*
- *Keep a ready supply of onions, fresh garlic and ginger root*
- *Try enhancements like Dijon mustard, vinegar, sherry or other cooking wines*
- *Stock lemons and limes in the refrigerator*
- *Use flavored vegetable cooking sprays*

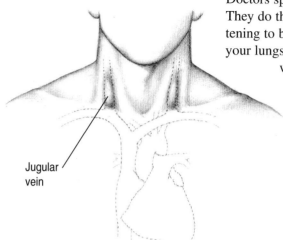

Jugular vein

*Your doctor can estimate the pressure of blood in the right atrium of your heart by observing the level of expansion of your jugular vein. Normally, the vein's bulge would not be visible above your collarbone if you were sitting down. The higher it appears to bulge above your collarbone, the higher the pressure in your right atrium. This finding gives physicians a good indication of the amount of blood circulating inside you. In conditions that cause congestive heart failure, blood volume often increases (see page 34).*

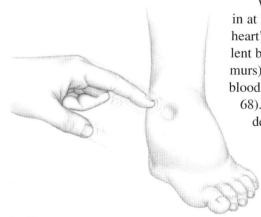

*Swelling of the foot, ankle, and leg can be severe enough to leave an indentation, or "pit," when you press on the area. This swelling (edema) is the result of excessive fluid in your tissues—often caused by congestive heart failure or blockage in a leg vein.*

## Listening to breath sounds

Doctors spend a lot of time listening through their stethoscopes. They do this because they can get a wealth of information from listening to breathing, heart, and blood vessel sounds. They listen to your lungs by placing the stethoscope on several areas of your chest while you breathe in and out.

In addition to listening with the stethoscope, your doctor may thump on your chest—a procedure that's called percussion. Percussion provides clues about where fluid may have accumulated between your lungs and chest wall, or near areas of the lungs that may have collapsed or become dense because of infection or inflammation. Tapping over these areas sounds dull, instead of producing a normal "hollow" sound.

From a heart-health standpoint, your doctor is mainly trying to tell whether excessive fluid has leaked into the air sacs of your lungs. This extra fluid makes a crackling sound in the stethoscope when you breathe in. These abnormal sounds (referred to as crackles or rales) provide clues to different types of disease. Crackles associated with increased fluid sound "wet," like many little bubbles popping. Other crackles sound like Velcro being pulled apart. These sounds raise a suspicion of scarring (fibrosis) in the lungs.

## Listening to heart sounds

When doctors listen to the heart with a stethoscope, they listen in at least four standard spots. They listen to the quality of your heart's valve sounds when they snap closed and for sounds of turbulent blood flow through the valves or other heart structures (murmurs). Murmurs can occur for several different reasons. One is when blood is forced to flow through an abnormally tight valve (see page 68). Another is when blood leaks back (regurgitates) through a defective valve. A murmur can also occur when blood follows an abnormal course through your heart—something that can happen when there's a hole in the ventricular septum or around an obstructing bulge caused by a condition called hypertrophic cardiomyopathy (see page 52).

Sometimes the cause of a murmur is not apparent. However, the causes of most murmurs can be determined by having you perform certain maneuvers. It's very normal to be asked to stand up, squat, or lie down as the doctor listens to your heart. The reason for this is that murmurs change in characteristic ways when you change your position.

Murmurs also change during different types of breathing, so the doctor may ask you to breathe in and out deeply, or to hold your breath and bear down as though you were straining during a bowel movement. Some murmurs can be heard more clearly in one position or another, so the doctor may ask you to roll onto your left side or to sit up and lean forward.

In special circumstances, the doctor may have you inhale a medication called amyl nitrite (AM-il NY-tryte). This briefly alters your blood pressure and heart rate so that certain murmurs can be characterized more completely.

Besides murmurs, doctors also listen for "gallops," which are extra sounds that give a galloping cadence to the normal noises your heart makes. The type of gallop that is heard may also help your physician tell the difference between abnormalities that occur while your heart relaxes from those that occur while it's contracting.

Other sounds—including whoops, clicks, snaps, knocks, and rubs—provide vital information about possible underlying heart and pericardial diseases. Some murmurs and sounds are "innocent," meaning they may be present even though you have no heart problems.

## Listening to blood vessels

The doctor may place a stethoscope over many different areas of your body to check the sounds of large blood vessels there. Vessels checked may include the carotid arteries in the neck, the abdominal aorta in the torso, and both femoral arteries in the groin.

When placing the stethoscope in these areas, your doctor is listening for whispering sounds called bruits (BRU-ees), which are made by abnormally turbulent blood flow. Like a river flowing over rocky rapids, your blood might make more noise as it goes through areas where flow is obstructed—such as those areas where plaque deposits have narrowed arteries. The presence of a bruit may indicate a degree of blockage (stenosis) at those sites.

*When doctors listen to your heart, they focus especially on areas that tell about the flow of blood through your heart valves. They also listen for murmurs, which may indicate turbulent blood flow caused by stenosis (narrowing or stiffening of the arteries) or regurgitation of a valve. Other sounds—such as gallops, clicks, rubs, or knocks—may indicate other types of heart problems.*

# Chapter
# 11 Common tests

**B** oth during and after your medical history and physical examination, your doctor may order a number of additional tests. Some, such as blood tests, are straightforward. Others may be more complicated. Knowing about them, what to expect and what information each test provides is important. It can eliminate some of your concerns about undergoing testing. In addition, it can help you become an active partner in your care. This chapter describes the tests you may encounter as you and your doctor continue the detective work necessary to diagnose your heart disease.

## Blood tests

Routine blood tests are used to rule out or help diagnose a wide variety of conditions. In most general examinations, blood testing includes a complete blood cell count (CBC) and an analysis of your blood chemistry. This testing can spot problems such as anemia (too few red blood cells) or levels of blood lipids (cholesterol and triglycerides) that are too high. Many other blood tests may also be advised, including thyroid studies, which assess how well your thyroid gland is working, and coagulation studies, which determine the rate at which your blood clots.

### How are blood samples taken?

It usually takes only a few seconds to draw a small amount of blood into a vial for testing. Sometimes special preparations, such as fasting overnight, may be necessary. Blood may be drawn from a tiny cut made in a fingertip and placed in a small container called a capillary pipette if only a drop or two is needed.

If more blood is necessary, the person drawing it (who is called a venipuncturist) places a tourniquet around your upper arm. This makes your veins bulge so they are easier to see and blood can be obtained more easily. The venipuncturist then selects a vein, cleans the skin over it with alcohol, and gently inserts a thin needle. Blood passes through the needle into an attached sterile syringe. When enough blood has been drawn, the tourniquet is released, the needle withdrawn, and the puncture site wiped again with an antiseptic. If blood is needed from an artery, a slightly different procedure is used.

## What do blood tests show?

The most common blood tests specifically done for heart disease measure blood lipid levels (cholesterol and triglycerides), cardiac enzymes, oxygen content, and prothrombin time (amount of time necessary for your blood to clot).

## Lipid levels

Lipid is a general term for fat circulating in your blood. The usual lipids measured are total cholesterol, high-density lipoprotein (HDL) cholesterol, and triglycerides (see page 172). Low-density lipoprotein (LDL) cholesterol values can be calculated from the three other cholesterol values by this mathematical formula: LDL cholesterol = total cholesterol – HDL cholesterol – (triglycerides divided by 5).

This formula provides a good estimate of the LDL cholesterol value. If a more precise measurement is needed, a blood test that specifically and more accurately determines your LDL level is used.

The lipids in your blood vary according to what you've eaten recently. That's why you often need to fast (usually beginning around midnight) if your blood will be drawn in the morning. Even with fasting, your blood lipids may vary because of fluctuations in how your body processes fats.

The laboratory test used to measure lipids isn't totally precise. It's accurate to within 2 to 5 percent of the actual value. Thus, two different analyses of the same sample of blood may give two slightly different values for lipids. That's why there's little reason to split hairs about small differences in measurements between two people or between two measurements from the same person.

Measurements from blood obtained from a vein in your arm are more likely to be accurate than measurements from a few drops of blood from your finger. A single measurement is also no guarantee that your cholesterol level is normal or abnormal. At least two sets of measurements that agree are needed before any conclusions can be made. If two measurements are widely different, a third measurement is needed. (To understand your blood lipid level measurements, see page 155.)

During your blood tests, your doctor will likely concentrate on your total cholesterol, LDL, HDL, and triglyceride measurements. In the future, measurements of just the protein portions of lipoproteins called apoproteins may become important in assessing your risk of heart disease.

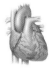

## HEALTHY HEART ♥ TIP

*Is heart disease in your future? A recently developed test may help doctors gauge your risk for coronary artery disease (CAD), even before symptoms appear.*

*The electron beam computed tomography (EBCT) scan reveals whether you have calcium in your coronary arteries, indicating that plaque may be accumulating. It can also detect the quantity of calcium; the greater the calcification, the greater your risk of blockage, which may lead to disease.*

*The scan isn't for everyone and can be overused. It may be helpful in some individuals without symptoms and multiple risk factors for CAD. Discuss this with your physician before undergoing the test.*

## Cardiac enzymes

Your blood may be tested for levels of enzymes that may indicate damage to the heart. Common enzymes doctors are concerned with include:

- Creatine kinase
- Lactate dehydrogenase
- Troponin-I
- Troponin-T
- Myoglobin

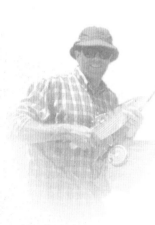

Cardiac enzymes may sound complicated, but think of them as chemical clues to your heart's health—particularly when a heart attack is a concern. For example, enzymes usually found in the heart may leak into the blood from damaged heart cells after a heart attack. Or they may be released at the earliest phase of a heart attack that is stopped by medical intervention or by your body working on its own. Sometimes these enzymes leak into the blood as you are about to have a heart attack, providing a warning of what's to come.

If you are experiencing chest pain, your physician may recommend testing your blood for these enzymes. If you come to an emergency room for evaluation of chest pain, the physician most likely will check these enzyme levels.

Cardiac enzymes are usually not elevated immediately after heart damage occurs. The reason is that it takes several hours for these enzymes to appear in your circulation. However, some of these enzymes may remain in your circulation for several days following an episode. That's why they're useful during several days after an episode of chest pain to detect whether a heart attack has occurred.

Even when a heart attack has been confirmed, cardiac enzymes may continue to be monitored. The reason is that doctors want to make sure that enzyme levels are decreasing. Enzyme levels that start to rise again may indicate ongoing or recurrent heart damage.

There are occasions, however, when cardiac enzymes are elevated falsely and may mimic a heart attack. This may occur more frequently in marathon runners, athletes with muscle injuries, people with chronic kidney insufficiency, and individuals with a genetic predisposition for elevated levels of certain enzymes. Most of the time, though, enzyme levels are very accurate indicators of heart damage, even at its earliest stages. Abnormal enzyme levels should be taken very seriously.

## Oxygen level

The measurement of oxygen circulating in your blood (or how saturated your blood is with oxygen) at various areas of your body helps your doctor determine whether:

- Your overall circulation is sufficient
- Your lungs are providing enough oxygen to your bloodstream
- Blood is being prevented from traveling through the lungs to pick up oxygen

Normally, the blood contains a lot of oxygen after it has passed through the lungs and picked up oxygen. Thus, the oxygen saturation of blood in the arteries leaving the left ventricle is high. Once the blood releases oxygen to the tissues, its oxygen saturation declines. That's why blood in veins returning to the heart has low oxygen saturation.

Oxygen can be measured in the arterial blood, which carries oxygen to your body's tissues, or in the venous blood, which returns to your heart and lungs. Where your blood will be drawn for this test depends on what information your doctor needs to know. If he or she wants to know the oxygen level in blood after it has received oxygen from the lungs, the blood must be drawn from an artery.

The procedure for testing arterial blood differs somewhat from a standard blood test. The person drawing the blood cleans the skin over the artery with an antiseptic and may inject a local anesthetic to numb the area. The typical sites where arterial blood is drawn are the areas where the pulses of the following arteries can be felt: the radial artery in the wrist, the brachial artery in the elbow, or the femoral artery at the groin.

When the area for drawing blood has been selected, the artery is punctured with a sterile needle attached to a disposable syringe that has been coated on the interior with oil to prevent air from contaminating your blood sample. After the blood sample is drawn, the needle is removed from the artery and the sample is transferred from the syringe into sterile tubes that are placed in a device that analyzes blood gases. You'll be asked to apply pressure to the puncture site and to rest quietly for 15 minutes before resuming normal activities.

The oxygen saturation of your blood can also be analyzed with a device called a pulse oximeter clip. It resembles a small clothespin and is placed on your finger or toe. The clip measures oxygen in your blood by assessing the redness of your blood when a light is passed through your skin.

The pulse oximeter clip is used during procedures such as angiography and surgery, during monitoring in an intensive care unit, or at any time when your physician believes that constant measurements of oxygen in your blood are needed.

If frequent measurements of blood oxygen are needed, blood may also be obtained through a catheter that is left in place.

## Prothrombin time and International Normalized Ratio (INR)

Again, these are ways to know how long it takes your blood to clot. Testing your prothrombin time is important when you're taking medications that prevent the blood from clotting. These medications are called anticoagulants. Although they are often referred to as "blood thinners," they do not actually "thin" your blood. They alter proteins in it that are responsible for clotting, and by doing so make your blood less likely to clot.

Anticoagulant medications are beneficial for people with a predisposition for abnormal blood clots or for people who already have blood clots. These are people with deep-vein thrombosis or pulmonary embolism (see page 125), dilated cardiomyopathy (see page 47), or mechanical artificial heart valves.

The most common anticoagulant is warfarin, which prevents the liver from using vitamin K to make certain proteins needed for blood clotting. Enough warfarin must be given to prevent abnormal clotting, but not so much that abnormal bleeding or bruising results. Excessive warfarin can cause bleeding. In fact, warfarin is the main ingredient in some kinds of rat poison.

Because individual responses to warfarin are not entirely predictable, people taking this medication must have their blood clotting monitored with a blood test that determines prothrombin time. The longer the prothrombin time, the more anticoagulated the blood is. Your prothrombin time is compared with the value that is considered normal in the particular laboratory where it was measured. Usually, the desired prothrombin time in people taking warfarin is 1.3 to 1.5 times the normal prothrombin time. Prothrombin times should be checked at least once a month, and sometimes more frequently, especially when warfarin treatment is started.

Prothrombin time is now expressed in a measurement called the International Normalized Ratio (INR). The INR is a way to standardize prothrombin time measurements made by different laboratories around the world. It is the most accurate measurement of anticoagulation with warfarin.

The desired INR for people with atrial fibrillation, a prior history of peripheral venous embolism or arterial embolism, or a history of reduced heart function is usually in the 2.0-3.0 range. The desired INR range for individuals with mechanical artificial heart valves is usually 3.0 to 4.0. It's important that your physician make frequent measurements of your INR until your values are relatively stable after repeated measurements.

After a stable pattern has been established, your INR may need to be checked only once per month or sometimes even less frequently. However, it's important to reassess your INR more often and establish stable readings any time you:

- Significantly change your diet
- Take new medication that interacts with warfarin
- Change the dose of a prior medication

## Electrocardiography (ECG)

Electrocardiography (ECG) is indispensable for evaluating many heart diseases. Since its introduction nearly a century ago, the ECG has advanced in its technique and its usefulness. By interpreting an ECG tracing, which is also called an ECG and consists of a series of waves, your doctor can diagnose several abnormal conditions that can affect your heart—including rhythm disturbances, a heart attack, or other abnormalities of the heart's structure.

## What is electrocardiography?

An electrocardiogram is simply a recording of the electrical activity of your heart. The so-called tracing can be displayed either on a strip of paper or on a monitor. It also can be recorded on tape or even transmitted over telephone wires. The equipment used to record an ECG is an electrocardiograph—the terminology is the same as for telegram and telegraph.

The electrical activity of your heart is detected by electrodes attached to your skin. These electrodes transmit your heart's electrical impulses to an electrocardiograph. Typically, the electrical impulses are recorded in the form of waves that are displayed on graph paper moving out of this machine at a set speed.

The graph corresponds to time horizontally. Vertically, it corresponds to the voltage or strength of your heart's electrical impulses. The recordings from each electrode represent the electrical forces from various areas of your heart. Each electrode is like a "command post" for a particular area of your heart, recording the impulses from its particular location.

Different waves represent the various areas of your heart through which tiny electrical currents are flowing, causing your heart to contract and relax. The main components of an ECG reading are the P wave, the QRS complex, and the T wave (see page 238).

The P wave represents the current in the atria, the QRS complex represents the current in your heart's ventricles, and the T wave represents the electrical recovery period of the ventricles. These components of the ECG can impart an enormous amount of information about your heart (see page A12).

## Understanding your ECG reading

The components of the ECG tracing—the P waves, the QRS complexes, and the T waves—sound like alphabet soup and can occur in seemingly endless patterns, shapes, and speeds. But each variation provides your physician with a wealth of clues about your heart's health, including information about:

- Heart rate
- Heart rhythm
- Whether a heart attack has occurred
- Inadequate blood and oxygen supply to the heart muscle
- Heart structure abnormalities

### Heart rate

The simplest piece of information the ECG can provide is the rate of your heartbeat at the time you had this test. If 10 QRS complexes are recorded on the ECG paper or monitor in 10 seconds, then your heart rate is 60 beats per minute. The ECG is seldom needed just for information about your heart rate. A check of your pulse will

### Is it an ECG or an EKG?

An ECG is sometimes referred to as an EKG. Both are the same test. The reason for the different names has to do with Willem Einthoven. In the Dutch language, electrocardiogram is spelled "electrokardiogram." Today, many doctors still say "EKG"—a historical reference to this test's Dutch pioneer.

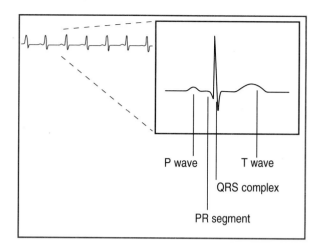

P wave

T wave

QRS complex

PR segment

suffice. An ECG may be helpful, however, when the pulse is difficult to feel or is too fast or too irregular to count accurately.

*The electrocardiogram—the reading taken by elctrocardiography—of each heartbeat consists of a series of "waves" that reveal much about the electrical impulses in different parts of your heart. The P wave shows the impulse as it travels through the atrium. Following the P wave is the PR segment, a flat portion that represents the time the impulse travels through the atrioventricular node. The QRS complex occurs as the impulse travels throughout the ventricles. The T wave is formed during the time the heart muscle recovers electrically in preparation for the next beat (see page A12).*

## Heart rhythm

The ECG is the most direct way to assess your heart's rhythm. It can distinguish normal sinus rhythm from all types of tachycardia, abnormally fast rhythms (see page 112). In addition, the ECG can distinguish normal rhythms from bradycardia, abnormally slow rhythms (see page 103).

Your heart normally beats in sequence: the atria first, and then the ventricles shortly afterward, at a speed that's usually between 60 and 100 beats per minute. Arrhythmias (see page 99) deviate from this pattern. An ECG, for example, might reveal a complete heart block when your heart's atria are stimulated normally but the electrical impulse is blocked from passing through the atrioventricular node to the ventricles. Therefore, the ventricles beat at a slow "back-up" rate that is different from the rate of the atrial beats.

On the ECG, this condition appears as P waves going at one rate and QRS complexes going at a slower rate, with no relationship to one another. All of the other arrhythmias discussed on pages 101 to 115 also have their characteristic patterns. This may sound complicated, but to a doctor experienced in interpreting ECGs, these patterns are readily understood.

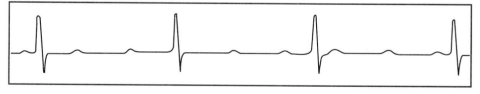

*Complete heart block, also called third-degree atrioventricular block, is the most severe form of heart block (see page 106). None of the impulses from your heart's sinus node are getting through the atrioventricular node to the ventricles.*

*This electrocardiogram shows what complete heart block might look like. Note that none of the P waves are followed quickly by a QRS complex, the jagged peak in the line. Instead, other parts of the conduction system may take over the task of producing a heartbeat, but at a much slower rate. You can see that the P waves and the QRS complexes are going at separate rates, unrelated to one another.*

## Detecting a heart attack

The ECG may provide crucially important information about whether you've had a heart attack. It can often distinguish between a heart attack that has already happened and one that's occurring when you are having the ECG. The patterns on the ECG can indicate which part of your heart (front, back, lower, or sides) has been damaged, roughly estimate the extent of the damage, and suggest whether damage has occurred throughout the full thickness of your heart wall.

How can an ECG do this? The reason is that injured heart muscle and scar tissue in your heart don't conduct electrical impulses normally. This causes the shapes of the QRS complexes and the T waves to change in characteristic ways that can help your physician make a diagnosis. Because of this, the ECG is an invaluable early warning system that helps people with chest pain get treatment more rapidly.

However, an electrocardiogram cannot detect all heart attacks. In some people who have chest pain indicating a heart attack, additional tests—such as measurements of blood enzyme levels—are needed to confirm that a heart attack has occurred or is occurring.

## Inadequate blood and oxygen supply to the heart muscle

Just because you're having chest pain or discomfort doesn't mean you're having a heart attack. Instead, you may be having angina or pain entirely unrelated to the heart. An ECG that is obtained during your symptoms may help make the distinction (see figure at right).

Inadequate blood and oxygen supply to a region of your heart muscle often changes the shape of an ECG tracing, particularly the segment between the end of the QRS complex and the end of the T wave. This can help your physician decide on further testing or treatment. Between episodes of inadequate blood supply to the heart, the ECG may be perfectly normal.

## Heart structure abnormalities

The ECG can provide clues to the presence of thickening (hypertrophy) of your heart muscle, to congenital abnormalities, or to enlargement of your heart's chambers. But in most cases, other tests are needed to confirm the diagnosis and to get more information.

The ECG is helpful in other ways. It can give information about potential health problems that aren't specifically related to your heart. Changes in the ECG tracing may indicate potassium or calcium levels that are too high or too low. This may suggest kidney problems or hormonal abnormalities. An ECG may also help detect

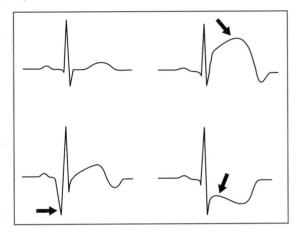

*The appearance of your electrocardiogram gives your physician important clues about certain heart problems. Here's what an ECG reading might look like in different circumstances:*

***Top left**. A normal heartbeat.*

***Top right**. The elevated portion (**arrow**) between the QRS complex and the T wave is a strong indication that heart muscle injury, such as a heart attack, is occurring.*

***Bottom left**. The deep early portion of the QRS complex (**arrow**) is evidence that a heart attack may have happened in the past.*

***Bottom right**. The lowered ST segment (**arrow**) suggests that blood supply to an area of your heart is insufficient. This might happen during an episode of angina or during an abnormal exercise stress test.*

side effects—or even toxicity—from medications you're taking. The reason is that certain drugs can alter the tracing in specific ways.

Like any other test result, ECG results are not always 100 percent accurate. Some rhythm disorders are so complex that they can't be diagnosed with certainty without further testing. The ECG may occasionally suggest coronary artery disease even when other testing shows no coronary artery disease. The ECG may appear normal when you do have such disease—particularly if you aren't showing any symptoms when you have the ECG. Nevertheless, because the ECG provides so much information at such a low cost and at no risk to you, it's considered vital to the understanding of your cardiac health in most cases.

## How is the ECG test done?

The ECG test is a simple one. Usually 12 to 15 electrodes are attached to various parts of your body, including one on each arm and leg, six across the left side of the chest, and often one or more at other sites on the chest, neck, and back.

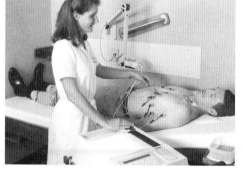

The electrodes are sticky patches that are attached to the skin while you're lying down. Because the electrodes are trying to detect very small electrical currents, good contact must be maintained with the skin. A conductive gel is used to improve this connection. The hair may be shaved off the chest in men, and the skin roughened with very fine sandpaper to ensure that the patch sticks.

After the leads are attached, the person performing the ECG test will record the information from the leads attached to you. You don't feel anything during the testing procedure. The actual ECG recording usually takes 30 to 60 seconds to complete. The test can be done in a hospital room or possibly your doctor's office.

*Undergoing electrocardiography is an easy procedure. Electrodes with adhesive on them are attached to your chest and limbs to record the electrical activity of your heart while you rest.*

Many hospitals and offices now have computerized interpretations of ECGs. Although this type of analysis has many benefits, computer programs raise a further possibility of error, no matter how sophisticated they are. ECGs should always be reviewed by a doctor to ensure that accurate and confident conclusions are drawn.

## Are there risks?

There is no pain or risk from ECG. The machine is only reading your heart's electrical impulses. It doesn't send any electrical impulses to your body. Nor is there a danger of electrical shock.

## Different types of ECG techniques

One of the problems with traditional ECGs is that because they are performed over only a minute or so, some sporadic rhythm abnormalities or other problems may be missed. Because of this, other ECG techniques have been developed to minimize the possibility that this test will miss an abnormality. These techniques include:

- Exercise ECG
- Ambulatory ECG
- Telephone-transmitted ECG and event recorders
- Signal-averaged ECG

## Exercise ECG

An exercise ECG test, often referred to as a "stress test," is one that's obtained while you walk on a treadmill or pedal a stationary cycle. Because higher heart rates make it easier to detect inadequate coronary circulation, abnormalities related to ischemia (insufficient blood and oxygen supply) are more likely to occur and to show up on an ECG during exercise. Also, some rhythm abnormalities are triggered by exercise, which makes them more likely to be detected. The exercise ECG test may also be used to follow your progress if you've had heart attacks or to assess the effects of various drugs or procedures on your health.

During an exercise ECG, the electrodes are attached to your chest and back. ECG recordings are taken before, during, and after you exercise. You start your exercise, whether it's on a treadmill or stationary bike, at a very relaxed pace. Every few minutes, the speed and incline of the treadmill (or the resistance on the bike) are increased to make you work a little harder.

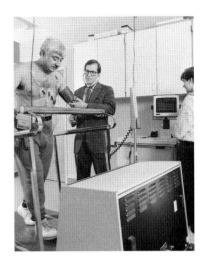

*An exercise electrocardiogram is obtained while you exercise ("stress test")—such as walking on a treadmill, shown here, or pedaling on a stationary bike.*

The doctor or nurses monitoring the test will ask you to rate how hard you are working according to the Borg Perceived Exertion Scale. They will encourage you to exercise until you're too tired to continue or until you experience any symptoms—such as chest pain or shortness of breath. The test is stopped once sufficient information is obtained.

If your heart's activity is normal during the exercise ECG test, there's a good chance that your heart will function normally when you exercise. The results will be useful for establishing exercise limits and developing a special fitness program. If the

### Borg Perceived Exertion Scale

During most types of exercise stress tests, you'll be asked to describe how hard you're working. One standard way of describing the amount of physical effort you're experiencing is to use the Borg Perceived Exertion Scale, shown below. This scale takes into account exertion, the physical stress you're feeling, and your fatigue. When you use the scale, think about your total feeling of exertion, not just one factor such as a sensation that your legs are getting heavier or that you're becoming short of breath.

**Borg Perceived Exertion Scale**

| | | | |
|---|---|---|---|
| 6 | | 14 | |
| 7 | Very, very light | 15 | Hard |
| 8 | | 16 | |
| 9 | Very light | 17 | Very hard |
| 10 | | 18 | |
| 11 | Fairly light | 19 | |
| 12 | | 20 | Very, very hard |
| 13 | Somewhat hard | | |

The scale ranges from "6," which indicates minimal exertion such as sitting comfortably in a chair, to "20," which corresponds to maximal exertion such as jogging up a very steep hill.

ECG shows any abnormalities, your doctor may recommend other tests that more accurately determine whether there are coronary blockages and where they are located.

## Stress tests at a glance

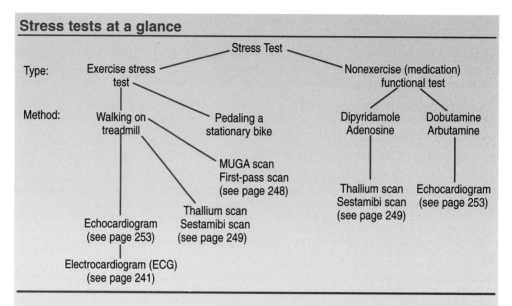

Stress tests are designed to examine how well your heart muscle functions, the adequacy of your coronary blood supply, or both. Many different kinds of stress tests are available. The type you will have depends on the questions that need to be answered, your ability to exercise, and the extent of abnormalities shown on your resting ECG. For example, an exercise test in which you walk on a treadmill while the ECG is monitored is useful if your physician suspects that you have coronary artery disease. A treadmill thallium scan shows the actual distribution of blood flow in your heart muscle. If you're not able to use your legs well (for example, because of arthritis), you may undergo an adenosine (or dipyridamole) thallium scan (see page 249). This isn't really a stress test, though the effect of stress on the heart is mimicked and similar information is obtained. Other stress tests, in addition to these, are occasionally done (for example, arm exercise can replace walking or cycling).

Undergoing an exercise ECG does carry a small risk because it involves stressing your heart. But the danger of suffering a heart attack during the test is remote—the odds are only 3.5 in 10,000. The risk of a serious heart rhythm problem occurring during the test is about 48 in 10,000. However, health professionals and equipment are standing by to monitor your symptoms and blood pressure continuously and to handle any emergency. The technicians, nurses, and doctors are trained to handle any situation that may come up, including the need for cardiopulmonary resuscitation if necessary. In fact, a medical facility is probably the safest possible place to have symptoms, because the problem can be diagnosed and treated appropriately and quickly. But problems rarely occur because doctors recommend these tests only for people in whom they believe the testing will be safe.

Even exercise ECG tests are not perfect and can yield either a false-positive or a false-negative result. It's always important to interpret the results of this and any other test in the light of other health information available about you. However, an ECG performed during exercise will correctly identify the presence of coronary artery disease in about 70 percent of people who have it. In addition, the test accurately rules out coronary artery disease in people who don't have it more than 90 percent of the time.

## Ambulatory ECG monitoring

Ambulatory monitoring of the ECG, which means your heart is monitored during your everyday activities, is used to detect heartbeat abnormalities that are intermittent. This is also called Holter monitoring, in honor of Norman Holter, who designed it in 1961.

Patch electrodes are attached to your chest and the ECG is recorded on tape or computer chip in a recorder that you wear for an entire day or two. You keep the recorder, which is about the size of a paperback novel, with you at all times during this test, including when you sleep. In most cases, you'll be asked to keep a diary of symptoms and activities so your doctor can correlate your experiences with the ECG obtained at that time. The recorded information can be played back and rapidly scanned by computer. Then, specially trained technicians and physicians analyze these data for heart rhythm abnormalities. The test also occasionally reveals evidence of inadequate blood supply to your coronary arteries.

Holter monitoring, like the usual ECG, is painless and there's no risk from the procedure. There is the slight inconvenience of keeping the recording device with you. You also need to keep an accurate diary to help relate your symptoms to the recording obtained of your heart at the time they occurred.

## Telephone-transmitted ECG

ECGs can be transmitted across telephone lines. If you need one, you'll receive a device that transmits ECG information across phone lines and be told how to use it. When a symptom develops, you dial a telephone number and transmit the ECG information to a monitor in the hospital or doctor's office. In the meantime, the device you have at home records the information, which can be played back later.

In this way, an ECG can provide information to help analyze infrequent symptoms. However, for this test to be effective, your symptoms must last long enough for you to dial the

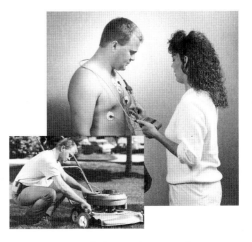

*A 24-hour ambulatory electrocardiogram, during which you wear a device called a Holter monitor, provides important information about the electrical activity of your heart as you go through your daily activities at home or work. Small electrodes stick to your skin and connect to a portable recording device worn on your belt (see photo inset). Every heartbeat is recorded for analysis later.*

### HEALTHY HEART ♥ TIP

*Children are more likely to smoke if their parents smoke—and the younger they start, the more likely they'll be heavy smokers later. Second-hand smoke is linked to increased risk of heart disease, cancer, asthma, infant pneumonia and respiratory failure. Parents: Lead by example. Don't smoke.*

telephone and make a transmission and, of course, the transmitter and a telephone must be handy when the symptoms occur.

If your symptoms are infrequent, sporadic, or otherwise hard to "capture" over the telephone lines, you may need to use another device called an event recorder. Like a Holter monitor, an event recorder is worn away from the hospital or testing site, and for a longer time—usually about a month. While it's best to wear it as much as possible, you can remove it briefly when you bathe, and so on.

When a symptom occurs, you push a button that tells the event recorder to "remember" what it recorded for several minutes before and after the button was pushed. Unless the button is pushed, the recorder simply monitors the heart rhythm. The signal from the recorder can then be transmitted over the telephone or taken to the doctor's office at your convenience.

A new type of event recorder is now available. Called an implantable loop recorder, it's the size of a pencil-top eraser and can be implanted under the skin of your chest. This monitor records your heart rhythm for up to 18 months. It's particularly useful in determining whether you have an abnormal rhythm during fainting episodes or "spells" that happen infrequently—about two or three times a year.

### Signal-averaged electrocardiography

Signal-averaged ECG is a noninvasive technique occasionally used to help identify people at high risk for ventricular tachycardia or ventricular fibrillation. During ventricular fibrillation, your heart cannot effectively pump blood to your body. This condition is the most common cause of sudden cardiac death outside the hospital.

Signal-averaged ECG uses a computer program to identify very low or weak electrical impulses in your heart that are undetectable on a regular ECG. The computer program amplifies the magnitude of these impulses. It then filters the recordings to eliminate "noise" from other sources—such as your skeletal muscles or even nearby machines. If certain tiny waves appear in the signal-averaged ECG, this may indicate that you're at a higher risk of a future heart rhythm abnormality and sudden death. If so, you'll likely need additional testing and preventive treatment. Frequently employed in the past, this test is not often used in today's practice.

## The chest X-ray

In medical practice, it's often necessary to see inside your body instead of just its surface. An X-ray film allows your doctor to do this without surgery and with minimal risk.

Although you may associate X-rays with broken bones, an X-ray can provide valuable information about your heart, lungs and other structures in your chest. In turn, this helps your doctor make a diagnosis about your condition. Many complex imaging tests have been developed in recent decades. But the chest X-ray is still a fundamental and important test in the evaluation and screening of heart disease.

## What is a chest X-ray?

A chest X-ray simply takes a picture of what's inside your chest: your heart and lungs.

An X-ray image is created by aiming X-rays at a region of your body (in this case the chest) and positioning a large piece of photographic film on the other side of you. Like any other film, once the X-ray film is developed, an image will show up. Parts of the film that received a large exposure to the X-rays will be dark. Those that received less will be lighter. This is like the negative in a picture taken by a regular camera: The parts of the film that received a lot of light rays (like a sunbeam reflected off pond water) appear dark. The parts that received little light (like a shadow) appear light.

The amount of X-rays that pass through your body and reach the film depends on the amount and type of tissues between the X-ray camera and the film. Because your muscular blood-filled heart is located between the two lungs filled with air, the silhouette of your heart is very conspicuous in the center of your chest. The heart will appear light on the film because fewer X-rays were able to pass through fluid or blood and reach the film. The lungs will appear very dark because they are almost transparent to X-rays, so the film behind the lungs gets a large exposure to the X-rays.

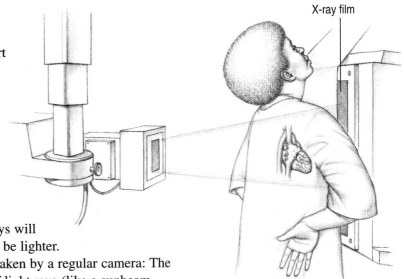

X-ray film

*A chest X-ray is obtained by passing an X-ray beam through your body. The rays penetrate different areas in different ways before they reach the piece of film. Parts of your body that let most of the beams through (such as your lungs) cause the X-ray film to turn dark when it's developed. Other areas, such as your heart (or especially your bones), block many of the X-rays, preventing them from reaching the film. These areas appear light on the developed film.*

## What do chest X-rays show?

The chest X-ray reveals several types of information that are important in assessing the cardiovascular system:

- Size and shape of your heart
- Calcium deposits
- Lung condition

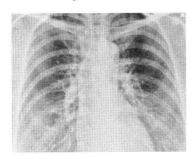 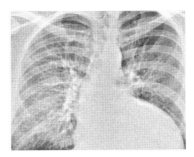

*The size of your heart is an important piece of information provided by the chest X-ray. The X-ray on the left shows a normal-sized heart. The X-ray on the right shows a heart that's conspicuously enlarged, a sign that it's not pumping efficiently.*

## Size and shape of your heart

Both the size and the shape of the heart can be judged on the chest X-ray, though individual parts can be distinguished only partially. Normally, the heart's width on a chest X-ray occupies no more than one third to one half the width of your whole chest. If your heart occupies half or more of this space, doctors consider it to be enlarged.

As the heart enlarges, it may change shape. The shape of the heart can provide a clue about what is causing the enlargement. A heart that is enlarged because of mitral regurgitation, for example, usually looks different from one that's enlarged because of mitral stenosis or aortic stenosis.

## Calcium deposits

Calcium is the main substance in your bones. It doesn't allow many X-rays to pass through, so bones appear very light on X-ray films. Sometimes calcium deposits can also occur in diseased or injured tissue. In the heart, calcium deposits can sometimes be found in diseased valves, coronary arteries with atherosclerosis, and damaged heart muscle or the pericardium—the sac that surrounds your heart.

Because they show up as light areas on an X-ray, calcium deposits within the heart image can be distinguished from other soft tissue on the chest X-ray. Their presence in the heart may be the first sign of a problem that requires further investigation.

## Lung condition

Chest X-rays can detect changes in your lungs that are related to abnormalities in the way your heart works. A weakly pumping heart, for example, results in back pressure in your lungs' blood vessels, causing them to swell and leak fluid into the lungs' air sacs. This condition is called pulmonary edema. Chest X-rays can detect this swelling in your lungs' veins. The reason is that X-rays do not pass through fluid as easily as they pass through air, so doctors can see fluid that has leaked into lung tissue.

## How is a chest X-ray done?

The chest X-ray procedure simply means a picture is being taken of your heart. It's straightforward and painless.

Before you have it, you'll probably remove your clothes and jewelry from the waist up and put on a hospital gown. Jewelry, zippers, and other items show up on the X-ray and could obscure parts of the image.

In most cases, you will be asked to stand against the plate that contains the X-ray film, roll your shoulders forward, and hold your arms up or to the side so that they don't interfere with the picture.

HEALTHY
HEART ♥ TIP

*With all the focus on no-cholesterol foods, you might think you'd be better off without any cholesterol at all. Just the opposite is true.*

*In fact, you can't live without cholesterol, which is one type of the fat-like substances (lipids) in your blood. Among other things, cholesterol helps insulate the nerves, produces certain hormones and helps your liver make bile acids.*

*But your body probably produces enough cholesterol on its own—which is why it makes sense to watch your dietary intake. Your liver makes about 80 percent of the cholesterol in your blood; about 20 percent comes from diet, from animal products, or foods containing them.*

The radiologist or technician will ask you to take a deep breath and hold it as the X-ray picture is being taken. Holding your breath fills your lungs with air. This helps your heart and lungs to show up more clearly on the X-ray. It also helps stop you from moving.

It's also useful to get a chest X-ray from the side. Most likely, a second picture will be obtained with you turned to one side against the X-ray plate.

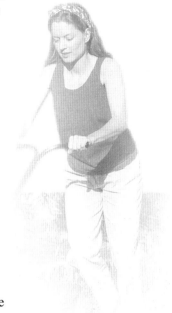

### Are there risks?

Although a small amount of radiation is involved in any X-ray, the risk of harm from a chest X-ray is very low and is greatly outweighed by the benefits of the image obtained. Great care is taken to use the lowest possible dose of radiation to produce the best possible image. No radiation remains in you after the X-ray.

The risk of X-rays can be put in perspective if you know that medical X-rays of all types account for only a little more than 10 percent of the total radiation exposure for the U.S. population. Other sources of radiation in the environment include radon, outer space, rocks, and soil. The amount of radiation from a chest X-ray is about the same as you might receive during a transcontinental airplane trip.

Women who have any chance of being pregnant when the X-ray is taken should tell their doctors. Although the risk of harm to an unborn child from an X-ray is very low, doctors take special precautions to minimize the baby's exposure.

## Nuclear scanning

Nuclear scanning techniques add a new dimension to the assessment of your heart and circulation. While a chest X-ray shows some of your heart's structure, nuclear scans show features of your heart's function and blood flow.

### What are nuclear scans?

When you have an X-ray, radiation passes through your body to produce an image. During nuclear scanning procedures, a tiny amount of radiation is introduced inside your body. It produces images as it radiates outward.

Briefly, here's how most nuclear scanning procedures work. Trace amounts of radioactive material (called radionuclides) are injected into your bloodstream. These "tracers" give off small amounts of energy (radiation) that are detected by special cameras, similar to Geiger counters.

The radiation "counts" are processed by a computer, and an image is produced showing how the material is distributed in your body. Depending on the tracer material and the specific type of scan, these procedures can tell your doctor a great deal about your heart muscle and blood flow.

## What do nuclear scans show?

There are many different types of nuclear scans. Collectively, they can provide a lot of information about your heart, including:

- Heart chamber size
- Pumping ability of the ventricles
- Blood flow to the heart muscle
- Blood flow in your lungs

Additional information can often be obtained from nuclear scanning by performing it in combination with an exercise stress test.

### Evaluating your heart's on-the-job efficiency

Doctors also monitor your heart's efficiency at its most basic job: the muscular contractions that pump blood through your body. The ventricles, the large lower pumping chambers of your heart, play a key role in your heart's efficiency. These assessments can tell doctors how well they're performing:

- *Ejection fraction.* This is the percentage (or fraction) of blood in the ventricle at the end of diastole (the phase of relaxation when the ventricle fills with blood) that is pumped out during systole (contraction of the ventricle). Normal is more than 50 percent.

- *Stroke volume.* This refers to the amount of blood the ventricle squeezes out with each systolic contraction. Normal is about 90 milliliters (about 3 ounces) for the average resting adult.

- *Cardiac output.* This is the amount of blood your heart pumps in 1 minute. Normal for a resting adult is about 5 liters (or about 5 quarts) per minute.

### Heart chamber size

A weakened heart enlarges, so an accurate measurement of the size of the pumping chambers (ventricles) is an important index of your heart muscle's strength. A type of nuclear scan called radionuclide ventriculography (ven-TRIK-you-log-ruh-fee) can provide this information reliably.

There are two versions of radionuclide ventriculography. One is called "MUGA" scanning (for *MU*lti*G*ated *A*cquisition). The other has a somewhat less interesting name. It's simply called a "first-pass study."

In both tests, a tracer is injected into your bloodstream. It is scanned as it passes through your heart. For the MUGA scan, the tracer stays in your bloodstream for several hours. For the first-pass study, it remains in the bloodstream only long enough to circulate once through your heart before it is eliminated. In both tests, a special scanner camera detects the radiation given off by the tracer as it passes through your heart.

A computer then uses this information to calculate the size and shape of your ventricles based on the amount and distribution of radiation emitted from them. An image is produced that can be studied by your doctor. In addition, numerical measurements can be made of the amount of blood in the ventricles.

### Pumping ability of the ventricles

Radionuclide ventriculography can also provide accurate and useful knowledge about the ventricles' pumping ability. To do this, the computer takes the information from the scan and then calculates the size and shape of the ventricles during systole (contraction) and diastole (relaxation). The difference between the size of the heart at these two points of time indicates how well the ventricles are squeezing.

A radionuclide ventriculogram can also determine whether all portions of the ventricular wall contribute equally to the pumping activity. Parts that move weakly may have been damaged by a heart attack. Or blood flow to these areas may be reduced because of coronary blockages.

## Blood flow to the heart muscle

When performed in combination with exercise or another form of stress, nuclear scanning tests can provide vital information about the flow of blood through your coronary arteries.

Radionuclide ventriculography again is useful to find out this information. Your heart is scanned before and during increasing stages of exercise. At each level of exercise, the pumping functions of all parts of your ventricle are examined. A normal heart will contract more vigorously during exertion. A heart in which one or more regions beat worse than expected during exercise likely isn't receiving enough blood to keep up with the muscle's increased need for energy. When the scan shows a region with poor function, your doctor can conclude that the coronary artery supplying that portion of your heart muscle is at least partially blocked.

Perfusion scanning is another nuclear scanning procedure to evaluate your coronary blood flow. It's usually performed in conjunction with exercise. Unlike the tracer used in radionuclide ventriculography, the tracer used for perfusion scanning does not remain in your bloodstream. Rather, it enters the cells of your heart muscle (myocardium) after it's carried there in the coronary arteries. During the scanning, an image is made of the heart muscle itself, not of the blood in your ventricle. If a portion of your myocardium receives less blood than the rest of your heart, less tracer appears in it and it shows up on the scan as a lighter area. This lighter area is known as a perfusion defect (see page A10).

Tracers commonly used for perfusion scans are technetium (in a form called sestamibi) and radioactive thallium. This is why the terms "sestamibi scan" or "thallium scan" are therefore often used synonymously with "perfusion scan." Sestamibi scans often can provide better images than thallium, especially in larger individuals.

The perfusion scanning is done after exercise and again after a rest period. Comparison of how your blood flows into (perfuses) the myocardium under these two conditions permits doctors to evaluate the health of your myocardium and the arteries that supply it with blood.

### Understanding your perfusion scan results

Perfusion scan results basically fall into one of three categories, although they may vary by location in your heart and by severity. Here's some help in interpreting your results:

1. *No perfusion defect found while you're resting or after you exercise.* Interpretation: Your myocardium and coronary arteries are normal.

2. *Perfusion defect found after exercise, but not at rest.* Interpretation: One or more coronary blockages are preventing sufficient blood flow from reaching your hard-working myocardium. After a rest period, the tracer eventually reaches the myocardium and enters the cells, so there is at least some blood flow to the region and there are living myocardium cells present.

3. *Perfusion defect after exercise and at rest.* Interpretation: An area of your heart muscle is now scar tissue because of a previous myocardial infarction (heart attack). The perfusion defect showed up because there's a blocked coronary artery and because there are no living myocardial cells at that site for the tracer to enter.

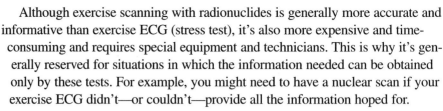

Although exercise scanning with radionuclides is generally more accurate and informative than exercise ECG (stress test), it's also more expensive and time-consuming and requires special equipment and technicians. This is why it's generally reserved for situations in which the information needed can be obtained only by these tests. For example, you might need to have a nuclear scan if your exercise ECG didn't—or couldn't—provide all the information hoped for.

Sometimes, health problems may prevent you from performing exercise-related tests needed to assess your heart's health. However, similar information may be obtained during a perfusion scan by using a medication (such as dipyridamole and adenosine) that mimics physical stress on your heart. Although this can be useful, a traditional exercise test remains the best option.

Neither the perfusion scan nor the radionuclide ventriculogram shows coronary blockages directly. Instead, they show only the effects of coronary blockages on the myocardium. Further testing, such as coronary angiography, is needed to actually see the location, number, and severity of the blockages (see page 261).

*A lung perfusion scan provides an overall picture of blood circulation throughout your lungs. The light patches in the lung images (**arrows**) are areas not reached by the tracer because of blockages in the pulmonary artery branches from clots. These clots are called pulmonary emboli.*

## Blood flow to your lungs

Blockages in arteries that supply your lungs are usually caused by blood clots, that is, pulmonary embolism (see page 128). A pulmonary embolus can be detected by a nuclear technique called ventilation/perfusion scanning—also known as lung scanning.

Lung scanning assesses blood circulation in your lungs. As with heart scanning, a radioactive tracer is injected into your veins. Then your chest is scanned. If there is a blood clot blocking blood flow through one or more branches of your lungs' arteries, the radioactive tracer will not be seen in that that area.

Lung scans are usually performed with another scanning technique that involves breathing in gas containing tracer material. The lungs are then scanned again. The adequacy of blood flow to all parts of the lung can be compared with the adequacy of airflow through the bronchi (airways). A blood clot would cause problems only with blood flow. Your airflow would be relatively unaffected. If this is the case, it may suggest other conditions for your doctor to focus on.

Lung scans are useful to assess whether certain symptoms such as chest pain or shortness of breath are the result of pulmonary embolism. A normal lung scan is reassuring because it means that it's unlikely pulmonary embolism has occurred. People who have a positive test result, however, may need to undergo pulmonary angiography to confirm the presence of a pulmonary embolus.

Recently, the ultrafast electron beam computed tomography (CT) scanner (see page 276) has been shown to be effective in detecting pulmonary emboli. In some medical centers, this is the preferred procedure to diagnose this condition. It is more accurate than the ventilation/perfusion scan.

## How is nuclear scanning done?

Nuclear scans may sound intimidating and complicated. Most of them, however, are fairly straightforward from a patient's perspective. Here's what to expect if you need one of these scans.

### Exercise perfusion scan

While you exercise on a treadmill or stationary bike, a small dose of the tracer material is injected into a vein in your arm. To reduce the possibility of nausea caused by exercising after a meal, you may be asked not to eat or drink for several hours before the scan. You may also need to stop taking certain medications before the test because some drugs can impair the test's accuracy.

Because you will be exercising vigorously during the test, wear comfortable clothing and shoes appropriate for brisk exercise. You may also be asked to wear a hospital gown. Before the test, you'll be connected to an ECG machine. An intravenous (IV) line will be inserted into a vein in your arm.

Usually you will exercise on a treadmill or a stationary cycle, just as you would during an exercise ECG. Your heart rate and blood pressure will be monitored, and it's normal for them to increase during exercise. If you have any symptoms—such as chest or arm pain, shortness of breath, or light-headedness—inform the technician. Adjustments can be made to the exercise test depending on your symptoms, blood pressure, ECG, or degree of fatigue. It's important to exercise for as long as possible. The reason is that it increases the accuracy of your test.

After you exercise nearly to your limit, the tracer material is injected and is carried to your heart in your blood. You then continue to exercise for 60 to 90 seconds more after the injection.

You then will lie under a camera that "takes pictures" of your heart from various angles. The camera detects the radiation being emitted by the radioactive tracer and reconstructs this into a computerized image. It is important to stay as still as possible while the pictures are being taken. This part of the test may last up to 25 minutes.

After the scanning is done, you can relax for several hours (typically 4 hours) and leave the testing center. When you return, you'll undergo a second scan, but you won't have to exercise again. This scan will then be compared with the first (see page A10). Because the size of a meal consumed before the second set of images may affect the quality of the images, ask the doctor what you are allowed to eat during your "time off." In some cases your doctor may want a third set of images taken the next day.

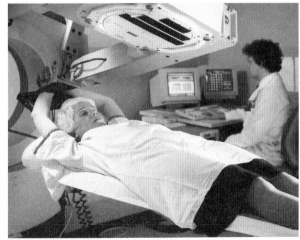

*A nuclear heart scan is obtained by a special camera that detects the radiation given off by the tracer material injected into you and carried to your heart. During the scanning, the camera moves at different angles while you remain still. The signals are used by a computer to construct an image of your heart and the blood flow to it (see page 248).*

## Radionuclide ventriculogram

To get a rapid and accurate assessment of your heart's size and function, this scan can be done while you're resting. Or it can be done before and during progressively harder exercise. For a MUGA scan (see page 248), the exercise is usually done while you are lying on your back and pedaling a bicycle wheel. For a first-pass study, you perform the exercise while you're upright.

Your doctor may ask you to stop taking any heart medications for a day or two before the test. But don't stop taking them unless you are specifically told to do so. You also may be advised to avoid eating a big meal several hours before the test.

For a MUGA scan, a small amount of your blood is drawn into a syringe containing technetium. In the syringe, the technetium attaches to your red blood cells. This coupling ensures that the technetium stays in your bloodstream and doesn't go into any of your body's other tissues.

About 10 minutes later, the blood containing the tracer is reinjected and the first scan is taken while you're at rest. For first-pass studies, the tracer is simply injected directly into a vein. Then you perform easy pedaling for 3 minutes. During the last 2 minutes, another scan is taken.

Then the exercise is made harder by increasing the resistance on the pedals. Again, you exercise for 3 minutes and another scan is taken while you exercise. There is no break between the stages of exercise. The test continues until you can no longer exercise. During the scanning, your ECG is recorded and your blood pressure is measured at each stage. No special care or precautions are needed once you finish the test.

## Are there risks?

Injecting radioactive material into your body may sound troubling. But the amount of radiation you're exposed to during testing is very low and very safe. In fact, the radiation exposure you receive during radionuclide heart scanning is comparable to that of a bowel X-ray taken after you swallow barium. The benefits of these tests far outweigh the risks of radiation exposure, and the doses used are safe. However, for women who are pregnant or breastfeeding, radionuclide scanning isn't used unless the information is vital and cannot be obtained by other means.

Adverse reactions to thallium, a tracer agent used in scanning, are possible but very rare. About a third of people receiving dipyridamole, a drug used to mimic physical stress on the heart, may experience headache, nausea, flushing, or dizziness. The drug could also possibly bring on chest pain and ECG changes. But your risk of heart attack while using dipyridamole is extremely low. However, you shouldn't take dipyridamole if you have asthma. A drug called aminophylline can be given to counteract the symptoms, but it's usually not necessary because the side effects often are gone by the time the scanning is finished. Adenosine produces similar side effects in most patients, but these effects are even briefer in duration than those caused by dipyridamole.

The exercise portions of these tests involve the same precautions that apply to the exercise ECG. The risk of heart attack or rhythm abnormalities is small. Physicians and other hospital staff equipped to deal with emergencies are always standing by.

# Echocardiography

Echocardiography, a procedure developed and refined during the past 40 years, makes it possible to "look" directly at your heart without penetrating your skin. This unique procedure is reducing the need for invasive, potentially risky tests such as cardiac catheterization.

## What is echocardiography?

Echocardiography is a special application of diagnostic ultrasound (sound too high-pitched for humans to hear). The concept behind the use of ultrasound is the same as that used in depth finders or fish locators on boats. In the case of echocardiography, ultrasound waves are sent out to and reflected (echoed) back from internal structures. The sound waves are sent into your body by a special microphonelike device called a transducer.

The transducer also detects the echoes bouncing back from the surfaces of internal structures, such as your myocardium (heart muscle) and heart valves. A machine (the echocardiograph) analyzes the waves to determine how far away the structures are from the transducer.

A computer calculates the time it takes the sound waves to travel to and from your heart and then reconstructs the shape of the heart on the basis of that information. The image (echocardiogram) of your heart is displayed on a video or television screen, and can be recorded on videotape or printed on paper.

The echocardiogram can be obtained in various ways and displayed in different forms, depending on the type of information needed about your heart. One type of display—called an M-mode echocardiogram—is very abstract and looks nothing like an actual heart. However, it's useful for measuring the exact size of various heart structures, such as the thickness of the myocardium or the size of one of your heart's chambers.

A second type is the two-dimensional (2-D) echocardiogram. As its name implies, it shows an image of your heart in two dimensions, as though your heart were sliced like a loaf of bread so that each slice could be individually examined. By changing the position of the transducer, doctors can see most parts of your heart and get a good impression of how well all of its parts are working.

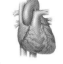

**HEALTHY HEART ♥ TIP**

*Your kids are couch potatoes, and you don't know what to do. Take heart: You can find plenty of ways to get them up and moving—and increase their chances of growing into heart-healthy adults.*

- *Lead by example, then invite your children to share in the exercise*
- *Plan family outings and vacations that involve outdoor activities such as hiking, bicycling or swimming*
- *Give them household chores that require physical exertion, such as mowing lawns, raking leaves, scrubbing floors and taking out the garbage*
- *Observe what activities appeal to them, then find out about lessons and clubs*
- *Stay involved in their physical education classes at school*

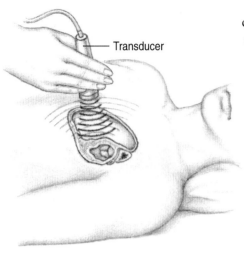

Transducer

*Echocardiography is done with ultrasound waves that reflect off (or "echo") the surfaces of your heart's structure. A computer uses this information to construct an image of your heart or analyze your blood flow.*

A third type of echocardiographic display is based on technology called Doppler ultrasound. When sound waves bounce off blood cells moving through your heart and blood vessels, they change pitch in a characteristic way. This change is called a Doppler shift—named in honor of an Austrian physicist and mathematician who lived in the early 1800s.

This effect is similar to that of a train whistle that sounds different when the train is moving toward you (sounds high-pitched), passes you, and then moves away (sounds lower-pitched). The change in pitch of the ultrasound waves bouncing off red blood cells can be measured, and the speed and direction of the flowing blood can then be calculated. Using Doppler signals, the echocardiogram can display both the sound and the visual information about blood flowing through your heart. During your echocardiographic examination, you may hear a pulsing "whoosh" sound. That sound is the echocardiograph's "interpretation" of blood flowing past the structures of your heart.

Doppler ultrasound is particularly useful to determine whether your heart valves are functioning properly. It can also measure pressure inside your heart and gauge the degree of narrowing or leakage of a heart valve.

A fourth type of echocardiographic display is called color Doppler. The echocardiographic computer does complex calculations of blood flow through your heart. These calculations are based on the Doppler shift. Then it displays the blood flow as colors on a 2-D image (see page A6). Each color represents a direction and speed of the blood flow. This technique is able to characterize further the way blood flows through your heart's valves. It can also detect abnormal blood flow—such as that created by a small hole in the atrial or ventricular septum.

Still other types of echocardiographic techniques can give more detailed and specialized information about your heart and how it's working.

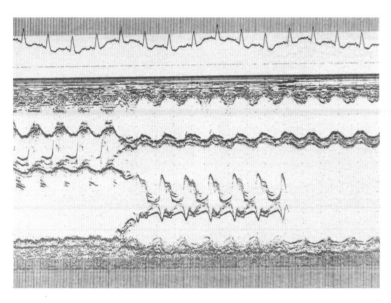

*One type of echocardiogram, called the M-mode echocardiogram, is an image that doesn't look anything like a heart. However, it's useful for making careful measurements of your heart's dimensions. The M-mode echocardiogram shown here is of a greatly enlarged heart that is not pumping vigorously. A condition called dilated cardiomyopathy caused the heart enlargement.*

## What does echocardiography show?

Echocardiography techniques enable doctors to accurately visualize and measure your heart's dimensions and shape, determine the myocardium's pumping ability, and measure pressures and gradients (narrowing) in valves and vessels. Echocardiography also makes it possible to visualize blood flow and valve leakage. With this technology, numerous aspects of your heart's health can be observed, including:

- Heart size
- Pumping strength
- Damage to the heart muscle
- Severity and type of valve problems
- Abnormal blood flow patterns
- Heart structure abnormalities
- Blood pressure in the lung arteries

### Size of heart

Weakened or damaged defective heart valves, high blood pressure, or other diseases can cause the chambers of your heart to enlarge (see page 50). The echocardiogram can reveal this enlargement and measurements can be made of important dimensions. Because the echocardiogram is noninvasive, it can be safely repeated to follow the stability or progression of a problem and help determine the need for treatment. Echocardiography can be used to determine how well the treatment is working.

### Pumping strength

The echocardiogram permits physicians to directly observe your heart muscle in motion. An experienced echocardiographer can tell at a glance whether the myocardium is pumping at full strength or whether it is slightly, moderately, or severely reduced in function. Measurements can also be made to determine ejection fraction, stroke volume and cardiac output (see page 49).

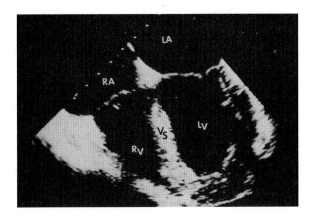

*This type of image is produced by two-dimensional (2-D) echocardiography. As its name suggests, it shows the structure of your heart in two dimensions—as though you were looking at a "slice" of the heart. This image appears on a TV monitor and is recorded on videotape so that your heart can be observed in motion. A 2-D echocardiogram gives an accurate view of the structure and action of your heart. RA, right atrium; LA, left atrium; RV, right ventricle; LV, left ventricle; VS, ventricular septum.*

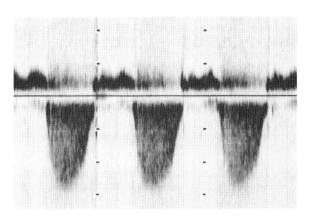

*These are Doppler signals. They indicate the velocity of blood flowing through a valve, which helps determine whether the valve is working normally. Doppler signals can also be processed by a computer to make color images of blood flow in your heart (see page A6).*

### Damage to the heart muscle

With an echocardiogram, doctors can determine whether all portions of the ventricular wall are contributing equally to the pumping activity of your heart. Parts that move weakly may have been damaged during a heart attack. Or they may be receiving too little oxygen because of blockage in your coronary arteries. Also, because the echocardiogram can show the myocardium, it's possible to see areas that may be thinner than neighboring areas and that do not thicken as expected during a contraction. These are all signs of damage in your myocardium.

### Severity and type of valve problems

Echocardiography is usually the best test for examining your heart valves (see pages A6, 253). One of the reasons is that it shows the anatomy of your valves and how they move during relaxation and contraction of your heart. Do they open wide to let blood flow through? Do they close fully to prevent leakage of blood? Are they misshapen by congenital defects, infection, deposits of calcium, or wear and tear? The basic echocardiogram can answer these questions.

The Doppler and color Doppler tests can also show whether blood is actually leaking back through a valve or whether blood flow is impeded by a narrowed valve outlet. In addition, these tests can help gauge the severity of problems detected. The Doppler tests are so sensitive that doctors now realize that most people normally have a tiny amount of back leakage through some of their valves. However, this tiny back leakage causes no problems and can't be heard with a stethoscope.

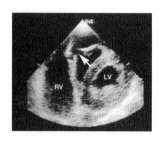

*The arrow shows a hole in the wall of the right ventricle (RV), as revealed by echocardiography.*

### Abnormal blood flow patterns

Doppler techniques can also reveal other blood flow abnormalities. For example, holes in the walls of your heart can be detected by a "jet" of blood flow seen on a color Doppler examination. Careful examination by 2-D echocardiography of the region where the "jet" is located may also reveal this defect.

### Heart structure abnormalities

Any test that can show the shape and position of the heart structure and patterns of blood flow in it can help evaluate conditions that produce structural heart problems. Congenital heart defects, for example, can be very thoroughly examined by echocardiography—revealing abnormalities in heart chambers, valves, and connections between the heart and major blood vessels (see pages 59 to 68).

Other structural abnormalities are also detectable by echocardiography. Overgrowth of the myocardium, which may occur if you have a condition called hypertrophic cardiomyopathy (see page 52), can be directly visualized. Doppler techniques can also disclose whether this overgrowth of the heart muscle is affecting blood flow.

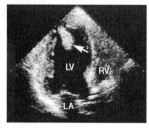

*Echocardiograph reveals a blood clot in the left ventricle (arrow).*

Echocardiography can determine whether a blood clot has formed in one of your heart's chambers. A clot here may break loose and lodge somewhere else in your body, causing other conditions, some of them serious. Finding a blood clot in the heart may be important in establishing the cause of a stroke or blockage in an artery elsewhere, such as your leg. This technique can also show whether you have clusters of infected tissue on a heart valve. This information can help your physician make a diagnosis of infective endocarditis, a condition that could cause infected tissue in this location (see page 70).

Echocardiography is also valuable in visualizing and evaluating the pericardium, the sac or membrane surrounding your heart. This is particularly true if it is diseased. It can detect small or large amounts of fluid between your heart and its sac (pericardial effusion; see page 133). This capability not only is important for making the diagnosis, but also is helpful for accurately and safely placing a needle or catheter through your chest wall to drain the fluid.

## Blood pressure in your pulmonary arteries

For many years, the only reliable way to determine the pressure in the pulmonary arteries was to thread a catheter through a vein and into a pulmonary artery. With the advent of Doppler techniques, accurate, noninvasive estimates of blood pressure are possible. The technique involves calculating the pressures that would be required to make blood flow at a particular measured velocity. Pulmonary hypertension—a condition in which lung blood pressure becomes dangerously elevated—can be detected and measured this way.

## How is echocardiography done?

Echocardiography usually is done in a cardiologist's office or laboratory, although the procedure can also be done at the hospital bedside with portable machines. But it can be performed in other settings—outreach clinics, emergency rooms and operating rooms. No special preparations are necessary before arriving for the test. In the laboratory, you remove your clothes from the waist up and put on a gown or robe provided for you.

You usually are asked to lie on your back or on your left side. Special gel or oil is applied to your chest to improve the transmission of the ultrasound waves. A technician or doctor moves a microphone-shaped transducer over your heart. Although the test is noninvasive and usually painless, the transducer occasionally must be held firmly against your chest. This pressure can be uncomfortable, especially over your ribs. The transducer is linked by a cord to the monitor screen and other electronic components.

You'll be asked to exhale and to hold your breath, because the air in your lungs can interfere with the image produced. The transducer will be moved to several sites on your chest to view your heart from different angles. A thorough echocardiographic examination may take from 15 minutes to more than an hour, depending on what your doctor is looking for.

*When you have an echocardiogram, the technician or doctor "views" your heart with a transducer held over your chest wall. Moving the transducer gives different views of your heart. An electrocardiogram (ECG) is monitored at the same time.*

## What may prevent standard echocardiography from getting a clear image of your heart

- **Pulmonary (lung) disease**
  Overinflated lungs (emphysema) from smoking
  Other causes of emphysema
- **Body shape**
  Obesity
  Emaciated patients or those who are tall and thin
  Spinal or chest wall abnormalities
  Breast implants or large breasts
- **Medical conditions**
  Prior heart or chest surgery
  Chest injury
  Use of ventilator

### Special echocardiographic techniques

A variety of techniques allow echocardiography to be used in different ways for different reasons, or to enhance the information the technology provides to your physician. These techniques include transesophageal echocardiography, exercise echocardiography, medication-induced stress echocardiography, and many others, such as contrast echocardiography, fetal echocardiography and intraoperative echocardiography.

### Transesophageal echocardiography

The development of this technique is an important advancement in the use of this technology. The reason is that it overcomes some of the limitations—such as body shape or weight—that prevent traditional echocardiography from taking a clear "picture" of your heart.

The name of the technique tells you how it overcomes these limitations. Transesophageal means "through (trans) the esophagus" (the tube that goes from your throat to your stomach). Traditional echocardiographic techniques view the heart through the chest wall. But with transesophageal echocardiography, the ultrasound transducer is attached to the end of a tube and inserted down your esophagus. Because the esophagus is close to your heart, having the transducer there provides a clearer picture of your heart structure and blood flow.

Transesophageal echocardiography requires some preparation. You'll be advised not to take anything by mouth—except medication—for 4 to 6 hours before the procedure to prevent nausea and vomiting. An intravenous (IV) line will be used to deliver a short-acting sedative. To help insert the transducer, the cardiologist or nurse will spray your throat with a numbing agent. You then swallow the end of the tube that has the transducer on it (this is easier to do than it sounds). Then the cardiologist gently manipulates the instrument to obtain the images needed.

The IV line may also be used to inject a small amount of saline (salt water) solution into your vein. After the fluid is injected into the bloodstream and circulates to the heart, it highlights the blood flow pattern in your heart.

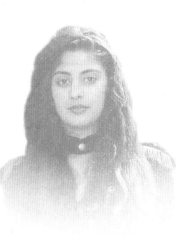

You remain partially awake during this procedure. One reason is that the doctor may ask you to hold your breath or to strain as if you were having a bowel movement. Straining alters the pressures in your heart chambers. Certain problems may show up when you do this that don't show up under normal conditions.

When the test is over, avoid eating or drinking—especially hot foods or beverages—for about 2 hours because your throat may be numb for a while. If you're given a sedative, avoid driving for 24 hours.

### Exercise echocardiography

Echocardiography can also be used while you're exercising to find out how well your heart works under stress. During this procedure, echocardiography is performed while you rest. Then you walk on a treadmill or pedal a stationary bike until you're at your peak exercise level, at which point you stop. Echocardiography is done immediately while your heart rate is still high. The cardiologist evaluates the overall response of your heart to exercise and whether all parts of the myocardium contribute equally to your heart's ability to contract under stress. If some areas of the heart don't contribute as much, this may suggest that coronary arteries to these areas are at least partially blocked. Exercise echocardiography can also be used to evaluate heart valve diseases.

## Medication-induced stress echocardiography

If you're unable to exercise for exercise echocardiography, a similar effect can be achieved by taking a medication to mimic the effect of stress on your heart. Typically, dobutamine, dipyridamole or adenosine is used. The medication is given through a vein. It gradually increases your heart's pumping capacity. The echocardiogram will show areas of your myocardium that don't respond to this stimulation. Lack of response to this drug-induced "stress" indicates areas of your heart that aren't getting enough blood supplied to them.

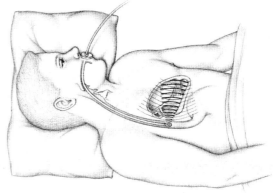

A technique with a long name—transesophageal atrial pacing stress echocardiography—is another option for patients who are unable to exercise. This involves swallowing a small flexible catheter. The catheter is positioned temporarily in your esophagus and attached to a pacemaker generator. The pacemaker generator is used to increase your heart rate. The simultaneous recording of the echocardiogram shows whether the myocardium responds appropriately to an increased heart rate. This technique can also provide indirect evidence of coronary artery blockage.

*During standard echocardiograms, the transducer is held on the surface of your chest. But sometimes, a clearer echocardiogram image can be obtained by inserting the transducer into your esophagus. This approach positions the transducer closer to your heart. Putting the transducer in your esophagus is easier than it sounds. Physicians will numb the back of your throat and give you a mild sedative to help you relax.*

## Additional echocardiographic techniques

Specific situations may call for the use of additional echocardiographic techniques. Contrast echocardiography is a procedure in which echocardiographic images are obtained as fluid known as a contrast agent—usually salt water or a protein solution—is injected into one of your veins. This technique is used to improve visualization of the walls of your heart and abnormalities of blood flow in the heart or blood vessels.

Fetal echocardiography can visualize the heart of an unborn baby and permit diagnosis of congenital heart disease before birth. Intraoperative echocardiography is useful for assessing heart function during surgical treatment—for example, during valve repair. Echo-guided pericardiocentesis is a procedure in which excess fluid in the pericardial sac is drained by a needle inserted into your chest. The cardiologist precisely positions the needle by observing its location on an echocardiogram.

Intravascular ultrasound is a technique in which a tiny ultrasound transducer on the tip of a catheter is inserted into one of your coronary arteries. Detailed images of artery walls and plaque inside arteries can be obtained by this type of study. Outreach echocardiography, another option, is used to transmit images from remote areas back to an interpretive center, saving patients a long trip in many cases.

Additional techniques are being developed to analyze blood flow within the myocardium and to reconstruct three-dimensional images of the heart from echocardiographic information. These procedures, however, aren't routinely available at most medical centers.

### Are there risks?

One of the chief advantages of echocardiography is that it gives information about internal structures and blood flow without having something enter your circulatory system. There are virtually no risks to having this procedure. There is no known risk associated with ultrasound waves passing through your body. Echocardiography also involves no X-ray radiation exposure.

During transesophageal echocardiography, there is a very small (0.02%) risk of developing an abnormal heart rhythm or having a minor injury to your throat. Exercise echocardiography and echocardiography performed with the use of medications to simulate exercise carry an extremely small risk of heart attack or rhythm problems. So do other exercise tests (see page 241).

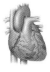

**HEALTHY HEART♥TIP**

*Sometimes doctors can correct congestive heart failure by treating an underlying cause. But when the problem can't be eliminated, the treatment is prescribed to prevent further damage to your heart.*

*Diuretics can increase the flow of liquids in your body. Often called water pills, diuretics make you urinate more frequently and keep fluid from collecting in your body. The drugs also decrease fluid in your lungs so you can breathe more easily.*

# Catheterization and angiography

Cardiac catheterization can help determine how well your myocardium and four heart valves are working. It also provides information about the condition of your coronary arteries. Although other tests provide valuable information about your heart, cardiac catheterization is the only test that can provide an accurate "road map" of the arteries whose job it is to supply the heart muscle with oxygen-rich blood.

## Understanding catheterization and angiography

Catheterization refers to any procedure in which a catheter (a long, thin, flexible tube) is inserted into your body. For cardiovascular problems, catheters are inserted into blood vessels or your heart. Sometimes the term "angiography" (angio means "blood vessel," graph means "record") is used to mean catheterization of the heart and blood vessels.

Technically, angiography refers to the injection of contrast material (dye) into a blood vessel through a catheter to enhance the vessel's appearance on an X-ray film. When dye is injected into an artery, the X-ray image is called an arteriogram. When it is in a vein, it's a venogram.

However, catheters are used to do more than angiography. Some catheters have miniature devices (sensors) at the tips that can measure oxygen in your blood. These also can measure pressure and blood flow within your blood vessels and heart. Some catheters are used to take a sample of your heart tissue—a biopsy. Catheters may be also used to treat coronary artery disease or valve disease (see pages 307, and 318).

Although other techniques, such as heart scanning and echocardiography, can provide a wealth of information noninvasively, some problems can still be detected only with catheterization techniques. In some situations, catheterization is used to confirm or add detail to problems identified by less invasive tests. However, since it involves placing a tube in a blood vessel or another part of your body, it's considered an invasive procedure and carries with it a degree of risk.

The term "cardiac catheterization" simply means that a tube (a catheter) is placed into your heart. Catheters can be placed into the left side, the right side, or both. Different kinds of information are obtained when the catheter is placed on the left versus the right, or when a catheter is put into both sides simultaneously.

Left-heart catheterization is usually done to measure the pressure inside the left ventricle. This information can be very important in assessing the severity of certain heart valve diseases or in diseases of the heart muscle—such as congestive heart failure and cardiomyopathy.

Right-heart catheterization is usually done to evaluate the pressures and blood flow through the right heart chambers and the lungs. This can provide information that's valuable in treating people with certain kinds of heart failure and those who have had severe heart attacks. The use of modified catheters with built-in miniature electronic sensors makes it possible to determine how much blood your heart is pumping and how certain drugs affect the function of your heart and circulation in areas of your body far from this organ. This type of catheter is sometimes left in place for several days if you are undergoing treatment in an intensive care unit.

## What does catheterization show?

There are several types of catheterization. Each type is used to obtain specific kinds of information. Types of catheterization include:

- Coronary angiography
- Left ventriculography
- Angiography in peripheral blood vessels
- Cardiac catheterization for congenital defects
- Pulmonary (lung) angiography
- Biopsy

## Coronary angiography

This procedure is one of the main uses of catheterization. It involves injecting a liquid contrast agent into your coronary arteries through a catheter. As the contrast agent fills your arteries, they become clearly visible on X-ray motion pictures and videotape (see page A9).

## Why not use angiography first to diagnose heart disease?

Angiography, which allows your doctor to see blood vessels, would seem to be the final word for diagnosing problems in your coronary arteries or the blood vessels. So why isn't it the first-line test used to diagnose all heart disease? And why do questions remain even after angiography is performed?

Some of the answers to these questions have already been discussed. Angiography is expensive, it requires special equipment and specially trained medical staff, and it carries some risk with it, though this risk is relatively small. There are other reasons, however. While angiography is an accurate test that provides extensive information, it doesn't always provide the specific information your physician is looking for. For example, abnormalities of the coronary arteries may be found on the coronary angiogram, but these abnormalities may not be the cause of your chest pain.

What the coronary angiogram does best is provide a road map to your blood vessels. Simply looking at a road map of a city doesn't necessarily tell you what the traffic patterns in the area are. To find out where the bulk of the traffic is, perhaps a satellite view of car exhaust gases would be useful. Similarly, to find out what the "traffic patterns" actually are for your heart's oxygen and blood supply, a thallium scan may provide more valuable information. In most cases, more than one test is needed to provide complementary information that puts the whole picture of your condition into focus.

Of course, it isn't really the coronary artery that is being seen, but the image of the contrast material in the hollow part (lumen) of your artery. If there are partial or total blockages of the coronary arteries by atherosclerotic plaque or blood clots, these show up as irregularities or places where the image of the contrast material cuts off.

### Left ventriculography

At the same time you undergo coronary angiography, you may often have a contrast agent injected into your left ventricle. This procedure, called left ventriculography, shows how well your left ventricle is pumping. This also reveals its shape and internal structures and whether there is any back leakage (regurgitation) through the mitral valve. If leakage is present, the contrast material can be seen flowing backward into the left atrium.

### Angiography in peripheral blood vessels

Angiographic techniques can be used to see blood vessels in other parts of your body—even those in your brain. It also can be used in the blood vessels to your legs or arms (performed there, it's called arteriography), the aorta and its main branches (aortography), and selected blood vessels to specific organs. Angiography in your brain is performed by neuroradiologists. Specialists called vascular radiologists perform angiography in many other areas.

### Cardiac catheterization for congenital defects

Other uses of cardiac catheterization include examining congenital malformations of the heart. It can be used to assess the degree of shunting of the blood through a septal defect (a hole in your heart) or through abnormal connections of the arteries (see page 66). It does this by measuring the oxygen in the blood in your heart.

Measuring oxygen is a useful way to assess whether blood is being shunted from the left side of the heart (where the blood has a high level of oxygen because it has just returned from the lungs) to the right side of the heart. If the amount of oxygen in the right ventricle is higher than the amount of oxygen in the right atrium, blood must have crossed from the left ventricle to the right ventricle through a hole in the septum.

Again, doctors can get much information about this condition and others from tests such as echocardiography. But catheterization can play a valuable role in confirming such a condition. It can provide more information about areas—such as certain blood vessels—that cannot be seen on the echocardiogram.

## Pulmonary (lung) angiography

Contrast material can also be injected through catheters to visualize arteries in your lungs. Pulmonary angiography is useful for determining whether there are any blood clots in these arteries or whether malformations exist in them. This procedure can also be used to show the condition of these arteries if you have certain congenital heart defects.

## Biopsy

Catheters are also used to obtain small amounts of heart muscle for microscopic inspection. This procedure is called biopsy. To obtain the tissue sample, a special catheter equipped with small jaws on its tip is usually inserted into the right ventricle through a vein. The jaws can be opened and closed by the cardiologist. At the right location, the tip is gently pushed up against the wall of your heart to take the specimen. More than one "bite" may be needed to ensure there's enough tissue for proper analysis. If you are having this type of biopsy, you won't feel the catheter when it removes the tissue sample.

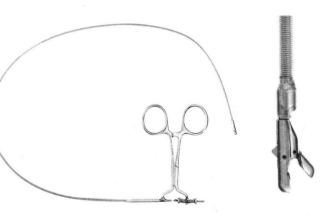

*The biopsy catheter, called a bioptome, is a thin tube with controls on one end. The other end has a small tip with "jaws" that can be opened and closed. The inset photo on the right shows the "jaws" greatly magnified.*

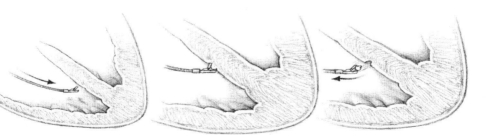

*A heart biopsy involves taking a small sample of tissue from your heart. To do this without surgery, a biopsy catheter is inserted through a vein into the right ventricle. Jaws on the tip of the catheter are opened, pushed gently against the inside of the heart wall, and closed tightly. Then, they are pulled back. The tiny "bite" of heart tissue taken by the catheter is examined under the microscope for more clues about your condition.*

A heart biopsy can help detect inflammation, abnormal protein deposits, or iron deposits that might explain cardiomyopathy (see page 46). It's also used to check for rejection of transplanted hearts (see page 301).

## How is catheterization done?

The answer depends somewhat on where the catheterization is performed. Here's what to expect.

### Catheterization in a cardiac catheterization laboratory

If the catheterization is not being done as an urgent procedure and you are otherwise healthy, you may not need to be hospitalized the night before the procedure. However, you'll still need to take special precautions at home. You'll be asked to take a bath or shower and to scrub the inside of your right arm at the elbow joint or both sides of your groin.

You'll also have to avoid eating or drinking anything after midnight, but continue to take your medicines (with only a small sip of water) unless you receive different instructions from your doctor.

At the testing site the following morning, technicians and nurses may draw blood and obtain an ECG if one hasn't been done recently. They will also discuss the procedure with you in detail, giving you a chance to ask questions about the procedure and to resolve any concerns you might have.

Although the catheterization itself takes only about 30 minutes, preparations are extensive. Before the catheterization, a technician will shave body hair off the small area where the catheter will be inserted through your skin. An intravenous (IV) line will be inserted into an arm vein. You will be given a sedative to help you relax, but you'll stay awake the whole time. Your family shouldn't expect you to return to your hospital room for 2 to 3 hours.

### The procedure

Catheterization is done in a specialized fluoroscopy (X-ray-equipped) suite that is similar to an operating room. The room has a fluoroscopy camera, monitors, and other equipment, but not all of it will necessarily be used during your procedure. The staff will place sterile drapes around you so that the catheters and other instruments do not touch anything unsterile. The people who will be with you in the catheterization suite include the cardiologist and an assistant, one or more technicians, and an anesthetist.

The staff will be wearing lead aprons to protect them from repeated exposure to X-rays. However, the X-ray radiation you'll receive during this procedure isn't harmful.

The X-ray table may be turned mechanically from side to side. Because of this, you may be secured to the table with straps around your waist, shoulders, and knees. The camera will also rotate about you. You will have ECG electrodes on your chest to monitor your heart. A blood pressure cuff on your arm will monitor your blood pressure.

Adults undergoing catheterization usually aren't given general anesthesia. You need to stay awake because the cardiologist needs your cooperation to get the best results. The cardiologist and other members of the catheterization team will explain to you what's being done and prepare you for the sensations you'll feel. You shouldn't experience pain or discomfort during this procedure.

To begin the catheterization, the cardiologist uses a local anesthetic to numb the site where the catheter will be inserted. This is usually at the groin, though sometimes catheters are inserted through your arm or wrist. When the area is numb, the cardiologist inserts a needle into the blood vessel and then threads a very thin guide wire through the needle. After withdrawing the needle, the cardiologist usually pushes a short tube called a sheath over the guide wire and places it into your blood vessel.

The sheath has a small one-way valve in it. This allows a catheter to be inserted through it, but prevents blood from leaking out if the catheter is removed. Once the sheath is in your blood vessel, the cardiologist can insert and remove many different catheters without using a needle.

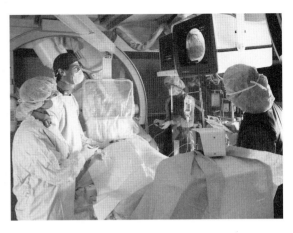

*The catheterization laboratory is similar in design to an operating room. It is equipped with X-ray imaging equipment. The catheterization team usually consists of one or two cardiologists, a cardiologist assistant, an anesthetist, an assisting nurse, and an operator for the imaging equipment.*

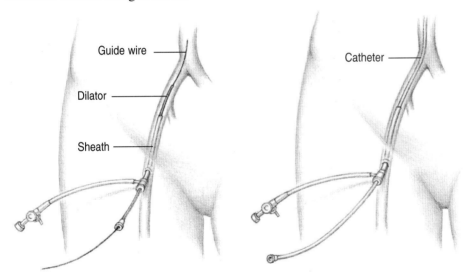

*Typical catheterization involves numbing a small area of your groin and inserting a needle into the artery. A very thin wire—called a guide wire—is inserted through the needle. Then the needle is pulled back and removed. The wire stays in place to maintain the pathway into the artery.*

*The illustration above left shows two short and narrow tubes (the dilator and the sheath) being gently pushed over the wire into the artery. The dilator is inside the sheath. The sheath, which maintains the open route to the artery, has a one-way valve so that no blood flows back out.*

*The illustration above right shows a catheter being inserted into the sheath, through the artery, and up to the heart and coronary arteries. If necessary, the catheter can be removed and another inserted without another needle puncture.*

So what does this feel like? Again, you shouldn't experience discomfort. You may feel pressure or the movement of the catheters where they're inserted in your body, but no pain. If you do, tell your doctor.

Instead of using a needle to make an entry into your body for the catheter, the cardiologist may sometimes make a small incision to expose one of your blood vessels. This is often done if the arm has been previously used for access to your circulation. The catheter or sheath is then inserted directly through a small nick made in the blood vessel. This is referred to as a "cutdown." If you have this procedure, it may take a little longer. You will also need several stitches in your arm.

A television screen shows an X-ray image of the catheter threading through your blood vessel. This helps the cardiologist position the catheter correctly. The X-ray machine can be moved mechanically to many different positions to get different views. A series of X-ray pictures will be taken. The pictures are taken by the X-ray machine, not the catheter.

Once the catheter is in position, the cardiologist uses it to perform whatever tests are necessary, such as measuring pressures or oxygen or injecting contrast material. The cardiologist watches the screen to see where the contrast material goes. If contrast material is injected into the left ventricle, you may feel a hot, flushing sensation all over your body for 15 to 30 seconds. This is normal and is usually only done once. You will also be asked to hold your breath, which helps to get a clearer image. In addition, you may have to hold your arms above your head or to the side in a somewhat awkward position. Again, this helps get a clearer picture of your heart.

The cardiologist may insert several catheters into various areas of your heart to evaluate different aspects of your heart and coronary arteries. In addition, different catheters may be needed to perform diagnostic tests, including drawing blood samples, injecting dye, and taking pressure readings in the heart chambers and the arteries. Catheters with specific shapes and bends and sensors, and specially shaped or bendable guide wires that fit inside the catheter, are used to move the tip of the catheter to the correct position.

You may feel your heart "skip" beats during the procedure, but this sensation is normal. You may also briefly feel flushed and warm all over, or become nauseated for a short time. These effects are common and shouldn't worry you. Occasionally, the heart slows down briefly or temporarily pauses after an injection of contrast material into a coronary artery. If that occurs, you will immediately be asked by the doctor to cough vigorously. This helps your blood circulate during the temporary slowdown. Immediately tell your doctor about any chest pain.

At the end of the procedure, the cardiologist removes the sheath and puts pressure over the site where it entered the blood vessel. This helps your body seal off the puncture site. Then you'll be moved to a recovery room, where pressure on the puncture site is maintained for about 15 minutes. A bandage and small sandbag may be placed over the site to keep pressure at this location. A tool called a vascular closure device may also be used to seal off the small hole left in an artery after the procedure. While vascular closure devices aren't used in everyone, they can be useful in helping some people get out of bed sooner after catheterization. There are several types of vascular devices. Some are simple plugs placed in or over the artery. Others involve using stitches to close the hole more directly.

How long you stay in the recovery room depends on bleeding and a number of other factors. After you leave, it's important that you avoid moving your affected arm or leg, raising your head, or straining the area for about 6 hours. You may also be told to drink a lot of fluid to help flush the contrast material from your system. Most people can begin walking 6 to 8 hours after the procedure.

## Catheterization in a cardiac care unit

Some types of catheterization are not necessarily done in a catheterization suite or laboratory. If you're a patient in a cardiac care unit (CCU), you may need a special type of catheter designed to measure pressure in your pulmonary arteries. This information helps gauge pressure in the left side of your heart and plays an important role in assessing your heart's function. This type of catheter is also used to measure blood flow through your heart, giving an index of how much blood your heart is capable of pumping. This is particularly important for people who have had a heart attack or who have heart failure.

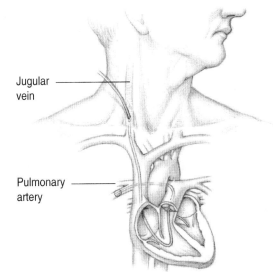

This catheter is usually inserted through the jugular vein in your neck or through the subclavian vein that runs under your collarbone. The area in which the catheter is inserted is anesthetized first to minimize discomfort.

This type of catheter goes by many different names. You might hear it referred to as a hemodynamic monitoring catheter, balloon flotation catheter, or Swan-Ganz catheter (in honor of its inventors). If necessary, it can be left in place for days at a time to monitor your heart's function continuously.

*A balloon-flotation (Swan-Ganz) catheter can be inserted through a vein, often the jugular vein in your neck. A small inflatable balloon on the tip "pulls" the catheter along as it floats in your bloodstream through the vein, heart, and pulmonary artery. This catheter is used for measuring pressures in the heart and pulmonary artery, and for assessing blood flow (cardiac output). It can remain in place for days at a time.*

## Understanding the risks

Catheterization is a procedure that provides detailed information about your heart that often no other test can. But since it's an invasive procedure (meaning that something enters your body), there are risks associated with it. If your physician has recommended this test, he or she feels the information obtained by this test outweighs the risks presented by it. Understanding what the risks are can help alleviate some of your concerns and help you become more knowledgeable about the decisions ahead.

One common but bothersome outcome of catheterization is having a small bruise develop around the puncture site. This is particularly common in elderly people with high blood pressure, who are especially susceptible to bruising. The bruise usually disappears in a few days or weeks. Infection at the puncture site is another concern, but it's extremely rare because of careful sterile techniques.

Other puncture-site problems can include the formation of a bulge in the artery, blockage of the artery, irritation of nearby nerve fibers (which may cause localized numbness or tingling that's usually temporary), or bleeding in the first few hours after the procedure. Another rare problem is an allergic reaction to the contrast material, which may develop abruptly. This can be treated with drugs that counteract the symptoms. Fortunately, most of these problems don't happen very often.

Some complications may be more serious, however. They may even require urgent surgical correction. If complications cause an obstruction of a coronary artery, for example, a heart attack is possible. Also, coronary angiography can result in irregular heart rhythms and cardiac arrest, which may require resuscitation. A blood clot or tear of the inner lining (dissection) extending from the aorta into a carotid artery may result in stroke. Keep in mind that the risk of a severe complication, such as a heart attack or stroke, is very small. The odds of one happening are between 1 in 100 and 1 in 1,000. Also, if these complications do occur, it's usually in a patient who is critically ill and in whom the catheterization was done under emergency conditions.

The risks for catheterization involving the arteries tend to be somewhat higher than those involving the veins because blood pressure is higher in arteries. Higher blood pressure makes bleeding and bruising more likely. Also, there's a greater risk of a blood clot forming in the artery and blocking downstream flow. In addition, there's a risk of perforating (poking through) the artery or causing dissection (a tear). There's also a chance that the right or the left side of the heart may be perforated. If this happens, blood can leak into the pericardial sac surrounding the heart, requiring emergency drainage. Fortunately, such events are rare.

## Electrophysiology studies

In certain situations, ECG and other related tests that assess your heart's electrical function are inconclusive. They don't provide all of the necessary answers in some cases or they may not be appropriate for certain problems. In these cases, electrophysiology studies are done in a hospital setting to find out exactly where the problem is and what can be done to fix or control it (see page A13).

Electrophysiology studies aren't used in everyone. Instead, they're typically used in people who have experienced light-headedness, fainting spells or syncope, a pounding or rapid heartbeat, or who were resuscitated from sudden cardiac death.

### What do electrophysiology studies show?

Electrophysiology studies are a type of catheterization in which electrode catheters (not the hollow catheter tubes just discussed) are inserted through blood vessels (usually veins) and into the heart's chambers—most commonly, the right atrium and right ventricle. These catheters allow impulses in various regions of the heart to be recorded. They can also measure how your heart conducts the impulse from one area to another. By determining where and when impulses occur, your doctor can construct a "map" of your heart's electrical wiring system.

The electrodes can pace the heart with a small electrical current, just like a pacemaker electrode (see page 332). Pacing the heart may help the mapping procedure. The current can also be used to induce or provoke certain abnormal heart rhythms so they can be observed. Abnormal heart rhythms that occur infrequently and without regularity usually can be reproduced in the electrophysiology laboratory. The doctor can then detect what may be causing the problem and try various medications during the test to see if they work.

A wide variety of heart rhythm medications are available (see page 368), but not every medication works equally well for different problems in different people. The technique of inducing arrhythmias during electrophysiology testing allows physicians to evaluate medications during the rhythm abnormality, helping gauge their effectiveness. If physicians can no longer induce the abnormality after you are given a medication, it's likely that the medication will prevent the "spontaneously" occurring rhythm abnormality in the future.

Testing different medications in the electrophysiology laboratory also enables the doctor to learn in a relatively short time which medications work best. However, the technique of using electrophysiology testing to assess the effectiveness of antiarrhythmic drugs is less commonly employed today. One reason is the emergence of new devices and new procedures. For example, cardiac arrhythmias identified by electrophysiology studies may be better treated with either an implantable defibrillator or catheter ablation. In general, these devices mean physicians now do far less "drug testing" with electrophysiology studies. However, they remain valuable testing options in many respects.

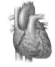

Electrophysiology studies don't always give a perfectly accurate answer. To make an appropriate diagnosis and prescribe treatment, information from the electrophysiology study must be considered with all the other available information. Since the test is invasive and manipulates the heartbeat, a degree of risk is involved.

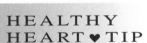

It's also worth noting that certain procedures may be done in conjunction with electrophysiology studies. For example, if a valid cause for a condition called tachycardia is identified, a procedure called catheter ablation may be performed. If this is necessary, your physician will discuss this with you ahead of time.

## How is an electrophysiology study done?

The procedure for an electrophysiology study is somewhat similar to that for catheterization. Electrophysiology studies are usually performed in a special suite or laboratory that has equipment to record your heart's electrical signals and to electrically stimulate the heart. There is also fluoroscopic (X-ray) equipment to view the position of the catheter electrodes in your heart. Like catheterizations, electrophysiology studies are done under sterile conditions. Medical staff in the room usually includes the electrophysiology cardiologist, an assistant, a nurse, a technician, and sometimes an anesthesiologist.

The preparations for an electrophysiology study are similar to those for catheterization. You'll undergo blood tests, X-rays, and an ECG before the test. You may be told to stop taking some of your usual heart medications for 2 or 3 days before the test—particularly anticoagulant medications that "thin" your blood. However, don't stop taking your medications unless you're advised to do so by your doctor. You may also need to fast before the test.

A small intravenous (IV) catheter will be inserted into a vein in your arm. This will be used to give you any medications needed during the test. General anesthesia isn't routinely used for the procedure, but you may be mildly sedated.

A technician will scrub and shave the area (usually the groin) where the electrode wires will be inserted. After a local anesthetic is injected into the area, the catheters are usually inserted through the femoral vein in the groin using the techniques described for catheterization (see page 265). During this kind of study, three or four catheter electrodes may be inserted simultaneously for the purposes of "mapping." Several of these may be inserted through the same vein, such as the femoral vein, which has plenty of room to accommodate several at once. Keep in mind that a catheter is about the diameter of a strand of spaghetti, whereas your blood vessel is about the size of your little finger. At times, both femoral veins are used for catheter placement. Another catheter may also be inserted through the right jugular vein in your neck.

During the electrophysiology test, the doctor may stimulate your heart with tiny electrical impulses. You cannot feel these tiny impulses, but they may trigger the arrhythmia causing your symptoms. In fact, you may feel the same symptoms that you had. Fortunately, you're in an extremely controlled environment with highly trained doctors and nurses available to relieve your symptoms promptly. In fact, this is the safest place for you to experience your symptoms, because the electrophysiology laboratory is both prepared and equipped to handle them.

When the electrode wires that sense your heart's electrical activity are in place, the doctor can see where the arrhythmia is occurring. This information is helpful in deciding how to treat your condition. The doctor can also test medications or other pacing procedures during the study to determine what treatment best controls your particular arrhythmia.

Because the doctor is not only diagnosing the arrhythmia but also testing various treatments, electrophysiology studies can be lengthy. Depending on the problem and the information discovered, a procedure may last less than an hour to more than 4 hours. You must lie flat on the procedure table during the whole time.

The table itself may be tilted to bring you toward an upright position. This maneuver helps test your heart's response to changes in position by detecting any rhythm or blood pressure changes. Straps around your chest will help you stay on the table.

When the study is finished, the electrode wires will be removed and pressure applied to the insertion sites. Because the puncture sites are small, sutures are not necessary. Recovery time is usually short.

## Are there risks?

As with other catheterization procedures, electrophysiology studies carry risk. In general, the risk of a complication is less than 1 in 100. There may be bleeding, bruising, blockage (blood clot), or infection at the site where the wires were inserted. There is also a small risk of perforation of the heart, tearing or separation of the lining of a blood vessel, or stroke. All of these are uncommon.

Electrophysiology tests also have risks that stem directly from the nature of the test. As mentioned, one of the goals of some procedures is to induce abnormal heart rhythms. In susceptible individuals, the procedure may result in severely abnormal heart rhythms, including ventricular fibrillation (see page 115). In this condition, the ventricles twitch in an uncoordinated manner and aren't able to pump enough blood to your body. If this occurs, prompt defibrillation and, possibly, resuscitation is required. As drastic as it sounds, the possibility of fibrillation is precisely why the electrophysiology laboratory is prepared and equipped to handle medical emergencies. A defibrillator (a machine that stops abnormally fast heart rhythm by shocking the heart electrically) is always available during the test.

If ventricular fibrillation occurs, you become unconscious and don't feel the shock from the defibrillator. If you experience markedly abnormal heart rhythms in which you stay conscious but require treatment involving a shock to the chest, you will be put to sleep briefly with a short-acting general anesthetic before the shock is administered.

## Noninvasive tests of your arteries and veins

Tests to determine the condition of the blood vessels and circulation don't necessarily require entering the arteries or veins with a catheter. A number of other noninvasive vascular tests can assess blood flow to different regions of your body and also provide specific information about the condition of arteries and veins, such as whether there's a blockage or other problems.

Many noninvasive tests are virtually risk-free and can be conveniently performed in either a clinic or a hospital. One consideration is that these tests don't provide the same degree of anatomic accuracy as angiography of the blood vessels. In some cases, however, they can provide more accurate details about blood flow than even angiography.

Sometimes the information a noninvasive laboratory test provides is sufficient to make a specific diagnosis and determine treatment. Other times, it will show that further testing is required. Often, these tests are used to follow the disease progression to assess the effects of treatment.

## Testing your arteries

Many diseases of the arteries are caused by partial or complete blockage of these vessels. A blockage in an artery has two basic effects on the circulation of blood through it. It decreases the flow of blood downstream from the blockage. In turn, this decreases the blood pressure below the blockage. The same effect happens when a garden hose becomes kinked (or blocked). The jet of water slows to a trickle because the pressure downstream from the kink is too low to push the water out rapidly. The pressure above the kink, however, remains high.

Many noninvasive vascular tests of arteries are designed to measure and compare blood pressure, blood flow, oxygen supply, and temperature at the sites of various vessels, including the carotid arteries. Comparing blood pressures above and below a blockage can help pinpoint its site and severity.

## Arterial blood pressure measurement

A blood pressure measurement in your arm—part of a routine physical examination—gives information about your overall blood pressure. For people suspected of having blockages in leg arteries, a blood pressure measurement in the legs is made and compared with that in the arm.

This test consists of putting blood pressure cuffs at various points along the length of your leg. Each cuff in turn is inflated to a point at which the blood flow downstream from the cuff is cut off. The cuff is then deflated slowly as a vascular technician determines the pressure at which blood flow resumes. Instead of using a stethoscope to hear the blood flow, as the doctor or nurse does when taking your

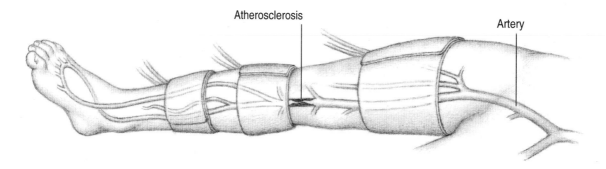

*Measuring the blood pressure at various sites in your leg is one way to determine whether you have a blockage in a leg artery. In this illustration, the blood pressure at the cuff closest to the waist would be about the same as the pressure in the arm. But the blood pressure at the cuff near the foot would be lower than the arm blood pressure because of the partial blockage of the artery near the knee that is caused by atherosclerosis.*

blood pressure, the technician uses a small microphonelike device—a Doppler ultrasound transducer (see page 254)—to "hear" blood flow. If the blood pressure is low when measured at your ankle but normal when measured at your thigh, it's likely that there's a blockage between those two sites, perhaps near your knee.

If the blood pressure is low at both the ankle and thigh, the blockage lies still farther upstream, perhaps near your groin or higher. If the blood pressure is reduced in both legs, the possibility of a blockage in the aorta—the main artery that branches to the leg arteries—must be considered.

Many other noninvasive procedures designed to analyze blockages in the arteries are based on the same principle, but with modifications to suit the specific problem. The same technique can be applied to determine whether a blockage is present in your arm, hand, or finger arteries—and where it might be.

Certain blockages in the arms may come and go, depending on the position of your arm. For example, some people are born with an extra rib that may actually crimp the artery under the collarbone. The effect of the compressed artery may be noticeable only when the arm is in certain positions. This condition is known as thoracic outlet syndrome.

### Pulse volume recording

This is a procedure that uses the blood-pressure-measuring technique but in a different way. In this procedure, a blood pressure cuff is partially inflated around a limb. The form of the pulse on the cuff is then measured. The shape of the pulse gives information about any blockage present upstream from the cuff. If the pulse is flattened, rather than showing the large difference between systole and diastole, then a blockage is present.

### Oculoplethysmography

This is used to check for blockages in the carotid arteries to the brain. Taking blood pressure measurements here requires ingenuity, since a blood pressure cuff can't be put around your neck or head. However, blood pressure can be assessed in your eyeballs. Because branches of the carotid arteries supply your eyes, an indirect measurement of blood pressure in the carotid arteries can be obtained by measuring eye pressure. By painlessly touching small pressure-measuring devices (similar to contact lenses) to the front of your eye, doctors can determine whether the pressure is lower than normal or differs between the eyes. If the pressure in one eye is low, there may be a blockage in a carotid artery.

It should be noted that other noninvasive but more sophisticated techniques—such as the previously discussed ultrasound scanning and color Doppler—are noninvasive options also capable of identifying narrowing of the carotid arteries in the neck. These not only add to information available about blood flow and possible blockages, but they may also enhance treatment. Recent advances in this technology

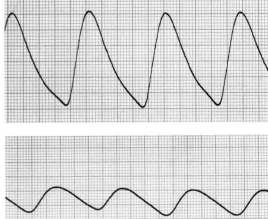

*The pulse volume recording in a limb with normal arteries (**top**) shows normal full pulsations. But the recording of a limb with a blocked artery (**bottom**) shows flattened pulsations.*

and other imaging equipment have made it possible in selected cases for vascular surgeons to repair a narrowing in your carotid artery without the need for conventional angiography.

**Strain-gauge plethysmography**

This is another noninvasive test involving measurements with blood pressure cuffs. For this, a blood pressure cuff is pumped up around your leg until it blocks the blood flowing in the vein below the cuff. It does not impede blood flowing to your leg through the arteries, however. This is possible because the pressure pushing blood through the arteries is much higher than that in the veins, so it's easier to block blood flow in the veins.

In this procedure, a special band called a strain-gauge plethysmograph is placed around your leg below the blood pressure cuff. This band detects tiny changes in the circumference of your leg. Because blood is flowing into your leg, but not flowing out because the vein is blocked, the leg gradually "fills up" and its circumference increases. The rate at which it "fills up" tells the doctor how efficiently (or inefficiently) blood is flowing through your leg artery. The test is painless and free of risk. It usually takes about 10 minutes to perform.

**Transcutaneous oximetry**

This is a noninvasive test that can help gauge the consequences of having a blocked artery. During this procedure, small electrodes are taped to your skin. The amount of oxygen that diffuses into them from your skin indicates how much oxygen the skin contains in that area. If blood flow into the capillaries of the skin is reduced (because of blockage upstream), then the amount of oxygen will be low. If the amount of oxygen is too low, skin ulcers, injuries, or surgical incisions in that area may be slow or impossible to heal.

Transcutaneous oximetry is useful in people with diabetes and others who may have disease of small distal vessels in their extremities. If you have a foot ulcer, normal tissue oxygen may predict good healing potential. Having low oxygen, a condition called tissue hypoxia, may indicate the need for surgical bypass or balloon angioplasty of diseased arteries to improve blood flow and promote healing.

Other noninvasive arterial studies can be performed in your upper extremities. These include taking segmental blood pressures in your arms and fingers while you're resting and exercising. Additional studies, some involving the previously discussed Doppler ultrasound, are also available to evaluate circulation in the very small vessels of your fingers. Testing the microcirculation in these tiny vessels can differentiate people with a condition called Raynaud's phenomenon (see page 40) from those who have fixed blockages of arteries to the fingers, a condition that increases the risk of gangrene in this area.

## Testing your veins

Most noninvasive tests of veins are designed to examine whether there's a blockage (usually caused by a blood clot) or problems with the valves in your veins (see page 129). The pressure in the veins is very low compared with that in the arteries, so techniques to measure pressure are not as helpful. This is why vein tests usually focus on blood flow through them.

A blood clot may occur in any vein in your legs, arms, abdomen and neck. The most common locations are leg and pelvic veins. A number of imaging techniques can be used to diagnose recently developed vein blood clots. So can more advanced scans, which will be discussed in the next section titled Advanced techniques to visualize your heart.

Noninvasive vein tests include the following:

## Doppler ultrasound

When used to study vein circulation, Doppler techniques can indicate whether a vein is obstructed (suggesting the presence of a blood clot) and whether the pattern of blood flow is normal. If it's abnormal, it may reflect damaged valves in the veins, which are causing venous incompetence (see page 129). Venous incompetence can cause chronic leg pain and swelling and may be the result of a previous blood clot.

To do a venous Doppler study, the technician places a hand-held Doppler transducer at various places on your leg, applying pressure above and below the instrument and listening to the whooshing sounds. The test is painless and takes about 15 minutes. The Doppler ultrasound is particularly valuable because it enables physicians to determine the amount of damage to the veins from a blood clot and the likelihood of future clots.

## Impedance plethysmography

This is a procedure very much like strain-gauge plethysmography, which is used to study the blood flow of arteries. For vein studies, however, the rate that the circumference of the leg decreases after the cuff deflates is measured. This gives an idea of how efficiently your veins are able to let blood flow out of the limb. If the veins are inefficient, meaning the blood doesn't flow out very fast, there may be a blockage.

In a variation of this test, the previously discussed strain-gauge plethysmography, a cuff may be used to find damage to one-way venous valves from a previous clot. In this test, your legs are elevated to drain most of the blood in your veins. Then you're tilted upright on a special table. If the veins suddenly fill with blood on standing, this suggests that your veins may not be working properly.

Another test involving the strain-gauge cuff looks at your calf muscle's ability to pump blood back through veins to your heart when you're standing. Strain gauges placed around your ankle measure its diameter while you're standing and after you've done 15 ankle flexes or deep knee bends. If your veins and muscle pump are working normally, the ankle circumference actually decreases with exercise. The reason is that there's less blood in your leg veins. Your muscle action has helped pump it back to your heart.

## Dual purpose tests for both arteries and veins

Some noninvasive tests are equally useful in your arteries or veins.

Duplex scanning is one of them. So named because it combines two different testing technologies, it can detect blockages in the arteries or veins. It can also evaluate a wide variety of other circulatory problems. For this test, the technician uses a combination of ultrasound imaging on a TV screen (like an echocardiogram, but focuses on the blood vessel instead of the heart) and the Doppler microphone device to measure blood flow through the vessel. Computers can interpret the signals and show the blood flow in color on a TV monitor. This allows your physician to study specific blood vessels for abnormalities in flow and structure. Duplex scanning is usually performed on the carotid arteries (see page A15) or vessels that supply the peripheral areas of your body, such as the arteries to the legs.

Doppler techniques can also be combined with impedance plethysmography to evaluate damage caused by blood clots in the veins located deep within the calf of your leg. Blood clots in this location can cause permanent damage to the vein and venous valves, which can lead to chronic leg pain and swelling, a condition called postphlebitic syndrome.

## Advanced techniques to visualize your heart

Although sophisticated diagnostic tests are available to study the structure and function of your heart, tests based on more recently developed technology may provide even more information about it. These procedures include:

- Computed tomography (CT)
- Magnetic resonance imaging (MRI)
- Positron emission tomography (PET)

### Computed tomography

Computed tomography, also known as CT or CAT scans, is an X-ray technique that's been extensively used to examine the brain and other organs. The image produced in a CT scan is generated by an X-ray beam that passes through your body. But this technology provides more information than an ordinary X-ray.

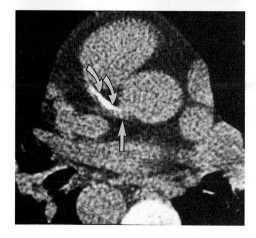

*An imaging technique called fast computed tomography (CT) can reveal fine detail in many structures of your heart. It can show portions of the coronary arteries and distinguish between those that appear normal (**arrows in top photo**) and those with calcium deposits (bottom, **white arrows**). Calcium deposits can indicate the presence of atherosclerosis and partial blockage of an artery.*

The reason has to do with how the image is gathered and processed. Part of the X-ray machine is rapidly rotated around your body so that images are obtained from all angles. A computer processes these images and combines them to make a detailed cross-section image of your body. By doing this, it shows body structures that cannot be identified on an ordinary X-ray. It also allows your doctor to view the internal structures of your body, including the heart, pericardium, lungs, and blood vessels, in cross section.

Because the heart is always in motion, special CT instruments have been developed that allow your heart to be seen clearly, rather than as a blur. These techniques are known as "cine CT" or "fast CT."

## Using CT scans to check coronary artery calcification

A great deal of attention has been given the technique of "scanning the coronary arteries" to detect calcium in them, an important indicator of coronary artery disease and, potentially, your risk of a heart attack.

Why is detecting calcium so important? The answer has to do with the nature of atherosclerosis. This is a chronic process of injury to your blood vessel walls and subsequent healing. Part of the healing process in the vessel (and in other body parts) involves depositing calcium in the injured area.

Calcium shows up well on X-rays because it's hard, which makes it difficult for X-rays to penetrate it. Physicians can assess your risk of coronary artery disease by taking advantage of this through a technique called coronary calcification CT—also known as EBCT (for electron beam computed tomography). Here's how it works:

A series of very high resolution X-ray exposures are taken of your heart. A computer reconstructs these multiple images into an image displayed on a computer. Physicians then examine these images for flecks of calcification in the areas where the three major coronary arteries are located within your heart. Increasing amounts of calcification are associated with the presence of atherosclerosis. In many instances, EBCT can detect atherosclerosis before significant blockage of the vessel occurs.

The EBCT scan holds potential as a way to detect heart disease early, enabling physicians and patients to take steps to prevent it from developing further. However, the test may not be valuable for everyone. Virtually all men over 65 in the United States—and women over 75—have some coronary calcification, meaning that the scan likely can't distinguish people with heart disease from people without it in this age group. For now, it appears that the test is best suited for patients at increased risk for atherosclerosis who are also young.

EBCT has other limitations. It cannot see the vessels clearly enough to substitute for coronary angiography, if that test is necessary. In addition, the value of the information it provides remains uncertain. If young patients are told they're at risk for heart disease, will this help reduce heart attacks? EBCT's role in detecting heart disease is promising and warrants more study. But for now, its role in preventing heart disease remains unclear.

The machine used to make a CT scan is large and the technology behind it may sound complicated. But from a patient's perspective, the procedure is straightforward and uncomplicated. The CT scanner looks like a giant doughnut. The ring of the doughnut contains the scanning equipment; it surrounds the part of your body being scanned. You lie flat on a movable table that slides into the doughnut's "hole." The machine directs X-rays in an arc through segments of your body. The procedure is painless. All you need to do is lie still. Sometimes a contrast material may be injected through a vein to enhance the image.

CT scans involve exposure to a small amount of radiation during the procedure. The benefits far outweigh the minor risk associated with this low level of radiation exposure.

## Magnetic resonance imaging (MRI)

Magnetic resonance imaging (MRI) is another technique that may be useful for investigating heart disease. Rather than using X-rays to produce an image, magnetic resonance imaging uses magnetic fields and radio waves. The machine can detect small energy signals emitted by the atoms that make up your body tissues, and can reconstruct images based on that information. The pictures produced with MRI are similar to those taken with X-rays, but they may be able to show slightly different tissues.

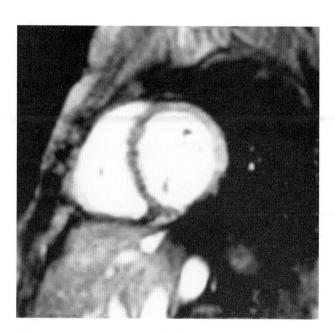

*Magnetic resonance imaging (MRI) is another technique that can show your heart's anatomy in greater detail.*

The procedure can be used to detect congenital defects and tumors and to evaluate ischemic heart disease and disease of your heart valves and pericardium. New research suggests that MRI can detect atherosclerotic plaques that are prone to rupture in your carotid artery, the thoracic aorta, and possibly even in a coronary artery. This technique hasn't been studied enough to make it a standard tool used by physicians. But in the future, it may enable cardiologists to diagnose diseases in people who are at high risk of having a heart attack or a stroke, and to initiate treatment before these happen.

This procedure does not use ionizing radiation as regular X-rays and CT do, and there are no known risks from MRI. Because the machine operates in a magnetic environment, certain patients cannot undergo scanning, including those with pacemakers or some other internal metallic objects. Patients with artificial heart valves can be scanned safely.

## Positron emission tomography (PET)

Positron emission tomography (PET) is a fairly new and expensive imaging technique that detects emissions from subatomic particles in your body. These emissions are detected by two different detectors placed on opposite sides of your body.

PET scans are used mainly to measure blood flow and the metabolism in tissues such as the heart muscle. This technique has a potential advantage of being able to characterize the way in which heart tissue actually uses energy. This may lead to new insights about heart cell metabolism and how oxygen is used to produce the energy needed to make the heart contract.

Equipment and materials for this procedure are expensive. This is why PET scans are now used primarily for scientific investigations.

## Putting tests in perspective

Despite the sophistication of testing procedures and the valuable information they can provide, it would be a mistake to think that tests provide the final answer in diagnosing heart disease. All tests have inherent differences in accuracy, and no test is 100 percent accurate, even under the best of circumstances. Remember, tests are not a diagnosis by themselves. Instead, they provide information that, when added to other information, leads to the diagnosis.

.Physicians' most important contribution to your health evaluation is not their ability to arrange for tests or to do them, but to select and interpret diagnostic tests as they apply to your problem. To do this, doctors must take into account all of the available data about you. They must know what each test can and cannot reveal, and how the test results relate to the actual disease. The care and skill that are applied in doing a diagnostic test and interpreting the results correctly determine how valuable a test is in leading your doctor to a diagnosis and to appropriate treatment.

Before moving forward with a diagnostic test, review with your physician what will be done with the test results. If the action is the same regardless of the test results, perhaps the test is unnecessary. The key question is what additional information the test will provide.

Keeping all this in mind, it's not surprising that occasionally even experts disagree about the best treatment for a condition. Situations in which a second opinion might be a good idea include:

- When a diagnosis is very serious
- If the treatment advised by your doctor is risky, experimental, or controversial
- If you may need to have a major surgical procedure

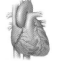

**HEALTHY HEART ♥ TIP**

*You may find yourself in an emergency room, intensive care unit or urgent care setting when doctors decide to do a blood test. Such seemingly innocuous exams can often confirm (or refute) suspicions about your heart that were raised in early evaluation.*

*The most common blood tests to confirm the existence of heart muscle damage use creatine kinase (CK) and lactate dehydrogenase (LDH). After a heart attack, these enzymes, usually found in the heart, may leak into the blood from damaged heart cells. Other tests measure the level of cardiac muscle proteins, specifically troponin T and troponin I. These proteins control the interactions between actin and myosin, which contract the heart muscle.*

Second opinions are also sometimes useful when the diagnosis is clear but the choice of treatments isn't. Often, several significantly different treatments are available for a specific disease. You may also want to get a second opinion if your treatment isn't working as well as you'd hoped, or if you feel that your doctor has not given you enough information about the diagnosis and treatment methods. Insurance companies often require a second opinion before treatment is undertaken.

Ultimately, the most important "second opinion" about any health decision must come from you. Only you know your priorities and what effect the test and treatments, each with its own risk and benefits, will have on your life. For a second opinion to be meaningful, you must be fully informed about your test results, just as your first doctor was fully informed about your medical history and symptoms.

If you want a second opinion, let your doctor know that you would like one to confirm the diagnosis or the appropriateness of the procedure. Your primary care doctor (family practice physician or general internist) is the best source of advice about whom to consult.

Many of the tests that have been discussed are highly specialized. Medicine today offers more extensive care and more innovative treatments than ever before. Knowledge about diseases and treatments is growing so rapidly that specialties and subspecialties have developed to manage this proliferation of knowledge. It should be clear that specialists are needed to perform many of the different diagnostic tests, and to interpret the data. It's reassuring to know that you and your family doctor have numerous sources for specialized assistance with the complex problems and decisions that may lie ahead.

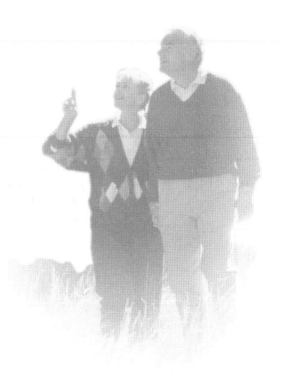

## Finding a cardiologist

To choose a cardiologist or another specialist, you have several options:

- The most useful and reliable option is a referral by a trusted family physician, general practitioner, or internist, or a referral by a subspecialist who has been treating you for a different problem.

- Another way to find a cardiologist is through a friend who has been satisfied with a particular doctor. Another is to choose a specialist with a good general reputation in your community.

- If you cannot find a cardiologist through your primary care doctor or referral by a friend, you can look to several directories for help. The 370,000 physicians recognized as specialists by the American Board of Medical Specialties (ABMS) are listed in many telephone directories throughout the country, noting the specialty or subspecialty. In addition, you may call the ABMS toll-free at 1-800-776-CERT (1-800-776-2378) to verify a doctor's certification.

- The following references can also provide information about a doctor's professional background. Look for them at your public library, medical society, or libraries at a hospital or university medical school:

American Medical Directory. This is a directory of physicians in the United States, Puerto Rico, the Virgin Islands, and certain Pacific Islands, and U.S. physicians temporarily located in foreign countries. This is published by the American Medical Association. It lists only physicians who belong to the AMA, whether board-certified or not. It provides such information as name, address, type of practice, and medical school attended.

ABMS Compendium of Certified Medical Specialists. This is published by the American Board of Medical Specialties. It lists physicians who are certified by the examining boards of recognized specialty organizations. It provides information such as a doctor's medical school and internship training, type of practice and hospital affiliation, and address and telephone number.

Directory of Medical Specialties. This is published by Marquis Who's Who. It provides, with a short curriculum vitae, information similar to that in the ABMS Compendium.

- Some hospitals have set up informational telephone lines staffed by people who can direct you to a doctor in your area. These lines are usually advertised in newspapers or on radio or television. In addition, university hospitals, medical schools, and medical societies can supply you with a list of affiliated cardiologists or other specialists.

# Part 5

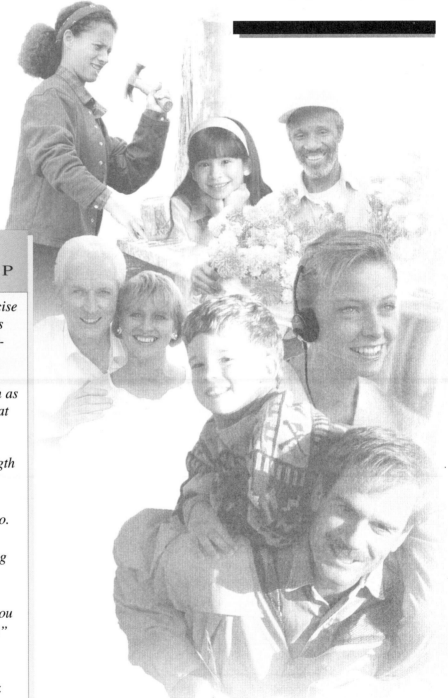

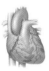

## HEALTHY HEART ♥ TIP

*As you age, you should exercise your heart and other muscles more than ever. Aerobic exercise is important, but you should also include body-strengthening activities, such as weight training. When done at least twice a week, weight-training exercises can help counteract muscle and strength loss that occurs naturally from aging.*

*There's another benefit, too. Since calories are burned in your muscles, weight-training exercises can also help you maintain a healthful weight. The more lean muscle mass you retain, the bigger the "engine" with which to burn calories. Think of it as having a V-8 engine instead of a 4 cylinder.*

# Treating heart disease

Once you discover you have some form of heart disease, you'll want to know what you can do about it. Medicine has made tremendous strides in the fields of cardiology and cardiac surgery, so that available treatment options now have a greater impact on the course of most cardiac illnesses.

Open-heart surgery was first performed about 45 years ago, heralding an era in which effective therapy would be developed for previously untreatable heart disorders.

Alternatives for treating heart disease now include a wide array of medications; complex surgical techniques; methods for using catheters to treat coronary artery disease, valvular disorders, and rhythm abnormalities; sophisticated implantable electronic devices to monitor and automatically treat both fast and slow heart rhythms; and procedures to replace a defective heart.

In many situations, more than one form of treatment is possible. Appropriate heart disease management entails selecting therapy that provides the best results for your particular medical problem while keeping risks, inconvenience, and expense to a minimum.

## Chapter

# Chapter

# 12 Emergency care

Numerous cardiac problems emerge without warning; in fact, silent coronary artery disease affects as much as 30 percent of the population. Yet it can be life-threatening if you don't get help immediately. In an emergency situation, your survival depends on the quick response of bystanders who may be in the vicinity long before medical attention arrives.

Because no one can predict when a rapid, life-sustaining response may be needed, everyone should learn the fundamental skills for dealing with emergencies in which spectators, not doctors, can mean the difference between life and death.

## When do you need an expert?

### Information to give the operator in an emergency call:

The location of the emergency. Provide as much useful information as possible, including the address, nearby intersections, or other landmarks. This information is vital—even "enhanced 911," which tells the operator where you're calling from, is ineffective if the telephone isn't at the precise site of the emergency.

Give the telephone number you're calling from. The operator may need to call you back. Briefly summarize the problem by describing what happened.

Tell how many victims need help and what their conditions are.

State what's being done for the victim. Let the operator hang up first so you're certain the operator has obtained all the necessary information.

Recognition is the first step in successfully treating most cardiac emergencies. As a rule, if you think there's a possibility a situation may require emergency medical help, don't hesitate: call 911 immediately. If it turns out it's not an emergency, you've done no harm. However, if you don't call an ambulance, contact a doctor, or get to a hospital during a real emergency, the consequences can be tragic.

Too often, patients don't seek help quickly enough after the first hint of symptoms. Luckily, community campaigns have educated the public about heart attack and the need for rapid action. This has increased the number of people who call emergency medical services for transport and shortened arrival time in the emergency room.

It's impossible to exhaustively list all the circumstances that warrant immediate attention. You should exercise your best judgment and common sense to determine when and how fast to move. Many emergencies are simple to identify, but others may be less obvious.

The key is recognizing the significance of symptoms discussed in Part 2, "What is heart disease?" Ultimately, "If in doubt, check it out" is a reliable rule of thumb.

The following table offers sound guidelines:

| Symptom | Suspected diagnoses | Possible associated features | Action |
|---------|--------------------|-----------------------------|--------|
| Chest pain, pressure, tightness, heaviness | Myocardial infarction (heart attack)<br>Unstable angina<br>Aortic dissection<br>Pulmonary embolism | Duration more than 15 minutes<br>Shortness of breath<br>Sweating<br>Pallor<br>Nausea, vomiting<br>Palpitations<br>Faintness | Any unexplained chest pain warrants immediate attention even if none of the other features are present. The presence of associated features increases concern. *Transport to emergency room; call 911. Give nitroglycerin if available.* Have patient chew an aspirin. |
| Loss of consciousness (syncope) | Serious arrhythmia<br>Stroke<br>Seizure<br>Extremely low blood pressure<br>Sudden cardiac death<br>Vasovagal syncope (fainting spell) | Palpitations<br>Fast or slow pulse<br>Convulsions<br>Sweating<br>Pallor<br>Chest pain<br>Loss of bladder or bowel control | Any unexplained loss of consciousness requires *immediate transportation to an emergency room; call 911.* The person should be positioned on the back with the legs and feet elevated. Evaluate for possible need to perform CPR.<br>The other features are important to note and discuss with the doctor. |
| Shortness of breath | Myocardial infarction (heart attack)<br>Sudden congestive heart failure<br>Sudden aortic or mitral regurgitation<br>Pulmonary embolism<br>Noncardiac causes, such as pneumothorax | Chest pain<br>Wheezing<br>Ankle and leg swelling (edema)<br>Palpitations<br>Fever<br>Calf or thigh discomfort | Any unexplained new or worsened shortness of breath warrants immediate attention; *transportation by ambulance to emergency room; call 911.* If the onset of symptoms has been more gradual, early evaluation is advisable but the level of urgency may be less. |

| Symptom | Suspected diagnoses | Possible associated features | Action |
|---|---|---|---|
| Sustained rapid palpitations, regular or irregular rhythm | Arrhythmia | Light-headedness Passing out Chest pain Shortness of breath | Without associated symptoms, urgent transportation (by car) to doctor's office or acute care facility is warranted. *If associated symptoms are present, transport to emergency room; call 911.* |
| Skipped beats or irregular nonrapid rhythm, or forceful heart beats | Arrhythmia Anxiety | Light-headedness Passing out Chest pain Shortness of breath | Usually does not require emergency evaluation. Make appointment with doctor. *However, associated symptoms, if present, require emergency room evaluation.* |
| Leg swelling | Congestive heart failure Deep/vein thrombosis (and possible associated pulmonary embolism) | Inflammation Redness Pain, tenderness Hot Shortness of breath Chest pain | Signs of inflammation may indicate thrombosis (clot) in leg vein. Rapid transport to doctor or hospital is recommended. *Shortness of breath or chest pain requires emergency evaluation.* Edema from heart failure usually is not sudden or an emergency but requires early evaluation and treatment. |

## What is sudden cardiac death?

In sudden cardiac death (or cardiac arrest), the heart stops beating and breathing ceases abruptly. The victim lies unconscious. This is distinct from actual death, in which the person experiences irreversible loss of brain function. It's critical to recognize and respond to sudden cardiac death because you may be able to avoid brain death. In other words, sudden cardiac death is potentially reversible.

Many instances of sudden cardiac death happen in people with other forms of heart disease who are already at high risk. However, as many as half occur in individuals with no previously suspected heart disease. In any case, if you witness sudden cardiac death and respond appropriately, you may give the victim a second chance at life.

Sudden cardiac death isn't the same as heart attack or stroke. The usual cause of sudden cardiac death is ventricular fibrillation. The heart ceases to beat effectively, which deprives the brain of oxygenated blood. Ventricular fibrillation almost never returns to a normal rhythm on its own, so if the victim doesn't receive immediate help, the brain will die.

Respiration is one function of the brain that stops during sudden cardiac death, which compounds the problem even further. Unless oxygenated blood returns to the brain in less than 4 to 6 minutes, potentially reversible cardiac death becomes permanent brain death. The technique for maintaining breathing and circulation is appropriately termed cardiopulmonary resuscitation (CPR).

A person who experiences sudden cardiac death as a result of ventricular fibrillation has the best chance of surviving if a bystander starts CPR within 4 minutes and if advanced life support begins within 8 minutes of collapse.

This is one reason why easy-to-use, public-access defibrillators have been installed in many public places, such as airports. Widely employed by trained emergency personnel, automatic external defibrillators are increasingly operated by nonmedical, minimally trained personnel such as security guards, spouses of cardiac patients, and flight attendants. Bystander-initiated automatic external defibrillation may soon expand throughout the whole country.

Of those who are resuscitated, about 40 percent will experience another episode within 2 years. They may need special interventions to minimize their future risk of death; but to have the opportunity for prevention, they must survive the initial episode. That's where CPR is vital.

## Cardiopulmonary resuscitation (CPR)

If CPR is performed properly and early enough, an estimated 100,000 to 200,000 U.S. lives could be saved every year. A bystander who can administer CPR until advanced cardiac life support begins is the most important lifesaving link in the emergency medical system.

CPR can be done by "anyone anywhere, using only our hands, our lungs, and our brains," according to the American Heart Association. It involves a sequence of actions that propels oxygen into a person's lungs and helps blood circulate through the body until more advanced medical care arrives.

You can't learn CPR by reading a book; you must practice the skills until they become automatic. Ideally, everyone should take this life-saving course from trained instructors who demonstrate how it's done, then supervise practice drills on mannequins that mimic victims of sudden cardiac death. Many organizations offer CPR courses, including the American Heart Association, the American Red Cross, local fire departments, community health services, and local hospitals.

Your skills in CPR may never be required. However, if they are, it may be the most important thing you can do for another person, whether a loved one or a stranger. If you live with or near a person who has heart disease and a possible predisposition to rhythm disorders, you especially should learn CPR.

CPR accomplishes two important goals in maintaining the brain's oxygen supply: It ensures that sufficient oxygen enters the blood in the lungs' circulation, and that oxygenated blood reaches the brain. You achieve the first goal by mouth-to-mouth breathing; the second with chest compressions.

How can the breath we exhale keep someone else alive? Fortunately, the air we inhale contains 21 percent oxygen, which is more than what enters the bloodstream. Consequently, we breathe out three fourths of the oxygen again when we exhale. That exhaled oxygen, breathed into a victim's lungs, is sufficient to keep the brain alive when the blood is squeezed out of the lungs and heart, through blood vcsscls to the brain, by chest compression.

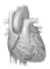

### HEALTHY HEART ♥ TIP

*Except for those with specific allergies and intolerances, everyone can benefit from the calcium and protein found in dairy foods. But dairy products can also deliver high amounts of saturated fat and cholesterol, which can eventually lead to heart disease. Try these healthier alternatives:*

- *Skim or 1 percent fat milk*
- *Nonfat or low-fat yogurt*
- *Low-fat or fat-free ice cream or frozen yogurt*
- *Reduced-fat, fat-free or part-skim-milk cheeses*
- *Low-fat or fat-free sour cream or cream cheese*

**Emergency signs of sudden cardiac death**

- Sudden loss of consciousness
- No breathing
- No pulse

**What to do**

- Assess the situation
- Call out for help. If someone responds, he or she should immediately call the local emergency telephone number (usually 911). If no other bystander is available, make the call yourself.
- Begin CPR

## Overview of CPR techniques

CPR involves a combination of mouth-to-mouth rescue breathing and chest compressions. It keeps some oxygenated blood flowing to the brain and other vital organs until appropriate medical treatment can restore a normal heart rhythm.

The American Heart Association, which sets guidelines for CPR, has an easy to remember way of describing the three basic rescue skills. They call it the ABCs of CPR:

- Airway
- Breathing
- Circulation

## Airway

For successful resuscitation, you must first open the airway, which may be obstructed by the back of the tongue or by the epiglottis (the flap of cartilage that covers the windpipe).

When someone's unconscious, muscle control diminishes. The tongue often drops to the back of the throat, impeding air passage to the lungs. When the head is tilted back and the lower jaw (chin) moved forward, the tongue and epiglottis rise. This technique usually opens the airway.

## Breathing

Mouth-to-mouth rescue breathing is the quickest way to get oxygen into a person's lungs. It must be performed until the person can breathe alone or until advanced medical assistance takes over.

If the victim has a heartbeat but isn't breathing, you must maintain an open airway and provide breaths (for an adult, once every 5 seconds, or 12 times a minute). If the person's heart has stopped, you must perform chest compressions along with the rescue breathing.

## Circulation

Chest compressions replace the heartbeat when it has stopped. Compressions help circulate some blood to the lungs, brain and coronary arteries. You must also perform mouth-to-mouth breathing any time you commence chest compressions.

## Performing CPR in adults and children older than 8 years

The following description of CPR reflects the procedures recommended by the American Heart Association. It should be considered a refresher for those who have taken a CPR course, since periodic review may be useful.

### Assess the situation and get help

1. **What to do:** Tap or gently shake the victim's shoulder. Shout "Are you okay?"

   **Reason:** You don't want to start resuscitative efforts on someone who may be merely sleeping soundly or intoxicated, or has only fainted.

2. **What to do:** Shout for help. If someone responds, have him or her call 911 (or other emergency number) for help. If you're alone, make the call yourself.

   **Reason:** CPR alone cannot save a victim of cardiac arrest. At the onset of cardiac arrest, more than 80 percent of nonhospitalized people with underlying heart disease have ventricular fibrillation, and defibrillation is their chance for survival. So, first, summon advanced cardiac life support, then start CPR. Basic CPR buys some time until medical rescue efforts begin.

### Airway

3. **What to do:** Position the victim on his or her back. The victim should be placed on a firm, flat surface—a bed or couch isn't firm enough—with the head at the same level as the heart. Kneel to the victim's side so that you're at a right angle to him or her. This should take no more than 10 seconds.

**Reason:** To produce effective blood flow to the brain, CPR must include compression of the chest between the rescuer's hands and a firm surface. On a soft surface, you can't deliver adequate compressions because of bouncing. Oxygenated blood won't reach the brain if the head is higher than the heart.

4. **What to do:** Lift the chin gently with one hand while pushing down on the forehead with the other to tilt the head back. Avoid completely closing the mouth.

   **Reason:** This maneuver opens the airway.

### Breathing

5. **What to do:** While maintaining the open airway, determine whether the victim is breathing.

   - Position your ear directly near the victim's mouth.
   - Look at the chest for movement.
   - Listen for breathing sounds.
   - Feel for breath on your cheek.

   **Reason:** Hearing and feeling are the only true ways to determine whether an unconscious person is breathing. If there's chest movement but you can't feel or hear the breath, the airway's still obstructed. You must diagnose this accurately—rescue breathing shouldn't be performed on someone who's breathing.

6. **What to do:** Pinch the person's nostrils while maintaining pressure on the forehead to keep the head tilted. Open your mouth wide, take a deep breath, and make a tight seal around the person's mouth. Breathe into the person's mouth two times initially. Give one breath every 5 seconds and completely refill your lungs after each breath. Always watch for the person's chest to rise with each breath.

   Each breath into the victim's mouth should take 1 1/2 to 2 seconds. Then allow the lungs to deflate.

   - Feel air going in as you blow.
   - Feel the resistance of the person's lungs.
   - Feel your own lungs emptying.
   - See the rise and fall of the person's chest and abdomen. (If rescue breaths don't inflate the lungs, repeat the obstructed airway sequence.)

   **Reason:** This step in CPR provides the lungs with oxygen.

### Circulation

7. **What to do:** Place two or three fingers on the Adam's apple (voice box) just below the chin. Slide your fingers into the groove between the Adam's apple and muscle, on the side nearest you. Maintain head tilt with the other hand. Feel for the carotid pulse in the neck for 8 to 10 seconds.

   **Reason:** This maneuver establishes the lack of a pulse. A pulse signals an effective heartbeat; if one's present, don't do CPR.

*If the victim isn't breathing, pinch the person's nostrils closed, make a seal around the mouth, and breathe twice into his or her mouth.*

8. **What to do:** Prepare to begin chest compressions by positioning your hands and body appropriately. First, locate the bottom of the sternum (breastbone) at the point where the lower ribs on each side converge. Second, place the heel of your hand approximately 2 inches up from the bottom of the sternum. Third, put the other hand on top of the first. Your shoulders should be directly over your hands, and your elbows should be straight and locked.

   **Reason:** Precise hand placement and proper weight distribution are essential for effective compressions without injuring the victim. Proper positioning also reduces your own fatigue.

9. **What to do:** Compress the chest smoothly and evenly, using the heel of your hand and keeping your fingers off the person's ribs. You must apply enough force to depress the sternum 1 1/2 to 2 inches at a rate of 80 to 100 compressions per minute. Use your weight to compress the chest vertically downward 1 1/2 to 2 inches.

   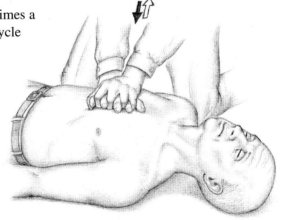

   *When administering CPR, check the victim's pulse on the same side you're working.*

   Between compressions, release the pressure and allow the chest to return to its normal position. To ensure your hands remain in the proper location, don't lift them off the chest.

   Count aloud to establish proper rhythm: "one-and-two-and-three-and-four-and" up to 15.

   **Reason:** This technique promotes the most effective blood flow. Half of the compression/relaxation phase moves downward to squeeze blood out of the heart, and the other half proceeds upward to allow the heart to fill. You may be tempted to "jab" downward and relax slowly, but that would be wrong. With each compression you want to squeeze the heart or increase the pressure within the chest so blood is pushed to the vital organs.

   Push down about 1 1/2 to 2 inches at a rate of 80 to 100 times a minute. The pushing down and letting up phase of each cycle should be equal in duration. Don't "jab" down and relax.

   After 15 compressions, breathe into the victim's mouth twice. After every 4 cycles of 15 compressions and 2 breaths, recheck for a pulse and breathing. Continue rescue maneuvers as long as there's no pulse or breathing.

10. **What to do:** Continue to ventilate properly. After every 15 compressions, deliver two rescue breaths.

    **Reason:** You must provide adequate oxygenation. Remember, you are maintaining the circulation in order to deliver oxygen to the body.

11. **What to do:** At the end of four cycles, each consisting of 15 compressions and two rescue breaths (which should take a little more than a minute), check for return of the pulse for 5 seconds. If there's no pulse, resume CPR. If

*If there's no pulse, begin chest compressions. Your hands should be located over the lower part of the breastbone, your elbows straight, and your shoulders positioned directly above your hands to make the best use of your weight.*

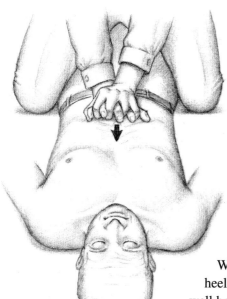

there is a pulse but no breathing, give a rescue breath every 5 seconds (12 per minute).

**Reason:** These actions establish whether pulse or breathing returns spontaneously.

### If the airway is obstructed

1. **What to do:** If you find your rescue breaths don't inflate the lungs, first reposition the head and try again to give rescue breaths.

   **Reason:** Improper head tilt is the most common cause of airway obstruction.

2. **What to do:** If the rescue breaths still don't inflate the lungs, give 6 to 10 abdominal thrusts below the diaphragm (the Heimlich maneuver).

   With the victim still lying down, straddle his or her thighs and place the heel of one hand on the abdomen's midline slightly above the navel and well below the tip of the breastbone. Place your other hand directly on top of the first hand. Press into the abdomen with quick upward thrusts.

   **Reason:** Such thrusts can force air upward into the airway from the lungs with enough force to expel whatever's blocking the airway.

3. **What to do:** Remove the foreign body from the victim's mouth or throat. Open the mouth, pull the lower jaw forward, and sweep deeply into the mouth along the cheek with a hooked finger. Dentures should be removed.

   **Reason:** You may now be able to remove the obstruction even if it hasn't been fully expelled from the mouth or throat. The hooked-finger sweeping technique avoids accidentally pushing the foreign body further back into the throat.

4. **What to do:** Open the airway and attempt to give 5 rescue breaths. Reposition the head with the head-tilt/chin-lift technique.

   **Reason:** By this time, you must make another attempt to get some air into the lungs.

5. **What to do:** Repeat the entire sequence until you successfully inflate the lungs. If the airway remains obstructed, alternate the maneuvers in rapid sequence: abdominal thrusts, finger sweep, attempt to ventilate.

   **Reason:** You must be persistent in trying to relieve the obstruction rapidly. As the person becomes more oxygen-deprived, the muscles will relax and maneuvers that were ineffective before may start to work.

*If the victim's chest doesn't rise when you breathe into his or her mouth, the airway is probably blocked. Try to dislodge the obstruction (such as a piece of food) by performing the Heimlich maneuver. Because the victim will be lying down, place your hands slightly above the navel and press upward, firmly and rapidly.*

*You will need to insert a finger into the victim's mouth to determine whether the obstruction has been discharged and to remove it from the mouth or throat.*

Remember, chest compressions without ventilation are useless, because there will be no oxygen to circulate. You must first open the airway.

**Performing CPR in infants and children**

There are special considerations for administering CPR in infants younger than 1 year and in children between 1 and 8 years. For infants and children, administer CPR for 1 minute before calling the local emergency telephone number (911).

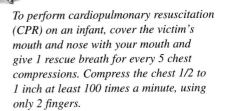

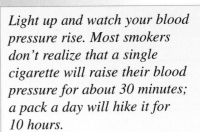

*To perform cardiopulmonary resuscitation (CPR) on an infant, cover the victim's mouth and nose with your mouth and give 1 rescue breath for every 5 chest compressions. Compress the chest 1/2 to 1 inch at least 100 times a minute, using only 2 fingers.*

1. **Infants (younger than 1 year).** To perform chest compressions on an infant, imagine a line drawn between the nipples. Measure one finger's width below that line. (These instructions are only guidelines because of the variations in sizes of infants' chests and rescuers' fingers.)

   Make sure your fingers are not below the breastbone. Compress the chest 1/2 to 1 inch at least 100 times a minute, using only two fingers, not the heel of your hand. Give 1 rescue breath for every 5 compressions.

   Do 10 cycles of compressions and rescue breaths, then check the pulse on the inner part of the upper arm. If there's no pulse, give 1 rescue breath and continue compressions with rescue breaths. Check the pulse every few minutes.

2. **Children (1 to 8 years old).** In children between 1 and 8, you'll position your hands for chest compressions the same as for adults, but use the heel of only one hand, not both. Compress the chest 1 to 1 1/2 inches 100 times per minute. Give 1 rescue breath for every 5 compressions.

   Do 10 cycles of compressions and rescue breaths, then check for the pulse in the neck. If there's no pulse, give 1 rescue breath and continue compressions with rescue breaths, checking the pulse every few minutes.

**When to stop CPR**

Once you start CPR, you're obligated to continue until the person regains pulse and breathing, another trained individual takes over, or you're too exhausted to continue.

Many states have "Good Samaritan" laws that protect professionals and laypersons who perform CPR in good faith. Most Good Samaritan laws shield laypersons from lawsuits if they perform CPR, even if they've had no formal training. Consider taking a course in CPR. This critical skill is easily learned with 3 hours of instruction and observed practice.

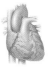

**HEALTHY HEART ♥ TIP**

*Light up and watch your blood pressure rise. Most smokers don't realize that a single cigarette will raise their blood pressure for about 30 minutes; a pack a day will hike it for 10 hours.*

*Although smoking doesn't cause persistent high blood pressure, smokers should check their blood pressure within 30 minutes of having a cigarette. If you're a regular smoker and you have high blood pressure after smoking, ask your doctor about treatment to lower blood pressure. Or better yet, quit smoking altogether.*

# Advanced cardiac life support

The emergency medical system is a team approach to handling emergency medical situations. It begins outside the hospital with people trained in CPR (basic life support), after which trained rescue personnel take over and use more advanced procedures and equipment for sustaining life (advanced cardiac life support).

### Intravenous (IV) catheter

Medications and fluids must be administered rapidly. Advanced cardiac life support personnel place an intravenous (IV) catheter to provide access to the circulation.

### Endotracheal intubation

Mouth-to-mouth ventilation is an indispensable stopgap measure, but the lungs receive far higher concentrations of oxygen with a tube inserted through the nostril or mouth into the windpipe (trachea).

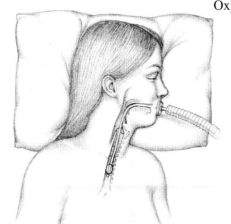

Oxygen can be pushed through the tube by repeatedly squeezing an inflated rubber balloon, which functions as a pump. The tube ensures that all the air goes to the lungs (not the stomach) and makes it easier to clear secretions from the lungs.

### Defibrillation

Defibrillation is the most effective way to stop ventricular fibrillation. Emergency medical personnel apply "paddles" or electrode patches to the chest that deliver a shock to the person's heart. This shock jolts the heart into a more normal rhythm mechanism, giving it a chance to regain control. Some defibrillator machines can interpret a person's heart rhythm and automatically render a shock when and if it's necessary.

The sooner it's applied, the more likely defibrillation will be successful. If ventricular fibrillation has caused sudden cardiac death and paramedics with a defibrillator reach the victim in time, about 25 percent ultimately can leave the hospital without evidence of brain damage. Effective CPR may provide the necessary time for a defibrillator to arrive on the scene.

*Oxygen can be administered best to someone who's not breathing through a tube inserted directly into the trachea (windpipe). The oxygen can be delivered by a ventilator machine or by a "bag" pump controlled by a caregiver. A small inflatable cuff at the end of the tube keeps the air from leaking backward, and it also prevents stomach fluids from getting into the lungs.*

#### *Automated external defibrillators (AEDs)*

Small, portable external defibrillators make it possible to shock people on-site, where they lie, instead of en route to or in an emergency room. These automated external defibrillators (AEDs) are widely available. The American Red Cross and the American Heart Association offer training in CPR and the use of portable defibrillators. For more information, contact a local chapter.

Rapid defibrillation holds the greatest hope for survival from cardiac arrest. In fact, the chance of withstanding ventricular fibrillation declines by approximately 10 percent for each minute that passes without defibrillation.

To make rapid defibrillation more available, the American Heart Association has developed a training program for lay rescuers that combines CPR instruction with training in automated external defibrillator operation.

AEDs automatically analyze the heart rhythm and instruct the operator with audible and visual prompts to press a button that delivers a shock. AEDs are becoming more available in many large public settings, such as airport terminals, high-rise buildings, gated communities, and sports arenas, for use by trained first responders, such as security guards and laypersons who may be immediately available in such settings. AEDs are being installed as standard equipment on commercial airlines in the United States and around the world.

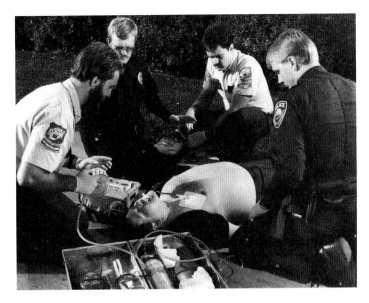

*Emergency personnel are trained to deliver an electrical shock to defibrillate the heart of someone experiencing ventricular fibrillation or other catastrophic heart rhythms.*

## External pacemaker

In contrast to ventricular fibrillation, in which a large electrical impulse must reset a disorganized heartbeat, sometimes a heart doesn't beat at all or beats too slowly to circulate blood effectively. A cardiac pacemaker is a device designed to deliver an electrical stimulus to the heart repeatedly, which causes it to contract.

It takes much less energy to contract the heart repeatedly than to defibrillate it. Pacemakers are useful when the heart rhythm is drastically slow or the heart has no rhythm at all. Most cardiac pacing uses wires inserted through veins and into the heart to supply stimulus directly to the heart muscle.

External cardiac pacemakers, however, use patches on the chest and back to transmit electrical stimuli to the heart. This external system is useful in emergencies, when inserting wire through a vein may be extremely difficult or time-consuming.

**HEALTHY HEART ♥ TIP**

*The more cardiovascular risk factors you have, the greater your chances of developing cardiovascular disease. In fact, if you have several of these elements, their effects don't simply add up, they multiply.*

*Risk factors include:*
- *High cholesterol*
- *Smoking*
- *High blood pressure*
- *Physical inactivity*
- *Obesity*
- *Diabetes*
- *Family history*

# Chapter
# 13
## Treating heart muscle problems

Treating congestive heart failure focuses on correcting the cause, if possible. When that's not feasible, treatment concentrates on optimizing the heart's performance. Many types of medical therapy can help relieve symptoms of congestive heart failure and potentially prolong life in those who have it (see page 366).

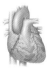

### HEALTHY HEART ♥ TIP

*People with blocked arteries— and chest pain that wasn't helped by medication—once had only bypass surgery to reroute blood flow around the blockage. These days, there are nonsurgical alternatives that open blocked arteries with less risk and expense.*

*Coronary angioplasty is probably the most common alternative. Done with local anesthesia, the procedure can take from 30 minutes to two hours and usually requires a hospital stay of only one day.*

*Angioplasty has about a 95 percent immediate success rate. In 10 percent to 30 percent of people, however, the treated artery narrows again within six months. If this happens, your cardiologist may recommend repeat angioplasty or perhaps bypass surgery.*

## Correcting the cause

When doctors can correct the cause of heart failure, the entire problem may be solved. For example, if a faulty valve hampers the heart's pumping efficiency, then repairing or replacing the valve may resolve the heart failure.

Likewise, if a section of the heart muscle doesn't get enough oxygen because of a blocked coronary artery, restoring blood flow to that region may improve the heart muscle function enough to reverse the deficiency. If the cause of the heart failure is a persistently fast heartbeat that produces inefficient pumping, correcting the heart rhythm problem may relieve the heart failure.

Because heart failure can stem from diverse sources, there are various treatments, depending on the specific problem that's causing the heart failure.

## Medications for heart failure

The basic principles for treating heart failure without a correctable cause focus on augmenting the heart muscle's pumping function, reducing the heart's work load, curtailing sodium and fluid retention that causes swelling (edema), decreasing the effects of adrenaline on the heart, and preventing thromboembolism (blood clots).

All of the potential beneficial effects must be weighed against the possibility of complications as a result of therapy. In addition, treatment with medications should be considered along with other options, from optimizing diet and activity to surgical intervention.

## Strengthening the heart's contractions: positive inotropic medications

In most heart failure cases, the heart doesn't pump enough blood to meet the body's needs, and the contractions are too weak. So it seems logical that strengthening the contractions would improve your condition.

Medications that increase the contraction strength of your heart muscle are called positive inotropic medications (ino means "muscle," tropic means "influencing"). Examples of inotropic agents include digitalis, dopamine, dobutamine, and amrinone.

Digitalis (from the foxglove plant) is one of the oldest medications available for heart failure; it was first used more than 200 years ago. Digitalis increases the strength of heart muscle contractions.

Digitalis seems to work best in people who have severe heart failure. It's also beneficial if you have atrial fibrillation because it slows the commonly associated rapid heart rate.

Despite the long history of digitalis use, its exact role and likely benefits still remain imprecise. Recent studies have been completed that systematically test the risks and benefits of digitalis in people with reduced pumping function of the heart. The results demonstrate that digitalis helps improve symptoms and reduces recurrent hospitalizations for heart failure, but has no benefit on overall survival.

Other medications have been developed to increase contraction strength, but they're given only intravenously. They are very useful for short-term use in people with advanced stages of heart failure who require hospitalization in the intensive care unit.

Unfortunately, there may be drawbacks to using certain inotropic agents. Like all medications, each inotropic agent has side effects. During drug-testing trials, taking some experimental inotropic medications on a long-term basis led to an even higher rate of complications and death than did the placebo (inactive) medication.

Although these specific inotropic medications have never been prescribed routinely, some doctors have speculated that standard inotropic agents that force a weakened heart to beat harder put an excessive work load on an already laboring muscle. This may actually accelerate its weakening process.

Thus, in the past decade, many doctors have expressed reservations about long-term use of inotropic agents other than digitalis. Nevertheless, these agents are practical in appropriately selected individuals and for short-term use.

### Is heart failure reversible?

Causes of heart failure that can usually be reversed:
- Heart valve defects
- Chronic fast heart rates (such as atrial fibrillation, supraventricular tachycardia)
- Metabolic abnormalities

Causes of heart failure that may be reversed:
- Severe high blood pressure
- Infections (myocarditis)
- Alcohol poisoning of the heart muscle
- Hemochromatosis (abnormal iron deposits in the heart muscle)
- Coronary circulatory abnormalities

Causes of heart failure that usually are not reversible:
- Idiopathic dilated cardiomyopathy
- Amyloidosis (abnormal protein deposits in the heart muscle)
- Extensive injury of the heart muscle from heart attacks
- Restrictive cardiomyopathy

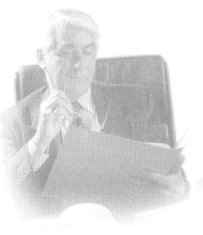

### Reducing the work load of the heart: vasodilators

Because there may be disadvantages to making a weakened heart work harder with inotropic agents, other medical strategies for treating heart failure have been refined. Here, the goal is to reduce the work load and increase the heart's efficiency.

A pump exerts more energy squeezing fluid (or blood) through narrow tubes (or arteries) than pushing the same amount of fluid through wider tubes. Thus, the main way to reduce the heart's work load in congestive heart failure is to widen or dilate the arteries with medications called vasodilators. Vasodilators were initially developed to treat high blood pressure, for which they're still prescribed.

Several types of vasodilators have been adopted for treating heart failure. The most widely used are the angiotensin converting enzyme (ACE) inhibitors. These medications decrease hormones in the circulation that constrict or narrow arteries and raise blood pressure. Studies and experience have demonstrated that ACE inhibitors and other vasodilators are effective for improving the heart's pumping efficiency, reducing symptoms, and increasing survival of people with heart failure. In fact, of the medications used for heart failure, vasodilator therapy was the first shown to prolong life and also to reduce symptoms.

### Reducing fluid accumulation: diuretics

One of the hallmarks of congestive heart failure is the accumulation of fluid (edema) in the legs, abdomen, liver, and lungs. Fluid accumulation may occur despite treatment with vasodilators and inotropic agents, especially in severe or rapidly developing cases of congestive heart failure. Thus, one treatment strategy is to reduce fluid accumulation by using diuretics.

Diuretic agents promote urine production by the kidneys. As the kidneys remove increasing amounts of water and sodium from the blood, the edema fluid is absorbed from the tissues back into the bloodstream and eliminated, which reduces swelling. Therefore, diuretics don't really treat the heart failure itself, but may reverse some of the effects, and relieve some of the symptoms of heart failure.

Diuretics can ease shortness of breath and swelling within hours or days, whereas other agents such as digitalis or vasodilators may take weeks or months. There are several types of diuretics, and they vary in potency and speed. Doctors sometimes prescribe a combination of diuretic agents.

### Reducing the effects of adrenaline: beta-blockers

Congestive heart failure is characterized by increasing levels of the circulating hormone adrenaline, which if chronically elevated may have an adverse effect on heart function. Beta-blockers obstruct the effects of adrenaline on the sympathetic nervous system. Although these agents have been routinely prescribed for other cardiovascular conditions for 30 years (hypertension, angina pectoris, and for heart attack survivors), they were initially regarded as inappropriate therapy for patients with reduced heart pump function. However, large clinical trials in the United States and Europe suggest that these drugs are safe and beneficial for this condition.

By preventing the adverse actions of adrenaline on the cardiovascular system, beta-blockers may avert progressive heart enlargement and decline in pump function, which often typify heart failure. Sometimes, cardiac function actually improves.

Like ACE inhibitors, these agents have been effective in improving the heart's pumping efficiency, reducing symptoms, and increasing survival of heart failure patients. If you have heart failure, your doctor will start beta-blocker therapy with a low dose and build up over a period of weeks.

### Preventing blood clots: anticoagulants

People with heart failure may be vulnerable to blood clots forming within the heart chambers or leg veins. Because the weakened heart pumps blood less vigorously, blood flow may be sluggish. This condition increases the chance of clot formation along the inner surface of the heart muscle. If a clot fragment dislodges, it travels through the circulation and may cause a stroke or other complications.

That's why many people with heart failure receive long-term oral therapy with anticoagulants (blood thinners). No adequate studies clearly demonstrate a benefit from a long-term anticoagulant, although it's logical to use them under certain circumstances (for example, in treating a large heart that contracts poorly). A common anticoagulant is warfarin.

Warfarin acts by preventing the liver from using vitamin K to produce clotting proteins. A blood test called the prothrombin time ("protime") measures the level of certain factors necessary for clotting. Your doctor once used the results of this test to determine how much anticoagulant medication you need. Prothrombin time has been replaced by the International Normalized Ratio, which takes into account differences in the strength of compounds used in the test itself.

Various medications can influence your prothrombin time, so check with your doctor before taking any new medications. Aspirin can increase the effect of anticoagulants (by inhibiting the natural clotting action of platelets). It can also cause irritation of the stomach lining, which may lead to internal bleeding. Thus, aspirin should usually be avoided while you're taking anticoagulants.

Rarely, large amounts of vitamin K from foods (such as green leafy vegetables) or vitamin supplements that include vitamin K may decrease the action of warfarin.

## Complications of therapy

Despite their potential, all heart failure medications have limitations. As already mentioned, some inotropic agents occasionally increase complications and death rates. You shouldn't take vasodilators if your blood pressure already is too low (systolic blood pressure less than 85 mm Hg), because vasodilators will lower it further. ACE inhibitors may lead to worse kidney failure in people with kidney disease.

You shouldn't take diuretics if your blood pressure is too low, because they'll lower it further by decreasing the volume of blood in the blood vessels. Furthermore, as diuretics eliminate excess fluid from the body, other substances go, too.

The most common chemical abnormality caused by some kinds of diuretics is a lowering of the body's potassium supply. Potassium maintains the electrical stability of the heart and nervous system; low potassium levels can lead to heart rhythm abnormalities. In addition, digitalis will more likely cause side effects (including some heartbeat irregularities) when potassium levels are low.

## Basic principles for treating congestive heart failure

1. Reduce the heart's work load:

   Maintain a comfortable activity level to help your body and circulatory system adapt and stay fit.

   Decrease physical activity during periods of worsened heart failure.

   Avoid isometric work (such as heavy lifting), which increases blood pressure (and decreases cardiac output).

   Curtail emotional stress.

   Lose weight if you're too heavy.

   Control high blood pressure.

2. Regulate sodium and water retention:

   Rest in bed during periods of worsened heart failure to enhance removal of water and sodium in the urine, then gradually increase activity.

   Restrict sodium in your diet.

   Limit fluid intake.

3. Medications:

   Decrease your heart's work load with vasodilators.

   Control sodium and water retention with diuretics.

   Improve pump function with inotropic medications.

   Prevent thromboembolism with anticoagulants.

   Block the effects of adrenaline on the sympathetic nervous system with beta-blockers.

4. Heart transplantation

Because of potassium loss, people taking certain types of diuretics must also take supplemental potassium. If you're taking a diuretic, it may be advisable to eat potassium-rich foods, such as bananas, cantaloupe, grapefruit juice, honeydew melon, orange juice, baked or boiled potatoes, avocado, flounder, halibut, prunes and prune juice, cooked soybeans, dates, and figs. Your doctor can measure the potassium level in your blood and advise if you need extra potassium.

Diuretics can also deplete magnesium. Low magnesium levels can lead to muscle weakness and irregular heart rhythms. Foods rich in magnesium include beans, nuts, poultry, fish, green vegetables, grains, and citrus fruits.

Beta-blockers shouldn't be prescribed if the blood pressure or heart rate is too low, as these drugs may cause a further decrease. There are other conditions in which beta-blockers aren't advisable, and their use requires a consultation with your physician.

## What should you do?

In the past, people with heart failure were told to rest and lead a sedentary life. This advice still holds true when you're experiencing episodes of severe heart failure. Increased bed rest during these incidents reduces the work load on your heart and also redistributes fluids in the body, thus helping the kidneys eliminate excess sodium and fluid.

These days, however, doctors encourage all but the most severely debilitated patients with chronic heart failure to continue regular activities within their comfort zone. If you're too sedentary you can get out of shape, which makes physical exertion seem even harder. You should not, however, engage in activities that make you constantly short of breath.

Rethink your diet. Limiting salt intake is essential. Unless you restrict sodium, medications may be ineffective. Periods of worsening heart failure often can be traced to eating sodium-containing foods.

You also need to limit fluid intake to no more than 2 quarts per day, which includes beverages, soups, puddings, Jell-o, and other fluid foods. By carefully monitoring fluid intake and daily weight, you can maintain fluid balance and lessen the use of diuretics. Overeating and being overweight add to your heart's work.

If you have trouble getting a good night's rest because it's hard to breathe, use pillows to prop up your head and avoid eating a big meal just before bedtime. If you have problems with frequent nighttime urination, your doctor may change your medication.

# Heart transplantation

In some situations, the heart becomes so weak that conventional medical treatment has little impact. You may need to explore the possibility of heart transplantation (see page A5).

Heart transplantation can significantly reduce symptoms and increase survival rates in some people with severe heart failure. Individuals receiving transplants at experienced medical centers have 1-year survival rates of approximately 85 to 95 percent, and heart transplantation is now considered a standard form of care for end-stage heart failure. Doctors perform about 2,300 heart transplantations annually in the United States.

## Selecting candidates

To optimally use the limited supply of donor hearts and to help ensure successful heart transplantations, doctors earnestly try to identify those who have the greatest need and will be most inclined to gain from transplantation.

People most likely to benefit are usually younger than 65 and have irreversible heart disease causing a life expectancy of less than 2 or 3 years. One difficult aspect of deciding who should be a heart transplant candidate involves estimating how long a person can live without a transplant and how the disease will progress during the waiting period.

The transplant candidate must be able to comply with medical recommendations, must be motivated for transplantation, and must not have major medical barriers, such as health problems that may preclude successful transplantation.

Contraindications to heart transplantation include pulmonary hypertension (high pressure in the arteries to the lungs), infection, noncardiac disease that significantly limits life expectancy or will be worsened by using immunosuppressive medications after transplantation, unresolved alcohol or drug abuse (including tobacco), extreme obesity, and inability to adhere to a schedule of medications and medical evaluations. These characteristics make it less likely that a heart transplantation will be successful.

## Water softeners and sodium

Did you know your tap water may be a significant source of sodium in your diet? Water naturally contains some sodium, but plumbing that directs drinking water through water softeners add even more. How much additional sodium depends on your water supply's "hardness," which is determined by mineral content.

Your local health department can provide information about the sodium and mineral content of your community's water supply. This will help you determine the total amount of sodium your tap water may contain after it has been softened.

You can estimate the amount of sodium (milligrams per liter) needed to soften water by multiplying the hardness of the water (grains per gallon) by 8. Add this figure to the amount of naturally occurring sodium in the water supply to determine sodium intake from tap water.

If you find that your tap water is significantly boosting your sodium intake, you may want to buy demineralized water for cooking and drinking or invest in a water purification system. Ask your doctor if you should be concerned.

Potential candidates for a heart transplant must undergo extensive testing to determine whether a heart transplantation is advisable. Exams include a careful assessment for evidence of infection, other diseases that would compromise the transplantation, and the likelihood that the immune system would reject a transplanted heart. Other organ systems must be healthy.

## Heart donation

Hearts for transplantation are in short supply because many still aren't aware of the vital need for organ donation. Nearly a third of patients waiting for a heart transplant die before a donor heart becomes available. That makes educational efforts a high priority.

No one wants someone else to die just to provide a heart for transplantation, but when deaths occur, families often find comfort in helping others through organ donation. A single donor may provide lifesaving organs (heart, lungs, kidneys, liver, and pancreas) for six or more recipients.

Families should talk about this issue before the situation arises. The decision to donate a loved one's organs is much easier if everyone knows beforehand what the person would want. Many states now have regulations that promote the process of seeking permission for acquiring donor organs.

When doctors recommend a heart transplant, they place recipients on a waiting list. Once you're on the list, you may have to relocate to within 2 to 3 hours of the hospital, although some institutions will transport you by air ambulance without requiring relocation. The hospital gives you a beeper so it can reach you anytime, wherever you are. You must have your suitcase packed and travel plans ready so you can get to the hospital immediately.

By law, heart transplantations are done on a "first-come, first-served" basis. The only exception is if you become so ill that you must be hospitalized in an intensive care unit that requires intravenous medications, a ventilator, or other life support devices. In these cases, you move to a higher position or category on the waiting list.

## The transplantation procedure and hospitalization

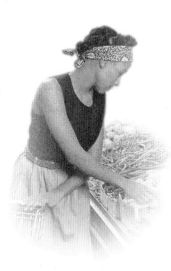

When a heart becomes available, tests establish the donor's blood type and whether there's evidence of infection, including human immunodeficiency virus (HIV), which causes acquired immunodeficiency syndrome (AIDS). Determining any hidden infections allows doctors to decide whether a heart is suitable and to plan preventive treatment against any infection the heart may carry.

Matching blood types helps prevent the body from rejecting the donor heart. If the blood type matches and the donor heart is healthy, the transplantation proceeds. The size of the donor heart should be fairly proportional to the recipient's body frame, but a precise match isn't necessary. Transplantation can occur between people of different sexes or races as long as size difference isn't extreme.

A nationally maintained waiting list uses a computer to match the next patient on the list with a compatible blood type and acceptable size range for the donor. If you're next and have the same blood type as the donor, you'll be advised to come to the hospital promptly for the heart transplantation. Once doctors remove the heart from the donor, it can remain outside the body for only 4 to 6 hours before transplantation must be completed.

Before the operation, you will have blood tests, urine samples, and a chest X-ray to ensure that all conditions are satisfactory. You will also shower with special cleansing soap to help prevent infection. Doctors will insert an intravenous (IV) catheter.

The heart transplantation itself is a straightforward procedure for skilled heart surgeons. After you're connected to a heart-lung machine, the surgeon removes your failing heart by making incisions in the atria, aorta, and pulmonary arteries, and connects the donor heart at these sites.

After the operation, you will be monitored closely in the intensive care unit for several days. As with most heart operations, you will require temporary supportive measures to speed recovery.

Drainage tubes inserted through the skin of the chest and upper abdomen during the operation remain in place for a few days to remove excess fluid or blood from the chest cavity. A breathing tube may be left for a day or so until you're able to take adequate breaths and clear secretions by coughing on your own. A catheter in the bladder simplifies urination and allows accurate measurement of your fluid balance. A nasogastric tube in your stomach removes stomach juices, since the intestines require time to begin working again.

Because you'll be temporarily unable to take water, food, or medications by mouth, these will be given through intravenous tubes. As a precaution, the surgeon will insert pacemaker wires that can be connected to a temporary pacemaker; if they aren't needed, they can be removed without another operation.

During your hospital recovery period (which lasts from 1 to 3 weeks), numerous specialists may participate in your care, such as a heart surgeon, cardiologists, and lung and infectious disease specialists. Specialized nurses, respiratory and physical therapists, pharmacists, and dietitians also are essential for the success of your transplantation.

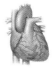

**HEALTHY HEART ♥ TIP**

*Heart attacks aren't always dramatic, chest-clutching events. In fact, many people waste precious minutes during a heart attack because they don't recognize the symptoms or they deny them. In addition, a heart attack also can be "silent," with no clues whatsoever.*

*Generally, though, a heart attack causes chest pain or pressure for more than 15 minutes. About half of all heart attack victims experience warning signs hours, days or weeks in advance.*

*The earlier the treatment is started, the better the outcome.*

## After the transplantation

Treatment after a transplantation includes medications to help prevent rejection of the donor heart. The body's immune system recognizes and defends itself against foreign substances such as disease-causing organisms (bacteria or viruses). It also perceives an organ from another person as a foreign substance and attempts to reject it. The medications suppress your immune system to minimize the chances it will attack the new heart.

Suppressing the immune system, however, reduces your body's ability to fight infection. Infection is one of the complications of transplantation, sometimes with types that usually don't occur in otherwise healthy people. The transplant team takes great care to prevent infections and to detect them immediately so they can be treated quickly.

For a while after the transplantation, visitors may be required to wear hospital gowns and masks to minimize the chance of exposing you to potentially infectious germs. After you leave the hospital, you may be advised to wear a mask in public places until your doctors think you're no longer at risk of infection.

Medications that suppress the immune system have other potential side effects, including high blood pressure, diabetes, kidney function problems, weight gain, and certain types of cancer. Doctors tailor medications and doses to meet your needs, and they monitor them closely.

## Possible complications of heart operation

Bleeding (hemorrhage)

Heart attack (myocardial infarction)

Stroke

Infection

Reaction to anesthetic medications

Heart rhythm abnormality

Prolonged dependence on a ventilator for breathing

Death

The chance of any complication is low, but it varies depending on the specific type of operation, the patient's overall condition, and the surgical team's skill. The odds of a complication should always be discussed thoroughly before any operation, and it should be weighed against the operation's anticipated benefits (or complications of not having an operation). No matter how low the risk of any operation or treatment, it will never be zero.

## Rejection

When the body's immune system attacks the donor heart, doctors say it's "rejecting" the organ. Rejection episodes may happen anytime after the operation, but most often they occur within the first few months.

Rejection is controlled by adjusting the immunosuppressive medications, which help prevent your immune system from rejecting your new heart. The level of medication in your blood, white blood cell counts, and other values must be monitored to check your response to the medications. Any doctor or dentist who treats you must be informed of the heart transplant and any immunosuppressive medications you're taking.

To detect rejection, endomyocardial biopsies are conducted at regular intervals after the transplant operation. Using a special catheter your doctor snips a tiny piece of tissue from your heart and checks it under a microscope for signs of rejection (see page 263). Biopsy specimens start on postoperative day 21, daily for 4 weeks, once every 2 weeks from 6 weeks to 3 months after operation, once a month from 3 to 6 months after operation, once every 3 to 6 months for 2 to 3 years, and once every 6 months thereafter.

## Long-term developments

Now that transplant recipients live longer, doctors find some problems that appear years after transplantation.

For one, the transplanted heart's coronary arteries may develop widespread narrowing. Because the nerves have been cut in the transplanted heart, recipients don't usually feel angina (chest pain) when their coronary arteries don't supply enough oxygen to the heart muscle. Therefore, doctors perform annual coronary angiography to look for possible narrowing of the coronary arteries.

Doctors also continue to examine patients for any evidence of tumor formation, especially of the lymph glands, because immunosuppressive medications may increase the chances of this occurrence.

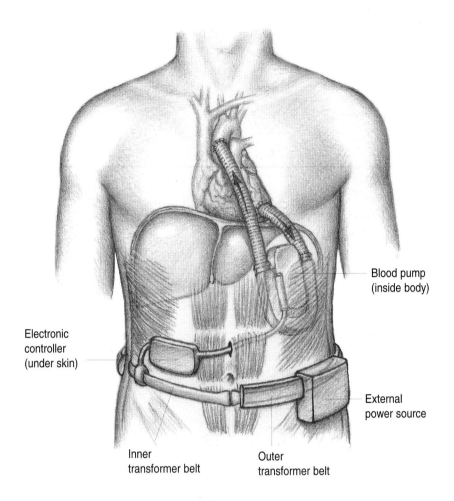

Blood pump
(inside body)

Electronic
controller
(under skin)

External
power source

Inner
transformer belt

Outer
transformer belt

*Here's one design of a totally implantable artificial heart. An external power source transfers energy from an outer transformer belt through the skin to an inner transformer. The energy then powers an artificial pump that draws blood from a person's damaged left ventricle and pumps it into the aorta, which distributes it throughout the body.*

## Artificial devices

Because of a donor heart shortage, researchers are studying the possibility of using artificial pumping devices or total artificial hearts to help people with severe heart failure who would otherwise be incapacitated or die soon.

Some people have received artificial hearts as a "bridge" to transplantation when their own hearts were unable to keep them alive until a donor heart was available. Other devices have been created that don't replace the human heart but rather help it to pump more effectively.

These devices are experimental and require outside power sources entering through the skin to help them work. This limits recipients to activities within range of the power source. Currently, however, a totally implantable electric artificial heart is being tested, one of the final steps before the device would be suitable for humans.

In addition, recent information suggests that the heart muscle of people with congestive heart failure may recover some of its function after time is spent on a left ventricular assist device.

## Operations for other heart muscle diseases

Hypertrophic cardiomyopathy (heart muscle overgrowth) causes symptoms because the muscle blocks blood flow from the left ventricle to the aorta. Medical treatment strives to reduce the obstruction's effect, promote efficient heart relaxation, and avoid rhythm disorders that may be associated with this problem.

Because the obstruction increases when the heart contracts, doctors use medications to reduce the heart's contraction strength. These medications, which include beta-blockers and certain calcium channel blockers, have the opposite effect of the positive inotropic agents. When rhythm problems are present, antiarrhythmic medications may be needed.

If medications don't adequately relieve the symptoms, doctors may want to remove the portion of overgrown heart muscle that's blocking blood flow. This procedure is called a myotomy-myectomy (myotomy means "cutting into muscle tissue," myectomy means "removing muscle tissue").

Myotomy-myectomy can be very effective for reducing symptoms, but it must be carefully considered because, like all surgical procedures, it carries certain risks. Some patients benefit from pacemaker treatment, even if they don't have a slow heartbeat, because it seems to help reduce the blockage's effects.

### Relieving congenital heart disease

Some congenital heart defects, such as a bicuspid aortic valve or a small ventricular septal defect, may be so minor that operation isn't necessary. Others, such as an atrial septal defect, a patent ductus arteriosus, or a ventricular septal defect, are straightforward abnormalities for which well-established surgical procedures are indicated.

Still other defects, such as transposition of the great arteries or truncus arteriosus, may be extremely complex. In these cases, deciding whether to operate and what type of operation to perform may require evaluation and treatment in a highly specialized surgical facility.

**Fixing the problem**

Operation for congenital heart disease conforms to one of three strategies:

1. **Palliation.** Doctors want you to experience few symptoms and live as long as possible without actually correcting the defect, because the defect can't be totally repaired. An example of a palliative procedure is the Blalock-Taussig anastomosis for tetralogy of Fallot (see page 61).

2. **Staged operations.** The operation corrects the problem partially and allows your heart and blood vessels to adapt or grow so that a second, more extensive reparative operation can be done in the future. For example, a two-stage procedure is one in which the pulmonary arteries enlarge in response to the Blalock-Taussig shunt in the palliative procedure so doctors can place a conduit (tube) between the right ventricle and the pulmonary arteries.

3. **Total repair.** Either the defect is corrected or a procedure reverses the effect of the congenital heart problem. An example of a complete repair is interruption of a patent ductus arteriosus.

(For more information on congenital heart disease, see page 59.)

# Managing valve disease

Disease can affect any of the four valves in the heart, but it's more common in the mitral and aortic valves on the heart's left side than in the tricuspid and pulmonary valves on the right. Valves may open incompletely (stenosis) or allow blood to leak backward (regurgitation). It's often difficult to select the best treatment because one can't always predict how valve disease and its effect on the heart muscle will progress (see pages A7 and A8).

## Observation

If the valve disease isn't causing symptoms or damage to the heart muscle's contracting function, your doctor may take a "wait-and-see" approach: continue with regular examinations to make sure the problem isn't worsening or producing a deterioration in the heart muscle's overall function.

## Medication

It's important to prevent or manage problems that can result from the disturbance in blood flow through damaged valves. One potential difficulty is infective endocarditis (see page 70). You should let your doctor or dentist know that you have a valve problem and that you need preventive antibiotics before any dental or surgical procedure that could introduce germs into your system.

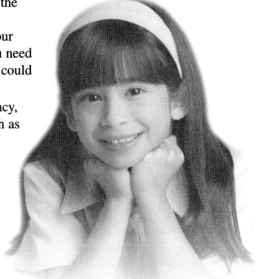

Because valve disease can reduce the heart's pumping efficiency, leading to heart failure symptoms, you may need medications such as digitalis, diuretics, or vasodilators to augment contraction of the ventricles, to prevent or control fluid retention, or to reduce the work load on your heart. Sometimes valve disease can also lead to heart rhythm problems, and you may need medication to help control your heart rhythm.

Valve problems cause abnormal blood flow through your heart, which may induce blood clots. Anticoagulant medications ("blood thinners") are used to help control this problem when valve disease is complicated by atrial fibrillation, heart failure, or blood clots.

Symptoms in people with some types of valvular heart disease signal that the valve problem must be corrected. Further observation or medications alone will be insufficient, and the valve and heart muscle's inadequate function will only continue to decline. With other types of valvular heart disease, your doctor may want to fix the complication—even if you have no symptoms—to prevent heart muscle deterioration and to prolong life.

In these situations, treatment consists of two basic strategies, depending on the nature of the valve problem: (1) altering the valve, or (2) replacing the valve. Altering the defective valve to improve its function can sometimes be done with catheterization procedures, but most often requires operation. Replacing the valve always demands an operation.

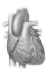

## HEALTHY HEART ♥ TIP

*HDL, LDL: What's the difference? High-density lipoprotein (HDL) is considered "good" because it helps remove cholesterol from arteries and prevent blockage. Low-density lipoprotein (LDL) is considered "bad" because too much LDL leads to cholesterol deposits in the arteries and, eventually, to atherosclerosis—a hardening of arteries that is the underlying cause of heart attacks and strokes.*

*Optimally, your LDL level should measure less than 130 mg/dL. If you have no risk factors for cardiovascular disease, an LDL level over 190 generally requires medication. With two or more risk factors, an LDL level over 160 may require medication. If you have coronary artery disease, your doctor may try medication and lifestyle changes to lower your LDL below 100.*

## Catheterization techniques (balloon valvuloplasty)

Catheterization can be used to widen heart valves that are stenotic (narrowed), which limits blood flow (see page A8).

Percutaneous balloon valvuloplasty (percutaneous means "through the skin" [with a catheter], valvulo means "related to the valve," plasty means [re]"shaping") is a procedure in which one or two balloons mounted on catheters are guided into the heart through blood vessels, positioned through the stenotic valve, and then inflated. This enlarges the opening through the valve and improves the blood flow.

As with any heart catheterization procedure, there are potential risks, in addition to the chance of causing further damage to the valve structure with balloon manipulation. In the right people, however, the risks are small compared with the probability of relieving symptoms promptly. In addition, patients stay in the hospital less time with valvuloplasty than with open-heart valve operations.

Balloon valvuloplasty has become the preferred method of treating properly selected people with symptomatic pulmonary valve stenosis or mitral stenosis. For mitral stenosis, doctors insert one or two catheters through the femoral vein (in the groin), threading them up to the right atrium of the heart.

The doctor punctures a sharp-tipped catheter through the atrial septum and passes the balloon catheters through the small hole, positioning them (with balloons deflated) midway through the mitral valve, then inflates them. The stiff leaflets that have become "stuck" to one another split open to allow more blood to flow through. When the catheter is removed, the tiny hole in the atrial septum seals on its own.

Mitral balloon valvuloplasty may not be appropriate if there's too much calcium buildup on the valve or if it's already allowing blood to leak backward. It's also not performed if there's a blood clot in one of the heart chambers, because of the risk of dislodging it. Under these circumstances, the valve must be replaced.

Doctors also use balloon valvuloplasty for aortic stenosis, but it's not the preferred approach because improvements are small and frequently last less than 1 year. Nevertheless, it may be useful if you have other illnesses that preclude an open-heart operation.

## Operation

Balloon catheter procedures aren't appropriate for some symptomatic individuals with mitral stenosis, for most people with aortic stenosis, or for anyone with mitral or aortic regurgitation. For these valve problems, doctors prefer operating on the valve.

### Valve repair

Many mitral regurgitation cases can be repaired: the surgeon can modify the original valve (valvuloplasty) to eliminate back leakage of blood. This procedure is most effective when mitral regurgitation is caused by chordae tendineae breakage, misshapen, billowy valve leaflets that don't close properly, or the tissue ring around the valve leaflets' base is enlarged (see page 69).

Doctors repair the valve by reconnecting the valve leaflets to their tethers or by cutting out sections of excess valve leaflet tissue so that valve leaflets close snugly. Sometimes repairing the valve includes "cinching" the surrounding ring of heart tissue to ensure the leaflets close adequately. This is called annuloplasty (annulo means "ring," plasty means [re]"shaping").

If your natural valve can be repaired, you'll usually have better and longer-lasting results, and you may not require additional medications such as anticoagulants that may be necessary with artificial valves. Surgeons can't repair valves that are very heavily calcified or that have been significantly destroyed by disease.

Some people with mitral stenosis undergo surgical revision called mitral commissurotomy, in which the surgeon cuts between the valve leaflets that have become "stuck" together. The natural separations between leaflets are called commissures, hence the name, meaning "to cut the commissure." Because percutaneous mitral balloon valvuloplasty is usually as effective as mitral commissurotomy, operations are being used less frequently.

### Which prosthetic valve is right?

| Situation | Recommended valve |
|---|---|
| Advanced age with limited life span expected | Bioprosthesis (tissue valve from human or animal) |
| Bleeding tendency | |
| Anticipated difficulty with anticoagulation (such as future pregnancy) | |
| Young age with long life span expected | Mechanical prosthesis |
| No reason to avoid anticoagulation | |

## Valve replacement

To replace a damaged heart valve, the surgeon removes it and sutures an artificial (prosthetic) valve at the site. This is the preferred treatment for aortic valve disease that needs treatment beyond medication. It's necessary to replace the mitral valve if the doctor decides that either repair or balloon valvuloplasty won't provide a satisfactory result (see page A8).

Mechanical prosthetic valves are constructed from metal and synthetic materials. They include ball valves, tilting disk valves, and double-tilting half-disk (bileaflet) valves. Bioprostheses are made from animal or human tissue. An animal tissue bioprosthesis usually comes from a pig's heart valve or the pericardium of a cow. Animal tissue valves are often called heterografts (hetero means "different," and in this usage it means "different from humans").

A human tissue bioprosthesis consists of a heart valve donated from someone who has died. These are called homografts (homo means [hu]"man"). Unlike heart transplants, the valves can be preserved and are no longer living tissue. They also do not cause rejection.

The key to finding the right prosthetic valve involves a careful discussion that emphasizes the advantages and disadvantages of certain valves, and an assessment of the risk of anticoagulation therapy. For example, mechanical prostheses are extremely durable, but patients need to take an anticoagulant (for example, warfarin) for the rest of their lives, because blood has a natural tendency to clot on the valve. This clotting could either plug the valve or result in an embolism.

The advantage of bioprostheses is that they rarely require anticoagulation. However, heterografts are not as durable as mechanical valves. About 30 to 50 percent of heterograft valves need replacing within 10 years after the first implantation.

Homografts may be more durable than heterografts, but there are fewer of them and they are used only to replace a defective aortic valve. In general, patients under 70 years old receive mechanical prostheses, while bioprostheses are preferred for those over 75 (between ages 70 and 75 is a "gray" area).

All prosthetic valves are prone to infection that is difficult to treat with antibiotics. Therefore, it's extremely important to take appropriate precautions before any dental or surgical procedure if you have a prosthetic valve.

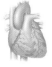

### HEALTHY HEART ♥ TIP

*Are you depressed? Studies show that 15 to 25 percent of people who've had a heart attack suffer from depression afterward. These people generally don't recover as well because they have trouble following their doctor's recommendations and making necessary changes in their lives.*

*Depression is common, correctable and underdiagnosed.*

*Cardiac rehabilitation programs help identify and treat post-heart-attack depression, and also provide techniques to control other emotions such as stress and anger—which may have contributed to your heart attack in the first place. Studies have shown that taking part in a cardiac rehabilitation program following a heart attack can improve your health and life expectancy.*

# Surviving heart attack and coronary artery disease

Coronary artery disease restricts the flow of oxygen-containing blood to the heart muscle, which can result in stable and unstable angina pectoris, heart attack, and sudden death.

Because coronary artery disease is so common in our population and because its consequences can be so serious, doctors continuously search for better ways to diagnose and treat it. In recent years, there have been many innovations in diagnosing and treating coronary artery disease. New medications, procedures, and operations that improve blood flow to the heart muscle can help minimize symptoms and lengthen life in people with coronary artery disease.

The initial and overriding treatment goal for all these problems is to balance the blood flow supply to the jeopardized heart muscle with the muscle's oxygen demand. What strategies and methods doctors use depends on the specific underlying problem causing the inadequate blood flow, the severity of symptoms, and the future risk posed by the coronary artery problems.

There are different strategies for stable angina, unstable angina, coronary spasm, and heart attack, which include medications, interventionist procedures with catheters, and coronary artery bypass operation.

## Medications

Medications that treat stable angina act either by promoting blood flow through the coronary arteries or by reducing the heart muscle's demand for oxygen, or both. This allows the myocardium to function better, even with a reduced oxygen supply.

Unfortunately, no medication reliably removes or dissolves the cholesterol plaques that clog arteries. Studies, however, suggest that some medications may lessen the severity of the blockage. Studies with statin, for example, indicate that these medicines may make the cholesterol plaques more stable and less prone to rupture.

Medications that increase the oxygenated blood flow to the heart do so mainly by relaxing the smooth muscle in the walls of the coronary arteries, allowing them to dilate as much as possible. This relaxation permits an increased flow of blood through the artery, but it doesn't eliminate the blockages from atherosclerotic deposits.

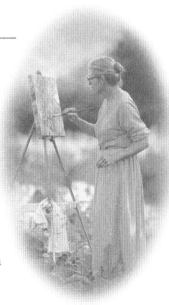

Medications that reduce the heart's demand for oxygen act in one of the following ways:

1. They slow the heart rate; the fewer times the heart beats per minute, the less oxygen it requires.

2. They decrease the vigor of heart muscle contraction; more forceful contractions require more oxygen. Unless the heart is already severely weakened, most people can tolerate some reduction in the intensity of their heart muscle contraction.

3. They reduce the size of and pressure inside the ventricles. The less pressure and stretch on the heart muscle of the ventricles, the less oxygen the muscle uses.

If you just have mild or infrequent angina spells, you may need only a medication to eliminate symptoms during sporadic episodes. This strategy is called "p.r.n.," from the Latin *pro re nata*, which means "according to circumstances."

Nitroglycerin pills dissolved under the tongue or nitroglycerin sprayed into the mouth when symptoms begin eliminates the chest discomfort in most people with stable angina. Discomfort usually ends within several minutes after taking the nitroglycerin, and may be all you need.

If you have symptoms that occur under predictable circumstances, such as climbing a flight of stairs, you may be advised to use nitroglycerin before the activity. Others with more prominent or frequent symptoms may benefit from taking medications regularly to try to prevent or reduce the frequency and intensity of chest discomfort or breathlessness. This is a prophylactic (preventive) medical strategy.

Other medications used to treat angina include nitrates, calcium channel blockers, and beta-adrenergic blockers. Nitrates (which include nitroglycerin and medications with a more prolonged effect) decrease the heart's demand for oxygen by reducing heart muscle stretch, and they increase blood supply to the heart muscle by relaxing the coronary arteries.

Calcium channel blockers interrupt the normal calcium flow through cell membranes in heart muscle and blood vessels. This produces dilation of the coronary and other arteries, and increases blood flow to the heart. It also diminishes the heart's demand for oxygen by decreasing blood pressure, heart rate, and the vigor of heart muscle contraction.

Not every calcium channel blocker produces these effects to the same extent. Calcium channel blockers vary according to whether they are short- or long-acting. Doctors now advise against certain classes of short-acting calcium-channel blockers for heart disease patients, unless they're used in conjunction with a beta-blocker. Beta-adrenergic blockers decrease the heart rate and blood pressure, and the heart's work load thus decreases.

You may need more than one medication to get the best effect. If symptoms progress, your doctor may recommend increasing the dosage of some or all of the medications. If symptoms are not adequately controlled by medications, further treatment may be required. Daily low-dose aspirin and reducing LDL cholesterol levels to less than 100 mg/dL are very important measures in all patients with coronary disease, even those with minimal symptoms.

The medical treatment for unstable angina—angina that's becoming more frequent, more easily provoked, or more intense or prolonged—is more urgent than that for stable angina. Unstable angina usually results from blood clot formation in a coronary artery that's partially blocked by atherosclerosis.

Unstable angina is usually triggered when a cholesterol-rich plaque ruptures to expose its contents to the bloodstream. Platelets, which are microscopic clotting disks present in blood, stick to the ruptured plaque and start the clotting process. Drugs that make platelets less "sticky," such as aspirin, can help in this situation.

A newer class of platelet blockers sometimes called "super-aspirins" are currently under investigation, and it appears they are particularly effective in individuals with unstable angina who are undergoing angioplasty. These drugs are sold under the generic names of eptifibatide, tirofiban, and abciximab.

People with unstable angina should be in the hospital so their condition can be evaluated and treated as soon as possible to try to prevent heart attack. Many patients with unstable angina require coronary angiography to determine whether they're good candidates for coronary angioplasty or coronary artery bypass operation.

Frequently, medical treatment (including nitrates, calcium channel blockers, and beta-adrenergic blockers) must stabilize the situation before angiography is done. Exercise testing (such as a treadmill electrocardiography test) isn't usually recommended in people with unstable angina, because it poses an additional unnecessary risk.

Even when doctors anticipate angioplasty or a bypass operation, they generally prescribe medications to people with unstable angina to reduce their immediate risk and stabilize their condition. Any medications directed at stable angina also may be used to treat unstable angina.

In addition, people with unstable angina usually receive oxygen in the hospital. Breathing oxygen allows the blood to release more oxygen to the heart tissues even when the amount of blood reaching the heart muscle has dropped.

In those with unstable angina, a thrombotic occlusion (total blockage due to blood clot) may develop in the coronary arteries at the site of an atherosclerotic blockage, which could lead to a heart attack.

## What about Viagra and heart disease?

Male erectile dysfunction is a common problem in the United States. Defined as "the inability to attain and/or maintain penile erection sufficient for satisfactory sexual performance," it affects between 10 million and 30 million men.

Male erectile dysfunction is particularly common in men after a heart attack or diagnosis of coronary artery disease. In many men, this is because they're afraid that sexual exertion will precipitate another myocardial infarction, although 10 to 15 percent comes from other causes. The introduction of a new drug, sildenafil citrate (Viagra), has been a major advancement in treating erectile dysfunction.

In general, Viagra's cardiovascular side effects in normal, healthy individuals are minor and come from the drug's dilating effect on the blood vessels. This can cause headache, flushing, and small blood pressure decreases. Still, it's important to emphasize that serious cardiovascular events, including a marked drop in blood pressure and even death, can occur in certain men.

You're at particular risk if you're taking nitroglycerin (Viagra should never be prescribed to patients receiving any form of nitrate therapy). In addition, if you've recently had an acute cardiac event (unstable angina or myocardial infarction), you should probably avoid Viagra. The drug is also potentially hazardous in patients with congestive heart failure and borderline low blood pressure, including patients on multiple antihypotensive drug treatment.

See page A10 and A11.

**Methods to restore blood flow**

(See page A10 and A11.)

1. Administering medications that dissolve blood clots (thrombolytic agents)
2. Opening the blocked area of the coronary artery with a catheter that has a balloon tip
3. Opening the blocked area of the coronary artery with an atherectomy catheter or laser-tipped catheter
4. Placement of a coronary artery stent
5. Emergency coronary artery bypass graft operation

Doctors reduce the tendency for blood clotting with anticoagulants and aspirin until they can treat the blockage with angioplasty or bypass operation. Administered intravenously, the anticoagulant heparin can be adjusted rapidly to provide just the right amount of "blood-thinning" effect. Aspirin decreases the tendency for platelets in the blood to clump together and cause clotting.

With coronary spasm, an abnormal tendency for the coronary arteries to constrict intermittently causes reduced supplies of oxygenated blood to the heart muscle. This may occur even when atherosclerosis isn't present, although the two conditions may coexist.

When treating coronary spasm, doctors primarily want to ease the arterial smooth-muscle spasm that causes the narrowing. Medications such as nitrates and calcium channel blockers relax the blood vessels.

A heart attack (myocardial infarction) occurs when a complete interruption in blood supply damages a heart muscle region. The usual cause is a blood clot forming inside a coronary artery at an atherosclerotic site. The goals for treating or managing a heart attack are threefold:

1. Reverse the blockage to allow blood flow to move into the heart muscle's jeopardized area. The resumption of blood flow is called reperfusion; it's done to salvage the heart muscle (myocardial salvage).
2. Eliminate symptoms (supportive care).
3. Monitor, prevent, and treat the complications of heart attack (intensive care).

## Medical treatment for heart attack

Heart muscle can survive longer than the brain without blood flow, but the duration is still limited. Unless blood flow returns within 30 minutes to several hours, the heart muscle will be irreversibly damaged. The jeopardized portion of the heart muscle will die, form a scar, and no longer contribute to the heart's overall pumping function.

For successful heart muscle salvage, your blood flow must be restored (reperfusion) before the heart muscle cells have been irreparably destroyed. A quick reperfusion after the onset of heart attack and its symptoms will ensure a better outcome, which is why it's so critical to get to the hospital. Prompt therapy can make the difference between heart muscle death and heart muscle salvage.

### Clot-dissolving medications (thrombolytic therapy)

The most common method for reperfusing heart muscle during a myocardial infarction is by using medications that dissolve blood clots (thrombolytic agents).

In the past, only pain medications and supportive measures were available to treat myocardial infarction. But thrombolytic agents—including streptokinase, urokinase, anistreplase, and tissue plasminogen activator (TPA)—have been a monumental step forward in preventing disability and death from heart attacks. With thrombolytic agents, damage can be prevented or minimized if you get to a hospital soon enough.

Doctors administer thrombolytic agents through an intravenous catheter. They can be given as soon as a heart attack is diagnosed based on symptoms and abnormalities on the electrocardiogram. You must have no condition that could cause a serious bleeding problem, such as recent injury or operation, recent stroke, very high blood pressure, or ulcer disease. Usually, the thrombolytic agent can be given promptly when you arrive in the emergency room.

About 80 percent of heart attack patients who receive a thrombolytic agent within 2 hours of symptom onset have reperfusion. Successful reperfusion reduces the size of the heart attack and helps preserve the heart's overall pumping function.

Benefits diminish for those who receive a thrombolytic agent later than 2 hours after symptoms begin. Much of the damage has already occurred, so there's less improvement even if the coronary artery opens.

An alternative to thrombolytic therapy for myocardial infarction is emergency angioplasty, known as primary angioplasty (see page A11). In clinical trials, primary angioplasty appears to be at least as effective as thrombolysis, particularly in patients who develop shock or very low blood pressure with a heart attack. Primary angioplasty requires skilled personnel and is not available in all hospitals.

## Supportive care

With heart attack, you'll usually require additional treatment, even if thrombolytic treatment succeeds. Other emergency tactics include oxygen, just as in cases of unstable angina. Nitroglycerin can also be given, either under the tongue or by vein, to decrease the heart's oxygen demand and improve blood flow through the coronary arteries.

Heart attacks can be very painful; you may need narcotics such as morphine. Medications such as beta-adrenergic blocking agents also may be helpful for reducing pain and enhancing survival, especially if you have high blood pressure or a fast heart rate.

Beta-adrenergic blockers make the heart beat more slowly and less forcefully, so it requires less oxygen. Inotropic agents and diuretics may be used if there's evidence of congestive heart failure, and occasionally calcium channel blockers are employed to decrease the heart's demand for oxygen. If blood pressure drops

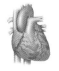

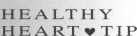
HEALTHY
HEART ♥ TIP

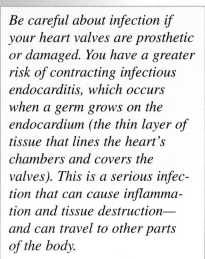

*Be careful about infection if your heart valves are prosthetic or damaged. You have a greater risk of contracting infectious endocarditis, which occurs when a germ grows on the endocardium (the thin layer of tissue that lines the heart's chambers and covers the valves). This is a serious infection that can cause inflammation and tissue destruction— and can travel to other parts of the body.*

*Ask your doctor about taking an appropriate antibiotic before and after undergoing certain dental procedures or other surgery where you may come into contact with germs. Treatment of infectious endocarditis may also employ antibiotics for extended periods to destroy all the germs and prevent further heart valve damage.*

too low, or if shock develops, medications that elevate blood pressure (vasopressors) and inotropic medications may be needed.

Because people with heart attacks possess a higher risk for blood clots inside their hearts near the dead heart muscle, they receive heparin, an anti-coagulant, to inhibit this tendency. Blood clots can re-form in the coronary artery at the sites where thrombolysis has already dissolved the original blood clot.

Thrombolytic medications dissolve blood clots that have already formed; anticoagulants prevent new blood clots from developing. Even when thrombolysis is unsuccessful or not done, anticoagulation may be advisable to prevent further coronary thrombi (blood clots).

People who've had heart attacks also are at risk for blood clots developing inside the left ventricle where the heart damage occurred. If blood clot fragments break off from this site, they may travel to other parts of the arterial circulation and cause complications such as stroke.

Like others undergoing prolonged bed rest, heart attack patients are at risk for blood clots in their leg veins. For all of these reasons, people who are hospitalized with heart attack receive anticoagulants.

## Intensive care: the cardiac care unit

Although all of the medications (thrombolytic agents, nitroglycerin, narcotics, oxygen, and anticoagulants) can be started in the hospital emergency room, an integral part of managing people with heart attacks is hospitalization in the cardiac care unit (CCU).

There are more than 1,200 coronary intensive care units in hospitals throughout the country. Since the development of CCUs in the past 30 years, heart attack survival rates have improved, even before the days of thrombolytic agents. Some experts credit CCUs with reducing in-hospital heart attack deaths by about 30 percent.

In the CCU, you're evaluated to determine whether you need further treatment after receiving the clot-dissolving thrombolytic agent in the emergency room. Even though thrombolytic agents may successfully dissolve the blood clot, they don't remove the underlying partial blockage by atherosclerotic plaque. Thus, you may have continuing risk of angina or even the recurrence of a blood clot and another heart attack.

You may undergo coronary angiography, which will help the doctor determine whether you need balloon dilation or a bypass operation. In most cases, coronary angiography and further treatment can be deferred for a few days or weeks until your condition has stabilized.

CCUs allow medical personnel to monitor you carefully and to respond quickly to complications that might occur after a heart attack. These complications include congestive heart failure, rhythm abnormalities, development of a ventricular septal defect, mitral valve regurgitation, ventricular aneurysm, rupture of the ventricular wall, clot formation, recurrence of angina or extension of the heart attack, pericarditis, and shock.

The CCU can manage these problems because it's staffed with a highly trained medical team whose members constantly monitor the electrocardiogram, the hemodynamics (pressures in the heart, circulation, and blood flow), and the oxygen level in the bloodstream. Specialized nursing personnel and medical technicians work around the clock. Emergency resuscitation equipment such as defibrillators and facilities for inserting emergency catheters and pacemakers are available.

Other equipment in the CCU helps the staff watch closely for early signs and symptoms of complications and administer prompt treatment when necessary. Continuous electrocardiographic monitoring allows around-the-clock heart rhythm observation. The electrocardiogram can usually be observed in your room and at a central panel of constantly watched monitors. The monitors often come equipped with automatic computers that can recognize problems and sound an alarm if ominous changes occur.

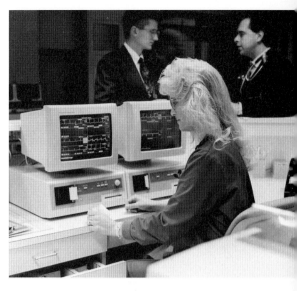

*In an intensive care unit, centralized electrocardiograms monitor all patients. Medical personnel use automatic computerized detection and human observation so they quickly know about any abnormality that needs immediate treatment.*

If you've had a heart attack, you're prone to heart rhythm abnormalities, including ventricular fibrillation. During the very early phases of a heart attack, doctors often give rhythm-controlling medications by vein to reduce the likelihood of a rapid dangerous heart rhythm or ventricular fibrillation. If uncertain rhythms develop, nursing personnel and doctors use medications and defibrillators as necessary.

Many, but not all, people who have had heart attacks—as well as others requiring hospitalization in CCUs (such as those with very severe congestive heart failure)—have a special monitoring catheter inserted through a vein and threaded into the heart and pulmonary artery. This is called a pulmonary artery catheter, or Swan-Ganz catheter (named after the inventors) (see page 267).

Used to determine the amount of blood the heart pumps per minute (cardiac output), this catheter measures pressures inside the heart and pulmonary artery. This gives medical personnel an early and sensitive way to determine the heart's functioning efficiency. The catheter constantly tells doctors whether there's any change in the heart's pumping function so they can start appropriate treatment.

The catheter is usually inserted through a needle puncture into a jugular (neck) vein, subclavian vein (under either collarbone), or an arm vein. A small balloon at the catheter's tip can be inflated to help it move through the vein circulation into the heart and out into the pulmonary artery.

After a heart attack, a slow heart rhythm may evolve or your electrocardiogram may suggest you're at risk for developing one. This potentially dangerous situation can be corrected by inserting a temporary pacemaker wire through the same spot used for the monitoring catheter. The electrode tip touches the right ventricle's inner wall, and the end of the electrode wire outside the body attaches to a small temporary pacemaker unit. This delivers stimulation to the heart muscle to make it beat at an acceptable rate (see page A14).

Slow heart rates often improve as the heart muscle begins to heal, and the temporary pacemaker can be eliminated. Sometimes the slow heart rate is permanent, or the risk of developing a slow heart rate in the future is high enough that you need a permanent pacemaker.

Besides emergency treatment, the CCU plays an important role in starting the heart attack rehabilitation process. In the hospital, you gradually increase your physical activity and start regaining your strength. Most CCUs also have a "step-down" area where close monitoring can be continued at a somewhat less intense level once you've recovered from your heart attack's immediate effects.

## Surgical and catheter treatment

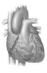

### HEALTHY HEART ♥ TIP

*Consider the valves in the heart as the body's workhorses. These pumps keep the blood flowing in one direction through the heart, and when they don't close properly, blood can ebb backward. This is called valve regurgitation, and it causes the heart to enlarge as it tries to accommodate this faulty flow.*

*Regurgitation can range from mild to severe. Some people notice no symptoms at all for years, but if the condition worsens they'll experience fatigue (especially during periods of increased activity), shortness of breath, edema (retention of fluid) in certain parts of the body such as the ankles, heart arrhythmias (abnormal heart beats) or angina pectoris (chest pain). See your doctor for appropriate treatment.*

Most cases of angina or heart attack result from one or more atherosclerotic blockages of the coronary arteries. It stands to reason that removing or reducing the blockage would solve the problem. If medications and lifestyle changes (such as diet, exercise, and smoking) don't heal you, your doctor may recommend coronary angioplasty or a coronary artery bypass operation to remove or bypass the blockage in your coronary artery (see page A11).

Doctors generally reserve angioplasty or bypass operation for people who don't get enough relief from medications alone or who've had an exercise (or other type of stress) test or coronary angiography that shows they're at higher risk for future heart attack or death. You'll have an elevated risk if you have decreased pumping function of the heart and blockages in all three coronary arteries or the left main coronary artery. (The left main coronary artery supplies most of the left ventricle, the main pumping chamber.)

### Coronary angioplasty

In coronary angioplasty, doctors insert a specially constructed catheter with a small balloon on the tip into an artery in the groin or arm. Then it's threaded into the coronary arteries and used to open the blockage. The complete name for this procedure is percutaneous (through the skin) transluminal (inside an artery) coronary angioplasty (blood vessel reshaping), or PTCA.

Not every coronary artery blockage accommodates treatment with a balloon catheter. Some blockages may be too long or in places that are difficult to reach with a catheter. In these cases, bypass operation may be advised. However, as doctors have gained experience with balloon catheterization, it has been used to treat increasingly complicated and severe disease.

## The PTCA procedure

Before the PTCA, you will have a chest X-ray, electrocardiogram, and blood tests. A member of the medical team who'll perform the PTCA will make sure you understand the rationale, procedural aspects and associated risks.

Don't eat or drink anything after midnight the night before your PTCA (although you may take medications ordered by your doctor with a small amount of water). You might also receive medications to decrease blood clotting or to relax the muscles in your coronary arteries. You won't need a general anesthetic for PTCA, but you will be given some form of sedation or medication.

On the day of the procedure, medical personnel insert an intravenous (IV) catheter and give you a sedative. They place small electrode pads on your chest to monitor your heart rate and rhythm, and wash your groin with an antiseptic solution. A sterile drape is placed over your body.

After administering a local anesthetic, doctors insert a short tube called a sheath into your leg artery. A guide catheter, which is a hollow, flexible tube, is placed into the sheath and moved to the narrowed coronary artery while doctors watch it on a televised X-ray image. You may feel pressure, but you shouldn't feel sharp pain in the groin area during the procedure.

The doctor injects a small amount of contrast agent (which appears on the X-ray image like a dye) through the catheter to see the exact location of the blockage. A smaller catheter with a tiny deflated balloon at the tip is inserted through the guide catheter until the balloon crosses the blocked area of the artery. The balloon inflates for 30 to 120 seconds and then deflates. This stretches the artery wall and increases the artery's diameter.

It's common to experience chest pain while the balloon is inflated, because it blocks the blood flow to an area of your heart for a short time. Tell the staff if this occurs. The pain usually disappears after they deflate the balloon. The doctor usually inflates and deflates the balloon several times.

The balloon catheter is removed, and more pictures (angiograms) are taken to see how blood flow through the artery has improved. The guide catheter is then extracted. The average procedure takes about 30 to 90 minutes. In many cases, a stent (wire-mesh tube) may be inserted into the coronary artery at the site of the dilated blockage.

During the recovery period, your electrocardiogram continues to be monitored for 12 to 24 hours. A nurse checks your vital signs, foot pulses, and PTCA site frequently. Tell your nurse about any discomfort, pain, or anything that bothers you after the PTCA.

After the procedure, the sheath usually stays in your leg artery for 4 to 24 hours. A salt (saline) solution with blood thinner (heparin) mixed in flows through the sheath to keep blood from clotting inside the sheath. You must not bend your leg at the hip or the knee until 6 hours after the sheath has been removed, so you'll be on complete bed rest for that time.

After the sheath is removed, pressure may be applied to the groin area for up to 6 hours to prevent bleeding and promote healing at the puncture site. Once the pressure's gone, you may sit up and walk around your room with your nurse's help.

Your doctor may prescribe medications such as nitroglycerin to relax the coronary arteries, calcium antagonists to protect against coronary artery spasm, or a combination of aspirin and dipyridamole to help prevent blood clots in the previously blocked coronary artery.

You will probably be released from the hospital 1 or 2 days after the PTCA. Many people return to work the next week. You'll be given follow-up instructions when you're released, and you may be asked to return 6 months after the PTCA for a follow-up evaluation, which may include angiography or an exercise test.

## Results of PTCA

More than 90 percent of PTCA procedures are initially successful. Successful PTCA reduces the blockage, improves symptoms, and does not lead to complications such as heart attack or emergency coronary bypass operation.

## Risks of PTCA

As with all procedures that involve inserting catheters into the coronary system, there are risks with PTCA. Catheter insertion can injure or puncture the artery, making operation necessary to correct the complications. Also, after the inside surface of the artery has been touched by the balloon, the risk of blood clots forming on the site increases slightly.

Occasionally the blockage is made worse, and coronary artery bypass grafting must correct the problem. The risk of death from PTCA is less than 1 percent; the risk of precipitating a heart attack or needing emergency bypass surgery is less than 3 percent.

Although PTCA reduces the amount of blockage in 95 percent of people, the procedure does have a disadvantage: About one third or more of the blockages return to their original severity in less than a year. The blockage causes a recurrence of angina, but only rarely (less than 5 percent of the time) does it cause a heart attack.

The chances of reblockage may be reduced by placement of a coronary artery stent. A second PTCA often resolves the problem, but coronary artery bypass grafting may be necessary. The use of stents, which are small, metal springs inserted into the coronary artery, have been successful in reducing the renarrowing rate to about 15 percent, or about half of that experienced with PTCA alone.

Despite these possibilities, the overall risks with PCTA are very low, especially considering the benefits that can be achieved.

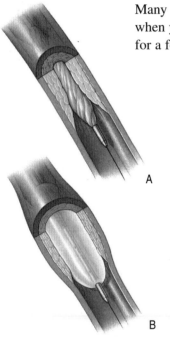

**Coronary angioplasty.** *Your cardiologist inserts a long, hollow tube (catheter) into a large artery in your groin (see page A11) or arm. The tube is guided to the narrowed coronary artery. Then a thinner, balloon-tipped tube is inserted into the first catheter and directed through the narrowing (**A**). The balloon is inflated (**B**), compressing deposits and widening the artery. Doctors also call this procedure balloon angioplasty, or percutaneous transluminal coronary angioplasty (PTCA).*

## Newer catheter techniques

Research on catheter methods for opening coronary arteries often deals with reducing blockage recurrence. Researchers have investigated medications that may decrease further atherosclerosis or blood clots at the dilation site.

Other dilating catheters have been studied, too, including a cutting or shaving type (atherectomy catheter), which actually shaves off and removes plaque from the inside of the artery, and laser-tipped catheters that "vaporize" blockages with a tiny laser beam.

If a coronary blockage is very calcified (hard, like a bone), doctors may use the atherectomy catheter. This simulates a miniature dentist's drill—the catheter consists of a metal cylinder about 1 inch from the tip containing a rotating disk that spins at 2,500 revolutions per minute.

The rotating blade nibbles away or shaves off the hard plaque while leaving the normal, softer material in place. The physician removes the catheter 4 to 6 times to discard the plaque fragments that are stored in the catheter's tip. Some microscopic abraded material passes through the heart muscle and is cleared from the circulation.

Using a catheter with a laser at the tip, doctors can focus rapidly pulsating beams of light that vaporize the tissue into gases that are dissolved in the bloodstream and eliminated in the body's natural waste system. Lasers may be useful in places where balloons are less desirable, such as in long, narrow spaces.

Coronary artery stents are small tube-shaped, wire-mesh scaffolds that can be inserted into a coronary artery at the site where a PTCA procedure has dilated a blockage. The small wire tubes (about the size of a ball-point pen spring) are simple devices that effectively prop open vessels that otherwise would close (see page A11).

Using stents in selected patients after PTCA has reduced the number of complications such as myocardial infarction or emergency coronary artery bypass grafting. Stents have also diminished the chances of blockage recurring (restenosis). Approximately 90 percent of those who undergo PTCA are candidates for placement of a stent, which is used frequently in place of angioplasty alone and, in many patients, coronary bypass surgery. Following stent placement, doctors often prescribe aspirin and other medications that reduce the chance of clotting.

Outside the coronary artery system, doctors use stents increasingly for conditions such as blockages in the arteries supplying the kidneys and the lower legs, and, more recently, in patients with carotid artery disease.

Although stents have many advantages, they aren't foolproof. Over time, repeat blockages within the stent occur 15 to 20 percent of the time, although that's only half the rate of repeat blockages with balloon angioplasty alone.

Nonetheless, this is a statistic that researchers are trying to reduce with new stent developments. Among the variations currently being studied are chemically coated stents to deliver drugs (e.g., anticlotting drugs) directly to the vessel at the obstruction site. One interesting research area involves radioactive stents, which may be helpful in controlling excess tissue regrowth into the stented coronary vessel.

Recovery after stent placement in the coronary arteries in general is short, and you'll be up and walking within a day of the procedure. There's a risk of developing blood clots in the stent; medications to prevent this usually include a combination of aspirin and either clopidogrel or ticlopidine, which is taken for 2 to 4 weeks following stent placement.

One new treatment called photoangioplasty uses a light-activated drug to shrink plaque buildup in arteries. A light is "piped" directly to obstructed leg arteries by a catheter with an optical fiber. It remains to be seen whether this will become more widely used in the future.

If you've had PTCA, you still need to reduce your risk for recurrence by quitting smoking, lowering cholesterol levels, maintaining a healthy weight, controlling diabetes and high blood pressure, and getting regular exercise. These measure are essential parts of your treatment programs.

## Coronary artery bypass grafting

Another way to manage a coronary blockage is to create a detour for the blood to go around it (see page A11). This is the principle of coronary artery bypass grafting (CABG). This type of operation was first done in 1969; doctors now perform about 300,000 bypass operations every year in the United States.

Bypass operation is usually appropriate in people who have a blocked left main coronary artery, those with disease in many vessels and poor function of the left ventricle (the main pump of the heart), and individuals with debilitating angina. For these people, a bypass operation can enhance and prolong life.

In a bypass operation, the surgeon reroutes blood flow around your coronary blockage site in one of several ways:

**1.** A saphenous vein is taken from your leg and used as a bypass tube or conduit. The saphenous vein isn't crucial for blood flow in the leg (it's the vein often involved with varicose veins and is "stripped" if necessary).

In this procedure, the surgeon connects one end of the vein to the aorta near where the coronary arteries normally originate, and the other end to the coronary artery downstream from the blockage. This allows blood to flow around the blockage from the aorta to the coronary artery.

**2.** A second technique for bypass operation involves one or both of two arteries that normally arise from branches of the aorta. These arteries are called the internal mammary arteries (also the internal thoracic arteries or ITA).

With this technique, the surgeon doesn't entirely remove the artery as in the previous procedure. Rather, the surgeon disconnects the downstream end of the artery from the inner part of the chest wall and reconnects that end of the artery to the coronary artery downstream from the blockage.

This procedure allows blood to flow through the aorta as it normally would, but it ends up in the coronary artery instead of along the inner surface of the chest wall. There are enough other arteries in the chest wall to supply an adequate amount of blood when the internal mammary artery is diverted.

Multiple saphenous vein segments from both legs can be used to bypass different blockages. Furthermore, one bypass graft can be adapted to bypass more than one blocked artery (sequential grafts).

Because the arterial grafts stay open more readily than vein grafts, other arteries from the body also may be used for heart bypass. Although it's not employed as frequently as the ITA, the forearm artery has been adapted quite well.

The hand's blood supply comes from two arteries that branch at the elbow from a large single artery. If both of these are open in the nondominant hand, the radial artery, or the one on the forearm's thumb side, can be removed and used for a heart bypass. Normally performed in patients who have a longer life expectancy, this bypass often lasts longer than the saphenous veins. It's also used when the leg veins have been previously removed for disease or other bypasses, or they're not otherwise satisfactory for use on the heart.

Another, smaller artery adapted for bypass supplies the stomach. The gastroepiploic artery requires opening the abdominal cavity, then bringing the artery through the diaphragm, the muscle that separates the lungs from the abdomen. This lengthens the operation, and the late results aren't sufficient to safely recommend this routinely. Again, this artery or other smaller arteries are more often used when the standard grafts aren't available or have been used before.

A more recent procedure—and one that has caught the attention of the medical profession and the public—is the minimally invasive heart bypass, or MIDCAB. This involves approaches that use a smaller incision, either vertical or horizontal, near the left breast. Part of the rib overlying the heart may be removed and the heart exposed through this small incision.

This procedure has undergone a rapid rise in popularity because it can be less painful and less expensive, and means a shorter hospital stay. Proponents believe it can be done as well as the standard operation and with the same results. There's no statistical information as yet on the success rates of these grafts, but early results indicate they're not as good as the standard operation.

In addition, patients who have this operation sometimes need subsequent procedures. Some feel that the pain with this procedure is, in fact, not less than with the standard operation and, if additional procedures are needed, it's not less expensive, either.

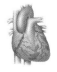

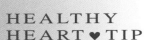

## HEALTHY HEART ♥ TIP

*People who experience chest pain at night may have variant angina pectoris, also called Prinzmetal's angina. This condition differs from typical angina in that it occurs almost exclusively at rest—usually between midnight and 8 a.m.—not after physical exertion or emotional stress.*

*About two-thirds of people with variant angina have severe coronary atherosclerosis in at least one major blood vessel. Many go through an acute, active phase, with cardiac events occuring frequently for six months or more. During this time, nonfatal myocardial infarction occurs in up to 20 percent of patients; death occurs in up to 10 percent.*

*Most people who survive this initial three- to six-month period stabilize, and symptoms and cardiac events tend to diminish. Long-term survival is excellent, ranging from 89 to 97 percent at five years.*

Some have recently advocated surgery through the standard median sternotomy incision, but without bypass. This reduces the expense and possible risks of the heart-lung bypass machine, but needs to be weighed against the risks of more frequent closure of grafts, and of operating on the beating heart.

In some patients, particularly older people with extensive atherosclerotic plaque in the aorta, the possibility of performing the operation without cardiopulmonary bypass is very promising. This technique has generated great interest. As in the case with the MIDCAB, doctors want to wait and see whether the late results justify the early enthusiasm. Nonetheless, it's likely that an increasing proportion of coronary artery bypass surgery will be done without the heart-lung bypass machine.

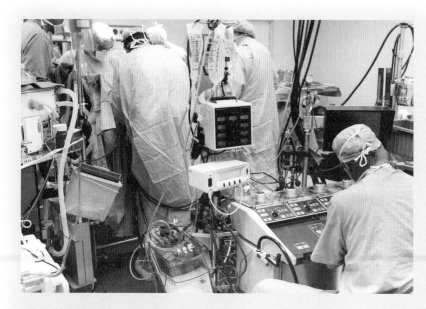

*A heart-lung machine (**foreground**) takes the blood returning to the patient's heart from all parts of the body, provides it with fresh oxygen, and pumps it into the aorta, which distributes it throughout the body. The heart and lungs are bypassed by this procedure, allowing the surgeon to operate on a motionless heart without blood blocking his or her vision.*

## The heart-lung bypass machine

During a coronary artery bypass grafting (open heart) operation, a heart-lung bypass machine performs the functions of the heart and lungs and keeps you alive while the operation occurs.

The machine takes blood that's returning from the body through your veins to the right atrium and diverts it into an apparatus that oxygenates the blood as your lungs would. After oxygenating the blood, the machine pumps it into your aorta downstream from the heart. From there it can flow to all of your organs (except the heart and lungs). No blood flows through the heart, so it can be stopped.

In coronary artery bypass grafting, this heart pause allows the surgeon to make the delicate maneuvers that are necessary without having to deal with a "moving target." In operations for congenital heart disease and valve disease, it allows doctors to open the heart and drain the blood so they can see what they're doing.

During the operation, the heart doesn't receive a continuous blood supply through the coronary arteries, although surgeons may intermittently allow blood to flow through them. To prevent the heart from suffering damage, it's cooled down while chemicals slow its metabolism and reduce its need for oxygen.

When the operation is completed, surgeons restart the heart with an electrical shock.

## The coronary artery bypass procedure

The events preceding and following coronary artery bypass grafting correspond to those with most cardiac surgical procedures. For the operation itself, doctors make an incision along the midline of your chest, through your breastbone.

For part of the operation, the functions of your heart and lungs will be assumed by a heart-lung bypass machine. Incisions are also made along the inside of your leg if surgeons intend to use a saphenous vein for a bypass graft. More than one bypass is usually needed, so you may have more than one incision in the legs.

Coronary artery bypass grafting usually takes 3 to 6 hours, depending on the complexity of your operation. The more bypasses that must be attached, the longer it will take. As many as 8 or 9 segments of arteries may be bypassed, but the average number is 4 or 5.

## Results of coronary artery bypass grafting

Coronary artery bypass grafting aims to restore adequate blood flow through the coronary arteries so you can enjoy a more productive and active life.

Coronary artery bypass grafting substantially improves symptoms in 90 percent of those who have it done, and it prolongs life in people with either left main coronary artery disease or blockages in 2 or 3 of the major coronary artery trunks, especially if the pumping function of the heart is also reduced.

In general, about 40 percent of those who have bypass operations show signs of a new blockage within 10 years after operation. Angina can recur in people with coronary artery bypass grafts for several reasons: Blockages can develop in the bypass grafts, new blockages can form in coronary arteries not originally bypassed, and there may be blockages in coronary artery branches that are too small to bypass.

Internal mammary arteries seem to stay open longer than saphenous vein grafts, so doctors increasingly tend to prefer them.

## Risks of coronary artery bypass grafting

If you're undergoing a scheduled operation for angina, you have about a 2 percent risk of dying from the operation, or about 8 percent if the procedure is done in an emergency situation, such as a heart attack, when your condition is unstable. Other complications may occur as a result of heart surgery and should be discussed with your surgeon ahead of time.

Risks are higher in older patients and in patients who experience heart failure due to large amounts of scar tissue as a result of previous damage to the heart.

## Preoperative autologous blood collection

If you're anticipating an operation, you can use your own blood for transfusions. Autologous blood is your own blood that's been collected and made available for you during operation. It's the safest blood product available for transfusion, because it eliminates the risk of transfusion-related diseases and reduces the risk of blood transfusion reactions.

When planning a surgical procedure, your doctor will discuss your blood needs with you, basing eligibility for preoperative autologous blood collection on your medical condition.

Safe and simple, the blood donation procedure requires about 1 hour of your time. You may donate 1 unit of autologous blood per week. You should donate the last unit of blood at least 72 hours before your scheduled surgical date.

Blood can be stored as a liquid for 5 weeks. Frozen storage techniques may extend the shelf life significantly for some blood components such as red blood cells and plasma.

# 16 What to expect before, during, and after a heart operation

Anyone anticipating a heart operation looks forward to relieving the problem. But fears and doubts naturally accompany any major surgery. For most people, knowing more about what to expect can ease some of the uncertain feelings. Don't hesitate to ask your doctor, surgeon, and others involved in your care any questions you may have.

Almost all types of "open-heart operation" involve some of the same steps before, during, and after the procedure. Procedures such as coronary artery bypass grafting, a valve replacement operation, repair of a congenital defect, and some operations for cardiomyopathy and pericarditis have many aspects in common. Some operations, such as heart transplantation, entail procedures that are unique to them.

## Timing of the operation

Most operations can be scheduled days or weeks in advance, depending on the medical urgency and on the surgeon's and your schedule. If the severity of the symptoms warrants emergency operation, it should done right away. If you've planned the operation electively for the future, discuss the possibility of donating your own blood ahead of time to use in case you require transfusion.

## The week or two before heart operation

Once you've scheduled your heart operation, your doctor will discuss with you some of the following standard instructions to prepare for the operation:

- You may be advised to not take aspirin or similar medications for at least 10 days before the procedure. These medications reduce the function of platelets, so excessive bleeding during or after operation is more likely to occur. Acetaminophen (such as Tylenol, Datril, Anacin 3, or Panadol) does not promote bleeding, so you can take it if needed.

- If you need an anticoagulant, you may be admitted to the hospital several days before your scheduled operation. During this time, your medication can be changed to a shorter-acting intravenous anticoagulant, which can be discontinued temporarily for the operation.

- Continue taking all other medications until reporting to the hospital, unless your doctor tells you otherwise.

- Report any signs of infection, such as fever, chills, and respiratory symptoms (including coughing or a runny nose), that occur within a week before operation.

## Preparations at the hospital

You'll probably be admitted to the hospital the afternoon or evening before the next day's operation. Sometimes, patients are asked to report to the hospital in the early morning the day of the operation.

To prepare for the operation, you'll have blood tests, a chest X-ray, and electrocardiography unless these were done recently.

Each hospital has its own procedure for giving you details about any final instructions or preparations. Usually, surgical team representatives (surgeon, cardiologist, anesthesiologist) visit with you and your family the evening before or the morning of the operation to discuss your procedure's scheduled time, perform a brief physical examination, and gather a medical history. You may be able to attend a class or watch a video about heart operation and what can be expected afterwards.

Family members should make sure they understand where they should wait during the operation and when they can expect information about the operation's progress. You and your family also will learn about the facilities and special monitoring in the intensive care unit where you'll spend the first few days after operation.

Your doctor will tell you which medications to continue taking up until the operation. Generally, medications for angina are allowed. Do not eat or drink anything after midnight on operation day because anesthesia is safer if it's given on an empty stomach.

Final preparations include shaving or removing most body hair (which can harbor bacteria) from your neck to your ankles and showering with a special cleansing soap.

You may receive medication to help you relax before going to the surgical suite. In a surgical preparation area, an intravenous (IV) catheter may be inserted. A small, flexible catheter slides over the needle and remains in the vein, but the needle is withdrawn. Anesthetics and other medications can be administered through the IV catheter. You are now ready for the operation.

## During the operation

You'll be given a general anesthetic to put you to sleep during the operation. The surgeon makes an incision and opens the chest. Depending on the type of operation, the opening is made lengthwise through the breastbone or crosswise between ribs.

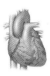

A heart-lung bypass machine (see page 324) performs the functions of your heart and lungs during operation, allowing the surgeon to make necessary repairs while your heart remains motionless.

A breathing tube, called an endotracheal tube, which will help you breathe while anesthetized, helps clear secretions from the lungs and decreases your heart's work load by assisting breathing. Inserted through the nose or mouth, the tube may remain in place after operation for a few hours or days, according to your need for breathing assistance.

Your family will be informed when the major part of the operation has ended, which is when you're taken off the heart-lung bypass machine and your heart resumes functioning on its own. You'll probably remain in the surgical suite for observation for another 1 1/2 to 2 hours before being moved to the intensive care unit (ICU). When you arrive in the ICU, a surgical team member will describe the operation and your condition to your family.

## What to expect in the ICU

While you're in the ICU, the health care team operates multiple monitoring devices which are very useful in determining how efficiently the heart performs. A catheter, inserted through a neck vein and threaded into the right atrium and ventricle and into the pulmonary artery, will measure blood pressure and pressures in the heart's chambers. The catheter also monitors the amount of blood flowing through the heart.

Tubes inserted through the chest wall during the operation drain excess fluid or blood from around the heart into a container on the bedside cart. A catheter removes urine from the bladder to assist the nurse in recording urine output.

A tube may be passed through your nose and throat into your stomach (nasogastric tube) to remove stomach juices and allow the intestines time to begin working again. You'll receive fluids, nutrition, and medications through the intravenous (IV) catheter in an arm vein. Throughout your stay in the ICU, all fluid intake and output will be closely monitored.

Your heart rhythm will be watched continuously with electrocardiography. Some people experience minor changes in heart rhythm after an operation. Many factors may contribute to these rhythm changes, including handling of the heart during operation, catheters used to monitor pressures within the heart, changes in potassium and sodium levels, and stress (the body's normal response to fear and anxiety). Some changes in heart rhythm may require temporary treatment with medications.

The endotracheal tube (or breathing tube) remains in place until you can breathe deeply and cough to clear lung secretions. Although the tube doesn't hurt, it can be uncomfortable. With the tube in place, you can't speak because it passes through the voice box, but nurses will help you communicate. The endotracheal tube is removed when blood tests show that you have enough oxygen in your blood and when you can cough up secretions. After the tube is withdrawn, you'll wear an oxygen mask and may have a raspy voice or sore throat for a few days.

To assist with recovery, you must breathe deeply and cough. Some types of movement will cause discomfort, but you'll receive medication to ease any pain.

A stay in the ICU won't be restful. Because of all the activity associated with monitoring your condition around the clock, you (and your family) may be distracted by equipment sounds and frequent visits from members of your health care team. Despite the commotion, the activity will enable your rapid recovery so you can safely leave intensive care.

How long you stay in the ICU varies, depending on the complexity of the surgical procedure. When doctors decide you no longer require the ICU's special facilities, you will be moved to a step-down area where close monitoring continues, but at a somewhat less intense level.

## What happens in the step-down area

Your heart rhythm will continue to be monitored with electrocardiography. Monitoring allows the doctor to evaluate whether any rhythm change requires treatment. Blood test results also help doctors manage your care.

Generally, you will wear an oxygen mask for the first day in the step-down area, and then as needed. The moisture from the oxygen mask helps loosen and clear secretions from your lungs.

Coughing is crucial to keep the airways clear and has several beneficial effects. It dislodges secretions that can block airways and prevent oxygen from reaching the air sacs, where it passes into the blood. If secretions block airways, pneumonia can develop more easily. Coughing also requires taking a deeper breath first, and this promotes re-expanding lung zones that were compressed during the operation.

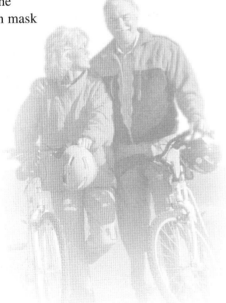

Nurses will help you turn in bed, cough, and breathe deeply. They also may continue chest physiotherapy—gentle thumping on the chest in different positions—to assist in clearing secretions.

You will be encouraged to increase activity levels gradually, even while monitoring continues. As your strength improves, extend the time you spend out of bed and walking. Short rest periods help as you get more active. Support stockings aid blood circulation in your legs.

Your fluid intake and output will be closely watched. Tell your nurse about any fluid you drink between meals. Urine output will be measured throughout your hospital stay to calculate the fluid balance in your body. Being neither too "wet" nor too "dry" is important for your recovery. You will be weighed each day as another indicator of the balance between your fluid intake and output. It's common to weigh more the first few days after operation because of the fluids given during the operation, but you will gradually lose the weight.

Your appetite may be poor for a few days. However, you need to consume enough liquid and food for nourishment and to promote healing.

You'll naturally feel emotional "ups and downs" during recovery. You will probably have both good and bad days after the operation. A degree of confusion is common during the first 2 or 3 days after surgery, and sometimes longer. This may reflect medication as well as the disruptive affect of sleep deprivation, and the multiple stimuli of the ICU. The entire health care team—cardiologists, surgeons, nurses, dietitians, and therapists—can offer support.

There's no standard length of stay in the cardiac surgical step-down area. Your surgeon determines when you no longer need special monitoring. Even after monitoring stops, you may need to recover further in the step-down area or general hospital unit.

# Restoring rhythm control

The heart's rhythm can malfunction in various ways. Depending on the nature of the problem, managing it may require medications, pacemakers, shocking the chest wall (defibrillation or cardioversion), internal cardioverter-defibrillator placement, operation, or catheter techniques to eliminate abnormal rhythms. This chapter discusses the different categories of treatment for abnormal heart rhythm.

## Medications

Drugs that treat rhythm disorders are called antiarrhythmics. Doctors use virtually all antiarrhythmic drugs to treat fast or irregular rhythms, except for atropine and isoproterenol, which they give intravenously in emergency situations to speed up slow heart rates.

Antiarrhythmic drugs act in different ways. Certain antiarrhythmic medications may be useful for one type of rhythm disorder, whereas others are appropriate for another. Conversely, two people with the same rhythm disorder may respond differently to the same medication. Choosing the correct medication requires an accurate diagnosis of the rhythm disorder and an understanding of its mechanism.

Most antiarrhythmic medications work by changing the heart's electrical behavior. Modifying electrical conduction alters the setting in which rhythm disorders can start or continue, thus minimizing their occurrence or severity.

Several principles of antiarrhythmic drug treatment are very important for both patients and doctors to understand.

All antiarrhythmic medications can cause side effects. Indeed, one of the most worrisome side effects of antiarrhythmic medications is their tendency to provoke rhythm disorders. Although an antiarrhythmic medication may benefit 9 out of 10 people, it may make 1 out of 10 worse.

Cardiologists have become aware more recently that medications given to help people may actually hurt them or increase their chances of dying. This was revealed in a study of antiarrhythmic medications in heart attack victims with rhythm disorders; people receiving certain antiarrhythmic medications had a higher death rate than those who were given inactive pills (placebos).

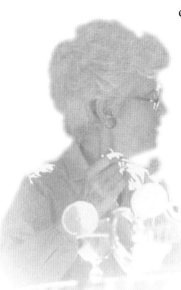

A medication must be thoroughly justified and its benefit documented before doctors prescribe it. There must be clear-cut reasons for you to use an antiarrhythmic medication, and you must be carefully observed for your response once you begin.

Not all rhythm disorders require treatment. Some rhythm disorders that cause symptoms such as palpitations pose less risk than the medication that might be used to treat them. Your doctor may encourage you to not worry about certain rhythm disorders such as premature ventricular contractions (a "skipped beat" an "extra beat" or a "hard beat"). Also, avoid factors that affect your heart rhythm and rate, such as tobacco, alcohol and caffeine.

A significant part of rhythm management is determining how successfully the medication does what it's supposed to do. Depending on the circumstances, effectiveness can be measured by (1) how the medication affects your symptoms, (2) how it alters your heart rhythm as observed on the electrocardiogram or monitor, or (3) how well the medication prevents your heart from being artificially stimulated into a rhythm disorder during electrophysiology testing. In some cases, this process can be lengthy and tedious, but it should be done.

No antiarrhythmic medication can work unless it's present in the bloodstream at adequate levels, which is why blood testing can be useful. If the rhythm disorder continues and testing shows the drug level is low, increasing the dose may help. The need for maintaining effective levels in the bloodstream means you must take the medication as prescribed. Avoid skipping doses unless instructed to do so.

## Pacemakers

An abnormally slow heart rate requires treatment (1) if it causes symptoms such as fatigue, shortness of breath, or faintness or passing out, or (2) if the heart rhythm poses a significant risk for symptoms developing suddenly in the future. The only effective treatment for a slow heart rate is a pacemaker (see page A14).

Pacemakers were originally designed to be used for one purpose: to maintain an adequate heartbeat when the heart beats too slowly or pauses. Now, more sophisticated devices not only keep the heart beating at an acceptable rate but also mimic a normal heartbeat by speeding or slowing the heart rate according to your needs and activity level.

### What is a pacemaker?

A pacemaker has two main parts: (1) a pulse generator that contains the batteries and electronic circuitry and (2) the wires (also called leads) that carry an electrical impulse from the pulse generator to the myocardium (heart muscle).

The battery, electronics, and computer chip sit in a waterproof, titanium casing about the size of 3 compressed silver dollars. Leads are made of flexible wires coated with a special insulating material such as silicone rubber or polyurethane, much like household electrical cord.

Programming and evaluation are a routine part of follow-up care. Your pacemaker will be evaluated postoperatively with a programmer and in the clinic. A programmer is a piece of computerlike equipment that's connected to a wand and placed over the pacemaker. The electronic circuitry sends and receives signals similarly to a television remote control.

## How does a pacemaker work?

At its simplest, a pacemaker can sense your heartbeat and respond accordingly. If it detects a heart rate that's too slow or if there's no heartbeat, the pacemaker emits tiny electrical impulses (too small to feel) that stimulate the heart to contract. If the pacemaker senses your heart's beating fast enough, the pacemaker will go "on demand" and stand by until you need it. The instant the heart goes too slow or pauses, the pacemaker begins pacing.

The pacemaker is programmed to know what heart rate it should accept as satisfactory or below which it should start pacing. Other functions can also be programmed, such as impulse strength and how sensitive the pacemaker should be in detecting your natural heartbeat. More sophisticated pacemakers offer additional functions, such as increasing the rate in response to exercise.

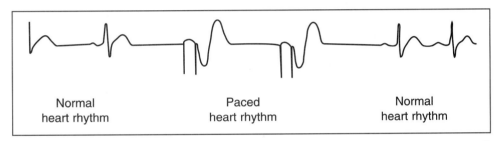

Normal
heart rhythm
    Paced
heart rhythm
    Normal
heart rhythm

*When your heart's natural pacemaker (called the SA, or sinoatrial, node) stops working properly, your pacemaker will begin pacing automatically. This forces your heart to contract at the right rate and speed.*

## Dual-chamber pacemakers

Two-wire, or dual-chamber, pacemakers consist of a pulse generator and wires to both the right atrium and the right ventricle. This type of pacemaker can sense when the heart's own pacemaker (the sinus node) fires.

In people with complete heart block, the message from the sinus node doesn't reach the ventricles because it's blocked at the atrioventricular node. With a dual-chamber pacemaker, however, the pulse generator senses the sinus node's message, which then causes the heart to contract by sending an impulse to the ventricle. This maintains the normal sequence of the heartbeat (the atrium beats first, followed by the ventricle), and the pacemaker can adjust its rate according to how fast the sinus node tells it to fire.

Your sinus node speeds up when you exert yourself. Thus, if you have a dual-chamber pacemaker, it will be "told" by the sinus node to stimulate the ventricles to beat faster, too. Heartbeat acceleration ensures that you can achieve a normal activity level.

Some people with a one-wire system (in which only the ventricle is stimulated) experience an uncomfortable feeling of neck throbbing, chest fullness, or faintness when the pacemaker paces (called pacemaker syndrome). Dual-chamber systems avoid these problems.

### Rate-responsive pacemakers

Some people don't have a normal sinus node that can be tracked by a dual-chamber pacemaker. If you have atrial fibrillation or an irregular or slow sinus node, you will probably benefit from activity-sensor-driven pacing. These features closely mimic the normal heart rates with activities.

Rate-responsive pacemaker models can sense physical activity, such as walking or climbing stairs, and alter the heart rate. When the sensor notes that you're sitting or at rest, it maintains a slower rate. Just as a normal heart speeds up during more activity and slows down during rest, the pacemaker changes its rate according to the activity it senses.

Sensor technology has expanded rapidly. Pacemakers may use one sensor or a combination, depending on the make and model. Each sensor or combination of sensors has the ability to increase the heart rate based on how active the patient is, and adjust according to the needs of the patient.

For example, one type of pacemaker senses the body's motion. When you begin to move rapidly, the pacemaker concludes that you're walking, running, climbing stairs, or doing some other exercise. The pacemaker raises the heart rate proportionately to the amount of activity it discerns.

Another pacemaker senses the depth and rate of breathing. When breathing becomes heavy and fast, this pacemaker concludes that you're exerting yourself and increases the heart rate.

Yet another pacemaker senses the temperature of the blood inside the ventricle. When you exercise, your blood temperature rises slightly because exercising muscle cells give off heat. This pacemaker increases heart rate as temperature increases.

Some patients need a feature that will shift from dual-chamber pacing to single-chamber ventricular pacing if the heart rhythm changes to atrial fibrillation. The pacemaker will adapt and record the event.

Technology has tremendously improved the diagnostic capabilities and amount of data pacemakers can store. Pacemakers have many special features that give additional information regarding the pacemaker, lead system, and special diagnostic functions.

### Pacemaker implantation

Installing a pacemaker is a fairly minor surgical procedure that takes about 1 hour. If you're not in the hospital already, you

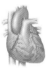

## HEALTHY HEART ♥ TIP

*You don't have to be a body builder or a marathon runner to improve your overall heart health. The key is the total amount of energy you expend, not the intensity.*

*Accumulate 5- to 10-minute intervals of moderately intense activity throughout the day by walking up hills, taking the stairs or mowing a hilly patch of lawn. These need total only 30 minutes to promote fitness.*

*In addition, you can boost your exercise total with household chores, shopping, gardening, running errands, working and other activities. Try getting up from a chair using only your leg muscles or raise and lower a milk jug several times as you carry it to the breakfast table.*

will be admitted the morning of or evening before your pacemaker implantation. You should not eat or drink anything after midnight. An intravenious catheter (IV) is inserted to administer fluids and medications. Your heart will be continuously monitored by electrocardiography before, during and after implantation.

Your chest will be cleaned with a special antibacterial soap, and shaved if necessary. A special X-ray machine is positioned over you to help your doctor correctly place the pacemaker lead wires. Surgeons numb the incision area with a local anesthetic, just below the collarbone, and may give you additional medications through the IV catheter to help you relax.

Tests will have ensured that the wires will be in the best location for pacing your heart. Doctors insert the lead wires into a vein under the collarbone and thread them into your heart's right side. Once they're positioned correctly, the wires are attached to the pulse generator, which is then positioned in a pocket beneath the skin and fat of your chest wall. The pacemaker is programmed so the stimulus is strong enough to pace your heart, but not so strong as to waste battery energy.

After the procedure, you can eat regular meals as tolerated. The pacemaker nurse or doctor will talk to you and your family about your pacemaker, providing information about checking your pulse, your activity level, your incision, and telephone monitoring for follow-up care and activity level.

Most people can be discharged from the hospital 1 to 2 days after implantation of the pacemaker system. Occasionally, same-day discharge is possible.

## Living with your pacemaker

Your incision may be mildly tender for several weeks. After the initial swelling goes down, you may feel or see your pacemaker's outline under the skin. You may shower or bathe 48 hours after your pacemaker implantation.

You'll be advised not to drive for 2 weeks after implantation to make sure the pacemaker works properly and to avoid any discomfort from hampering your driving skills. You should avoid, for 1 month, vigorous above-the-shoulder activities, such as golf, tennis, swimming, bicycling, bowling, and lifting anything that weighs more than 15 pounds. These activities may compromise the pacemaker lead's stability as it becomes securely attached to your heart's inner wall.

Contact your doctor if you experience increased swelling, redness, or drainage from the incision or a fever above 100 degrees Fahrenheit.

Fortunately, you don't have to do much to ensure the pacemaker works correctly. Activities that emit strong electromagnetic fields, such as arc-welding, may interfere with your pacemaker's function and should be avoided. In addition, you should forgo contact sports or shooting a shotgun or rifle from the shoulder where the pacemaker's positioned. Airport monitoring devices don't harm pacemakers, but they may cause the metal detector to sound. Airport security personnel know about this and can help. Microwave ovens don't affect modern pacemakers.

### Replacement

Because pacemakers are battery-driven, they eventually wear down. You can't always predict when this will happen, because it partly depends on how often the pacemaker actually paces versus stands by. If your pacemaker has to stimulate your heart only occasionally, the batteries will last longer. However, if it has to prod your heart most of the time, the batteries will wear out sooner.

Pacemakers generally last about 8 years, depending on the make, model, and frequency of use. The battery status, as well as the pacemaker function, can be monitored by telephone, so you usually don't have to make frequent office visits. You'll be provided with a special telephone monitoring system so you can send an electrocardiogram and special signals over the telephone to a central monitoring office. These transmissions are recommended every 2 to 3 months.

When the pacemaker begins to send signals of a weakening battery, you'll be told to schedule an appointment to replace the pulse generator. Although there's no reason to delay, replacement doesn't usually need to occur right away since there's lag time built in.

Doctors restore your pacemaker by replacing the entire pulse generator; they also check the original leads, which are generally satisfactory for continued use.

## Pacemaker precautions

Do not arc-weld. Electromagnetic fields may interfere with your pacemaker function.

Don't do mechanical work on a running car engine where small electromagnetic fields are present.

If you undergo magnetic resonance imaging (MRI), inform the doctor or medical staff beforehand that you have a pacemaker, because this procedure can pose serious problems for your pacemaker.

If you're scheduled for any type of operation in which electrocautery controls bleeding, your doctors should take precautions to ensure normal pacemaker function throughout the operation.

Carry your pacemaker ID card with you at all times. Know the company manufacturer.

# Defibrillation and cardioversion

Some fast or chaotic heart rhythms can't be effectively treated with drugs. Rhythms such as ventricular fibrillation cause such catastrophic consequences (for example, sudden cardiac death) that there's no time to begin medication. Others, such as atrial fibrillation, may not respond to medicines. Fortunately, an alternative form of treatment is available for these conditions.

## External defibrillation and cardioversion

Administering an electrical shock to the heart through the chest wall can convert a fibrillating heart to a normal rhythm. When used in people with ventricular fibrillation, this procedure is called defibrillation. In people with less severe rhythm disorders, it's termed cardioversion (conversion of cardiac rhythm to normal).

Defibrillation and cardioversion are thought to work by momentarily stopping the heart and the chaotic rhythm. This often allows the normal heart rhythm to take over again.

The size of the electrical shock ranges from 20 joules to 400 joules, which registers thousands of times stronger than a pacemaker stimulus. A shock of this magnitude can cause your entire body to twitch vigorously. When used for defibrillation of ventricular fibrillation, you're unconscious and unaware of the shock.

When cardioversion is done electively, you're put to sleep first for 2 or 3 minutes with a short-acting general anesthetic agent. Elective cardioversion refers to cardioversion not done in an emergency; you schedule it ahead of time. Although you can survive and function with atrial fibrillation, restoring normal rhythm by cardioversion is worth trying when atrial fibrillation is recent or of unknown duration. When atrial fibrillation is longstanding, it rarely responds to cardioversion and is usually managed with medications.

For at least 3 weeks before attempted cardioversion of atrial fibrillation, doctors generally prescribe warfarin to prevent any clot formation inside the fibrillating atria that might be dislodged by the shock and cause complications such as stroke. Alternatively, your doctor may use heparin intravenously to prevent a clot and a transesophageal echocardiogram to make certain that no clots have formed in the atria prior to starting the procedure.

Before the cardioversion, you should not eat for 8 hours. An intravenous (IV) catheter is placed in your arm and you breathe oxygen through a face mask. A short-acting anesthetic is given through the vein, which puts you to sleep for 2 to 3 minutes. During that time, doctors administer the electrical shock. If necessary, they may give two or three shocks.

After the cardioversion, you wake up and are monitored for several hours before you can leave. You may be somewhat drowsy, so you should arrange transportation home ahead of time. If warfarin was used, it should be continued for another 2 to 4 weeks. Whether you continue taking antiarrhythmic medications after cardioversion should be decided by you and your doctor according to the likelihood that the arrhythmia will recur.

If standard external cardioversion isn't successful, catheters can be placed in the heart to allow internal cardioversion, which usually works. Whether or not to do internal cardioversion depends on the severity of symptoms and other medical conditions.

Most defibrillations and cardioversions are done in a hospital or by an ambulance team. With adhesive patches applied to the chest wall, the device can sense the type of arrhythmia. The defibrillator then delivers a shock in an appropriate fashion. Although machines and computer chips aren't infallible, this device improves the odds for people who require emergency defibrillation.

In addition, a special type of defibrillator now enables individuals untrained in interpreting electrocardiograms to administer lifesaving defibrillation in an emergency.

## Implantable cardioverter-defibrillator (ICD)

People who have survived a cardiac arrest caused by ventricular fibrillation or have episodes of ventricular tachycardia risk recurrence. Those with ventricular tachycardia also may experience serious symptoms such as loss of consciousness, and may progress from ventricular tachycardia to ventricular fibrillation.

These sudden death rhythms account for an estimated 400,000 fatalities each year. Medication may reduce the risk of recurring ventricular fibrillation or ventricular tachycardia, but a safety net may be desirable in case these rhythms occur despite the medications.

Implantable cardioverter-defibrillators may provide that protection. ICDs have been 99 percent effective in averting abnormal rhythms. Your cardiologist or electrophysiologist will evaluate to see if medications or a combination of medication and ICD is the best way for you.

Like pacemakers, implantable cardioverter-defibrillators are battery-driven devices implanted in the body. They've become smaller in recent years and are now about the size of a bar of soap, whereas a pacemaker is more the size of a pocket watch. Previously, implantable cardioverter defibrillators were placed beneath the skin and muscle of the abdomen, but they can now be fitted conveniently beneath the skin under the collarbone. Technologic advances should further reduce the size of future devices.

Like pacemakers, wire electrodes attach the ICDs pulse generator to the heart, with the attachment site and type of electrodes varying. Usually a combination of wires is used. Some wires, inserted through veins into the inside of the heart, sense your heartbeat. They also can be used for pacing, just like a regular pacemaker, should the need arise. Inside the ICD is a battery, a microchip and related electrical circuits.

Occasionally wires may be attached to the outside of the heart, including patches that are sewn onto the surface of the heart. These deliver a shock to the heart when it's required.

New models don't need electrode patches affixed to the outside of the heart, but instead use electrodes that go under the skin of the chest near the heart. Electrodes that emit the shock usually are positioned inside the heart. Careful testing determines which specific internal cardioverter-defibrillator design and which lead placement will give the most reliable response.

The implantation procedure parallels that for placing a pacemaker, except that doctors do additional testing to make certain the device detects and treats the ventricular arrhythmia. Normally, you'll be discharged from the hospital on the day following implantation.

### How does ICD work?

The implantable cardioverter-defibrillator monitors your heart rhythm at all times. It can pace like a pacemaker for slow heart rates, rapidly pace for tachyarrhythmias, and give smaller cardioversion or large defibrillation shocks. When ventricular tachycardia occurs, it attempts to convert the rhythm by painlessly pacing the heart with short rapid burst patterns the EP physician has programmed.

If several of these attempts are unsuccessful, or if the chaotic rhythm of ventricular fibrillation develops, then the ICD automatically charges to shock the heart. This is similar to the conventional external defibrillator, but the internal device has an advantage because it's always ready to deliver a lower energy shock when needed. The specific electrical therapy used is based on the presenting rhythm and any results of an electrophysiologic test.

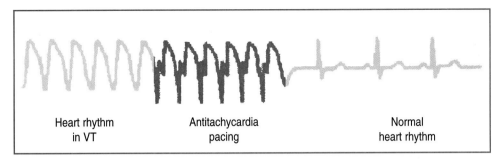

Heart rhythm in VT      Antitachycardia pacing      Normal heart rhythm

*People surviving cardiac arrest caused by ventricular tachycardia (a rapid, regular heartbeat also known as VT) may benefit from an implantable cardioverter defibrillator. The ICD paces the rapidly beating heart into a slower, more normal rhythm.*

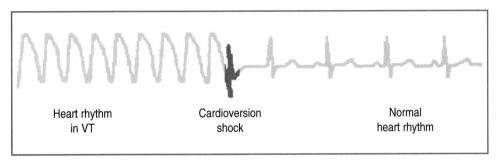

Heart rhythm in VT      Cardioversion shock      Normal heart rhythm

*Sometimes an ICD needs to make a bold statement to the heart, shocking it momentarily so that the heart can resume its normal rhythm. This is called cardioversion, or converting the cardiac rhythm to normal.*

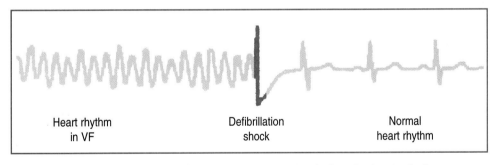

Heart rhythm in VF      Defibrillation shock      Normal heart rhythm

*When ventricular fibrillation (VF) occurs, it's imperative for the heart's chaotic rhythms to receive corrective measures immediately. One benefit of an ICD is that the device is always on hand, ready to deliver a life-saving shock.*

The ICD will record and save each event and therapy. When you return for evaluation, your doctor can retrieve these data from the device's programmer, which is a computer-type device with an attached wand that's placed over the ICD. Special signals that send and receive information work like your TV remote control.

## How does it feel?

Shocks may be sudden and painful. They have been described as a "kick in the chest." However, the discomfort lasts only a fraction of a second and doesn't cause lingering pain or damage. Generally, the pain relates to your symptoms before therapy started. If you feel light-headed, you may be only vaguely aware of the shock. It is not unusual to be briefly surprised, confused, and anxious immediately after a shock.

## When you receive a shock

If you receive one shock or pacing therapies, but then feel well and recover immediately, you may call and report this to your health care provider, although it isn't mandatory.

When you call, you'll be asked about activities and symptoms before the shock and how you're recovering. If you feel fine, but a little anxious, the phone call may be all you need. Keep a diary, since this can then be compared with data obtained from the programmer.

If one or more therapies occur or you don't feel well, ask someone near you for help. You may need to call 911 or your ambulance service. If CPR and other lifesaving activities are required, they should be started immediately.

## Implantation procedure

The implantation of an ICD is similar to that of a pacemaker. During the procedure, however, you are briefly put to sleep. After implantation you will return to a monitored cardiac area and typically stay only 1 or 2 more days in the hospital.

After surgery, you will have some pain over the ICD incision area. You may shower or bathe 48 hours after implant. Discomfort for several days is normal. After the swelling goes down, you may still be able to see or feel the outline of the ICD and the lead(s).

## Restrictions after implantation

As comfort permits, continue with your normal activities. This includes mild exercise, light work, and sexual activities.

For 4 weeks:

- Avoid vigorous above-the-shoulder activities or exercises.
- Avoid golf, tennis, swimming, bicycling, bowling, or vacuuming.
- Avoid lifting anything weighing 5 pounds or more.
- Do not play contact sports. The impact from contact sports could harm you or the ICD.

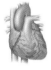

### HEALTHY HEART ♥ TIP

*You've probably felt light-headed when you rose too quickly. The feeling's caused by the effects of gravity.*

*Anytime you stand from a sitting or lying position, your blood pressure drops slightly because your body is adjusting to gravity by increasing the tone (constriction) of your blood vessels and by increasing your heart rate.*

*If your blood pressure drops too much, however, you can faint. Usually, there will be other circumstances, such as an excessive dose of blood pressure medication; disease of the autonomic nervous system, including complications from diabetes; or an uncommon disorder called Shy-Drager syndrome. See your doctor to be sure.*

- Monitor strenuous exercise programs. To help ensure your safety and prevent unintended shocks, your physician must evaluate any new programs. You may need a treadmill exercise test before discharge.

## Other precautions and assurances

- Carry your ICD identification card with you at all times. Know the ICD's manufacturer.

- Household appliances such as microwave ovens won't interfere with ICD function.

- Household tools can be used if they're grounded and in good repair.

- You can walk through security devices in stores and buildings without fear.

## Should you drive?

Although the ICD is life-saving, it doesn't prevent loss of consciousness that may occur with ventricular fibrillation. For this reason, your physician may recommend that you not drive for 6 months.

After that, your specific cardiac events, rhythm, and tolerance to the rhythm and therapy will be evaluated. Depending on your heart rhythm, your doctor may advise you not to return to driving. It takes between 5 and 15 seconds for the ICD to detect, charge, and deliver a shock. Consequently, activities such as driving put everyone at risk if you experience ventricular fibrillation.

## Follow-up and replacement

Outpatient evaluation appointments are scheduled every 3 to 6 months, more often when replacement time approaches. During each visit, medical personnel obtain tachy event data (shocks and fast pacing therapy), battery status, and pacemaker information from the ICD programmer.

ICDs last about 4 to 6 years. New models are smaller and last longer than previous devices. When replacement time arrives, you will likely be scheduled within a few weeks. This does not need to be done urgently, although there is generally no reason to delay. The ICD will continue to function normally during this time. During replacement the original leads are checked, and the ICD (the entire generator) is replaced. This can usually be done as an outpatient procedure.

## ICD precautions

- Tell your physician, dentist, and all medical personnel about your ICD.

- Do not allow airport security to use a hand-held metal detector because it contains a magnet. Ask to be searched by hand. The metal detector will not harm the ICD, but it may set off the alarms and temporarily interfere with proper functioning of the ICD.

- Medical procedures such as diathermy, lithotripsy, and radiation therapy should be discussed with the EP physician (electrophysiologist) before the procedures. Magnetic resonance imaging (MRI) is not recommended for ICD patients.

- Whenever you have ANY surgery in which cautery will be used, your doctor must contact the cardiologist or EP physician. Cautery used during surgery may interfere with ICD function. Temporary reprogramming may be needed before and after the procedure.

- Do not arc-weld. Stay 10 to 12 feet away from anyone who is arc-welding.

- Strong electromagnetic fields, high voltage, strong electrical current, or industrial equipment may interfere with ICD function. Ask your physician about specific situations.

- Cellular phones should be carried a minimum of 6 inches (15 centimeters) from the ICD. Use on the ear opposite to the implanted site.

# Surgical and catheter treatment

Some fast rhythm disorders don't respond adequately to medications and aren't appropriately treated with internal defibrillators. For example, some people have atrial fibrillation that causes the ventricles to beat exceedingly fast despite the use of medications. This fast rate can be extremely uncomfortable or even potentially dangerous. Other people have fast rhythms that emanate directly from the atrioventricular node.

Some people have an abnormal "bridge" (in addition to the normal atrioventricular node) that electrically connects the atrium with the ventricles. This allows electrical impulses to travel from the atrium to the ventricle without going through the atrioventricular node. This condition, called Wolff-Parkinson-White syndrome (WPW), can predispose you to exceedingly rapid and potentially dangerous heart rhythms.

If medications don't work in any of these situations, other approaches are available.

## Surgical treatment

The "bridge," or accessory pathway, in WPW can be disconnected by a surgeon's scalpel. Operation has been a solution for this condition for several years, but now it has been largely replaced by catheter techniques.

Under some circumstances, rhythms such as ventricular tachycardia emanate from a specific heart muscle site. If other means fail, removing that site surgically may prevent the rhythm from happening over and over again. A surgical treatment called the "maze" procedure can treat atrial fibrillation in patients who have significant symptoms despite medical therapy.

## Catheter ablation

Nonsurgical techniques with a special "ablation" (ablation means "elimination" or "removal") catheter have been perfected so that they're often used to treat WPW, rapid atrial fibrillation, or fast heart rates originating from the atrioventricular node, atrium, and ventricles.

Using special electrophysiologic studies, specialists can determine where the accessory pathway is located in people with WPW (a technique called mapping). Doctors insert a special catheter so that it lies close to the pathway and then pass radio frequencies through it. The tip of the catheter heats up and destroys the precise area of the heart that contains the abnormal tissue bridge (see pages A13 and 112).

If the atrioventricular node behaves abnormally by transmitting electrical impulses to the ventricle too quickly (such as during rapid atrial fibrillation) or by initiating fast heartbeats, it can also be selectively damaged by radiofrequency ablation to slow the heart rate.

Catheter ablation procedures have been effective in managing these selected problems. Depending on the cause of the fast heart rate, radiofrequency ablation procedures may result in complete heart block, requiring a pacemaker. For example, to control the heart rate in people with rapid atrial fibrillation, radiofrequency ablation causes complete heart block in more than 90 percent of cases. The regular paced rhythm is a vast improvement over the symptomatic fast heart rates that were previously occurring. However, ablation of the bridge in WPW very rarely causes complete heart block.

Catheter ablation can also eliminate atrial or ventricular tissue that may be responsible for arrhythmia. Electrophysiologic testing and mapping localize the abnormal tissue, which is then ablated with radiofrequency energy. This approach can treat atrial tachycardia, ventricular tachycardia, atrial flutter, and atrioventricular nodal tachycardia. Catheter ablation of the atrium in patients with atrial fibrillation is still under investigation and a subject of considerable research interest.

## Should all palpitations be treated?

Cardiologists and other physicians often discuss how to handle "minor" problems. A good example would be palpitations—the awareness of heartbeat irregularities caused by "flip-flops" or "skips" in the chest.

Although palpitations can signal a potentially serious heartbeat problem or hint at significant irregularities in the heart muscle, valves, or coronary arteries, most palpitations that aren't associated with other symptoms—such as light-headedness, blacking out, shortness of breath, or chest discomfort—don't pose any problem for your overall health.

Still, doctors often investigate symptomatic palpitations (or certain types of frequent extra beats observed on an electrocardiogram) for various types of heart disease. They generally want to be sure that palpitations aren't the "tip of the iceberg" (that is, whether more serious rhythm problems are also present).

Even if there's no underlying problem, palpitations can be an uncomfortable nuisance if they occur frequently or seem strong, and they can provoke high anxiety in some people. Consequently, it seems reasonable that some palpitations should be treated with antiarrhythmic medications that may suppress them and reduce or eliminate symptoms.

Several factors must be weighed in deciding the best way to approach this perplexing condition.

How bad are the symptoms (barely noticeable, a nuisance, or virtually disabling)? What are the chances the rhythm abnormality will become

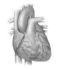

**HEALTHY HEART ♥ TIP**

*Is a cholesterol-lowering medication right for you? Your doctor should evaluate all your risk factors, then help you decide. If you already have heart disease, then your goal will be "secondary prevention," or lowering your risk for subsequent heart attacks or strokes.*

*There are three types of medications that can provide an extra degree of secondary prevention. These include:*

- *Statins. Also called HMG-CoA reductase inhibitors, this drug class includes atorvastatin, fluvastatin, lovastatin and simvastatin.*

- *Beta-blockers. Often prescribed to prevent angina attacks, these drugs slow the heartbeat, decrease blood pressure and reduce the heart muscle's contraction strength.*

- *Aspirin. Aspirin acts on the blood's circulating platelets to limit clot formation. Clots can initiate heart attacks.*

more serious or symptomatic in the future: slight ("no chance" doesn't exist in medicine) or highly probable? What's the likelihood of a medication helping the symptoms: low or high? Most important, what's the chance a medication will create new problems—a side effect or even worsening of the heart rhythm?

Traditionally, doctors attempted treatment even if the symptoms were minor, even if they were unlikely to get worse, and even if the medication might not be very effective. Their rationale was "it can't hurt to try." However, new information about the possibility of side effects has raised major questions about that approach. As it turns out, in some people it can hurt to try.

One medical study, called the Cardiac Arrhythmia Suppression Trial (CAST), examined the effects of various antiarrhythmic medications on patients with certain types of rhythm abnormalities occurring after a heart attack. The study was intended to discover whether reducing extra beats after a heart attack would promote long-term survival and which of several medications might best accomplish that.

The study found that in less than 1 year, nearly three times as many patients who received medication died of severe heart rhythm abnormalities as those who didn't receive a medication. And more than three times as many died of heart problems not caused by rhythm abnormalities as those who received no rhythm medication. As this trend became apparent, the study was discontinued so that further patients would avoid the risky treatment.

The CAST study results don't mean that antiarrhythmic medications play no useful part—they have been effective in treating certain rhythm disorders. But medications must be used cautiously and only when they are clearly required.

General guidelines for their use:

Don't use medications if your heart rhythm abnormality is benign (if your risk of future problems isn't predictably increased) and doesn't produce symptoms.

Try to tolerate the palpitations to avoid the risk of medications if your heart rhythm abnormality causes palpitations but is benign.

If you can't tolerate the palpitations use medications with the lowest possible risk. Fortunately, low-risk medications, such as beta-blockers, are often effective.

If your heart rhythm abnormality is "prognostically significant" (which means it may suggest future problems) or malignant (with a high risk of dangerous developments in the near future), use the most effective medication (or an implantable cardioverter-defibrillator) based on appropriate testing.

# Treating circulatory problems

The many types of vascular problems that can jeopardize the circulatory function of the heart and blood vessels were discussed in Part 2. A wide range of therapeutic options is available. This chapter discusses the typical treatments for each of the general categories of vascular disease.

## Atherosclerosis

Atherosclerosis is the slow, progressive deposit of hard plaque on the inner walls of arteries. This creates areas of narrowing that impede the flow of blood. Arteries to the heart (coronary), legs and brain (carotid) are most commonly involved.

Virtually everyone in Western societies eventually develops some degree of atherosclerosis. However, this shouldn't be viewed as a normal part of aging. Rather, you should consider atherosclerosis as the price of an easier lifestyle, richer food, and less physical work.

Intermittent claudication is the discomfort you may feel in your leg muscles when walking with reduced circulation. A program of regular walking can significantly increase the distance you can walk without distress. Such a walking program stimulates the formation of collateral vessels. Collateral vessels are like small side-roads that bypass a narrowed main road.

Although collateral vessels will not return circulation to normal, they may reduce symptoms enough to eliminate or delay the need for more aggressive treatment. Walking also produces a "training effect" by improving muscle efficiency; the leg muscles can per-form more work with the blood supply they receive.

### Medications

Your doctor may recommend aspirin or Plavix, an aspirin substitute, to reduce the likelihood that platelets will clump at atherosclerotic sites, form a blood clot, and cause further block-age. A medication called pentoxifylline tends to make red blood cells "softer" and the blood better able to flow through narrowed areas. For some people with claudication, this medication allows them to walk moderately greater distances.

Another medication, cilostazol, approved last year by the Food and Drug Administration, can widen leg arteries somewhat. This drug also decreases the ability of blood platelets to clump together. These mechanisms allow people with intermittent claudication to walk somewhat farther before leg pain occurs.

### Surgical treatment

With severe symptoms, blockage severe enough to threaten muscle or skin tissue survival, or hampered function of the organ supplied by the blood vessel, a bypass operation or a surgical "coring out" (endarterectomy) may be required. In suitable candidates, opening the blockage with a balloon catheter is possible, just as with the coronary arteries. Other types of catheters that use laser energy or mechanical devices to open the artery may be used in certain circumstances.

## Arterial thrombosis and embolism

Just as in the coronary arteries, blood clots can develop at other atherosclerotic sites. They can rapidly block a vessel (thrombosis) or break into fragments and block branches of vessels farther downstream (embolism). This results in a sudden cessation of blood flow to the areas supplied by the artery and branches.

With sudden blockage, there's no time for collateral arteries to develop. The body can't compensate for this blood flow reduction, and you require emergency medical attention.

Treatment may involve dissolving the blood clot with a thrombolytic agent (similar to the thrombolytic medications in myocardial infarction) or removing the blood clot surgically. The clot must be eliminated within a few hours or the tissue supplied by the blocked artery may die, and amputation may be necessary.

*A blood clot that has lodged in an artery can often be removed by passing a catheter beyond the clot and inflating a small balloon at the tip of the catheter. When the catheter pulls back, the clot is dragged to where it can be readily removed.*

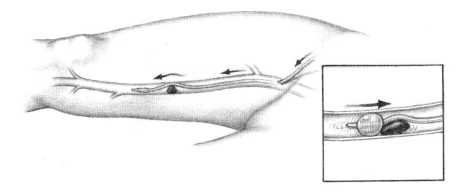

### Medications

Thrombolytic medication that dissolves the clot may be given through a catheter directly to the affected area. If you've had arterial thrombosis or embolism or are at risk of their development, you'll receive blood thinners (anticoagulants) to reduce the likelihood of blood clotting and future problems.

## Surgical treatment

The surgeon can remove a clot in an artery by making a small opening upstream from the blockage and passing a balloon-tipped catheter past the blood clot (the clot is soft). Once the balloon is downstream from the blood clot, the doctor inflates it and pulls the catheter back to the opening in the artery. The balloon pulls the blood clot upstream where it can be removed. Occasionally, it's necessary to replace or bypass the blocked vessel.

## Aortic aneurysm

Bulging in the aorta (aortic aneurysm) usually occurs in the abdominal portion of the aorta but may also be present in the chest or other arteries (especially the legs). (See page 121, A15). Aneurysm carries a risk that the aorta may rupture.

With a small aneurysm and no symptoms when it's discovered, your doctor may recommend careful monitoring at regular checkups to determine whether it's enlarging. Generally, you won't require treatment until the aneurysm reaches a size at which the possibility of rupture is significant. For an abdominal aortic aneurysm, you should seriously consider operation when the diameter is 5 centimeters (about 2 1/2 to 3 inches), when a smaller aneurysm enlarges rapidly, or when symptoms occur.

### Medications

Drugs have no specific value in aortic aneurysm, except that treating high blood pressure is prudent. By reducing blood pressure, beta-blockers theoretically will slow the aneurysm's expansion rate, which means they're frequently used—particularly for those with aneurysms of the thoracic aorta.

Doctors can only reduce the risk of rupture by repairing the bulge surgically before a rupture occurs. Once the aneurysm bursts, it may be too late to do anything, because rupture is often fatal within minutes to hours. Emergency operation is the only hope for survival at that point.

### Surgical treatment

The operation for an aortic aneurysm is safe and fairly uncomplicated. It consists of replacing the area of the bulge, where the arterial wall is weak, with a tube made of synthetic material. With time, the blood vessel's normal lining cells grow into the tube's inner surface, producing a durable conduit for blood to flow through. It may be possible to introduce grafts by a catheter, avoiding the need for a large abdominal incision, a method currently under investigation.

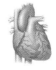

**HEALTHY HEART ♥ TIP**

*When someone's experiencing a heart attack, quick thinking becomes crucial. Here's what to do:*

- *Call 911. Describe symptoms such as shortness of breath or chest pain to ensure the emergency team will send someone trained in cardiac life support.*

- *If the victim is unconscious, begin CPR. If you don't know how, a dispatcher can instruct you until help arrives.*

- *If you live in a rural or large metropolitan area, you may get to the hospital faster by being driven. If you think you're having a heart attack, ask someone to drive you. Never drive yourself.*

- *Chew aspirin. Aspirin discourages blood clotting, which helps blood flow through a narrowed artery. When taken during a heart attack, aspirin can decrease death rates by about 25 percent.*

# Aortic dissection

Dissection of the aorta, in which the layers of the aortic wall separate from one another, is a medical emergency (see page 122). Not only does it cause pain, but there's also a risk of impending death if the tear should go completely through the wall.

Once doctors establish the presence of dissection with tests such as computed tomography, echocardiography, magnetic resonance imaging, or aortography, an emergency surgical procedure is usually advisable. Occasionally, some specific variations of aortic dissection may be treated with medication alone.

## Medications

If blood pressure is high in the aorta, the likelihood of extending the tear increases. Therefore, the first treatment focuses on keeping the blood pressure low by using intravenous medications. Narcotics may be required for pain.

## Surgical treatment

Operation for aortic dissection consists of either replacing a portion of the aorta where the tear originated with a synthetic material, or "tacking down" the tear with a suture so that blood can no longer force its way through the opening. If repairing the dissection involves replacing parts of the aorta where vessels branch off to the brain, arms, kidneys, or other organs, the surgeon must disconnect the branch vessels and reconnect them to the synthetic tube.

# Arteritis (inflammation of the arteries)

Inflammation in arteritis (itis means "inflammation") can result in obstruction of the arteries, which reduces the supply of blood reaching the affected areas or the formation of arterial aneurysms.

## Medications

Doctors usually treat inflammatory conditions of the arteries with medications that reduce inflammation. The most potent anti-inflammatory medications are corticosteroid drugs, which are related to cortisone. The side effects from these medications are minimized by giving them in the smallest dose needed to control symptoms adequately, and decreasing or discontinuing them as the condition resolves.

**HEALTHY HEART ♥ TIP**

*Damaged hearts that need improved blood flow may be candidates for a new procedure called transmyocardial revascularization (TMR). In TMR, doctors use a laser to cut a series of channels in the heart muscle to increase blood to the organ.*

*To do this procedure, surgeons make an incision on the left side of the chest and insert a laser into the chest cavity. Then they shoot holes through the heart's left ventricle between heartbeats and press a finger on the holes on the outside of the heart. This seals the outer openings but lets the inner channels stay open, which allows blood to flow through the heart muscle.*

*How this works is not yet known. Another new technique is being developed to create the channels by running a laser catheter into the chamber of the left heart, thus avoiding open-heart surgery. This procedure is still experimental.*

## Surgical treatment

Some types of arteritis may cause blockage of the vessels, even after the active inflammation has been treated or has resolved. Occasionally, you may need an operation to bypass or open the blockage.

# Arterial spasm

To treat arterial spasm, doctors must first determine whether there are any provoking factors. Some medications, such as ergotamines used for treating migraine headaches, may aggravate arterial spasm. Cold temperatures can intensify Raynaud's phenomenon.

## Medications

As with coronary spasm, treatment may include medications that prevent the smooth muscle in the artery wall from overcontracting. Thus, vasodilators are the preferred medications.

# Venous thrombosis

Venous thrombosis is best treated by preventing it. If you've had thrombosis before or if you're at greater risk of developing it because of prolonged bed rest, immobility from operation or other diseases, or injury to the legs and leg veins, you should be concerned about preventive measures.

## Prevention

People in these situations, such as those in the hospital recovering from operation or a heart attack, often receive anticoagulants until they're able to get up and move around. Anticoagulants are given temporarily in low doses—usually small injections of heparin under the skin twice a day. This dosage minimizes the risk of a blood clot forming inside a vein, yet it's low enough to avoid most blood-thinning complications, such as a tendency to bleed or bruise.

Support stockings work well for individuals confined to bed or who have had damage to leg veins. The stockings help prevent blood pooling in the veins and thus reduce the chance that blood will clot.

## Medications

If venous thrombosis does develop, you'll require full doses of anticoagulants. Treating deep-vein thrombosis of the legs requires hospitalization so that heparin can be given in full doses, intraveneously or by injection.

After about 5 days of effective heparin therapy (measured by tests that monitor the blood's ability to clot), your treatment will switch to warfarin. Treatment for deep-vein thrombosis with warfarin, taken by mouth, usually continues for 3 to 6 months.

People on anticoagulation therapy must have periodic blood tests to measure the prothrombin time ("protime") to make sure the blood's tendency to clot has been reduced enough, but not too much.

Because deep-vein thrombosis may lead to venous insufficiency, in which the veins can't adequately return the blood to the heart, measures to reduce this consequence include the use of support hose and periodic leg elevation.

## Pulmonary embolism

If a thrombus (clot) in the leg's deep veins breaks loose, the blood carries it through the veins into the heart and out into the pulmonary arteries, where it lodges and obstructs blood flow to a portion of the lungs. Depending on the size of the pulmonary embolism, the results may range from no symptoms, to chest pain and shortness of breath, to shock and death (see page 128).

### Medications

For pulmonary emboli that do not immediately threaten survival, doctors prescribe blood thinners to prevent the embolism from getting worse. You must be hospitalized and given heparin, after which you're treated with warfarin for 6 months to a year.

For more extensive pulmonary embolism, medications to dissolve the clot have been shown to improve blood flow and promote survival.

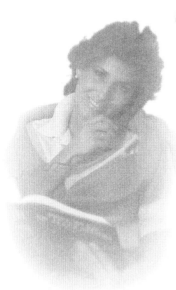

### Surgical treatment

For particularly life-threatening pulmonary emboli, an emergency operation may be required to remove the blood clot from the lung arteries. In patients with recurrent emboli or at risk of recurrences, a device called an umbrella is inserted into the vena cava on the end of a catheter. It acts as a filter preventing blood clots from escaping into the heart.

## Pulmonary hypertension

This general term refers to conditions that raise the blood pressure in the arteries to the lungs but not in other arteries, Regardless of the cause, pulmonary hypertension is seldom completely reversible if it causes symptoms such as breathlessness, chest pressure, or blacking out.

## Medications

Vasodilators improve pulmonary hypertension in some people, but they rarely normalize elevated blood pressure in the lungs completely and must often be used in high doses.

Vasodilators should be started in the hospital during careful monitoring with a pressure-measuring (Swan-Ganz) catheter in the pulmonary artery. Some people with pulmonary hypertension may become worse if the vasodilators lower their "regular" blood pressure more than their pulmonary blood pressure.

The most effective vasodilator for the treatment of this condition is also the most complicated to administer. Called epoprostenol, it must be continuously dispensed into a vein, which means you must have a permanent venous catheter inserted by a surgeon and then use a portable intravenous pump 24 hours a day.

Nevertheless, this medication improves the quality of life in most patients by lowering pulmonary blood pressure, reducing symptoms, increasing exercise capacity, and extending life span. Although patients with all of these conditions may benefit from cardiac rehabilitation, it's best to check with your health insurance provider, since rules about reimbursement for valvular heart disease, cardiomyopathy, PTCA or coronary bypass surgery vary widely.

A blood thinner (warfarin) increases life span in some people with pulmonary hypertension. Your doctor may also recommend oxygen use on a continuous basis, because a low oxygen level in the bloodstream can be one of the consequences of pulmonary hypertension.

## Surgical treatment

On rare occasions, people with pulmonary hypertension may have a large thrombus (clot) in the pulmonary artery (presumably from an old pulmonary embolism), even though they don't have a specific history of pulmonary embolism. In a year, an estimated 0.1 percent of the approximately 600,000 people in the U.S. who have a pulmonary embolism develop pulmonary hypertension due to blood clot persistence.

Thus, about 600 individuals annually might benefit from a procedure called pulmonary thromboendarterectomy, in which surgeons remove blood clots as well as the artery lining. The surgical risk is high, with a 5 to 10 percent chance of operative mortality. But if successful, the operation can return pulmonary blood pressure to near normal and markedly reduce the patient's symptoms. Lung or heart-lung transplantation may be considered for people with severe pulmonary hypertension.

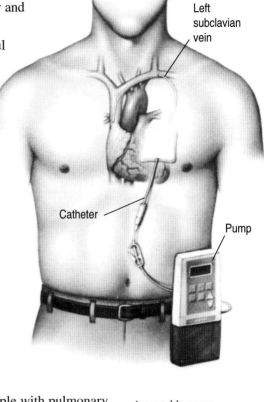

Left subclavian vein

Catheter

Pump

*A portable pump attached to the patient's belt delivers epoprostenol by means of a catheter that enters the blood circulation at the left subclavian vein. This is the most effective treatment for pulmonary hypertension. It's also the most complicated to administer.*

# Chapter
# 19 Dealing with pericardial complications

The pericardium or sac that surrounds the heart (see page A16) can develop a variety of diseases, most often caused by inflammation, accumulating fluid, or stiffness. The pericardium can come under attack for reasons that range from virus to cancer, and produce symptoms such as sharp pain, fever, dizziness, or shock.

## Pericardial effusion and tamponade

Excessive fluid accumulation in the pericardial sac surrounding the heart (pericardial effusion) can make the heart's pumping task more difficult and lead to tamponade, a condition in which the heart is compressed in the sac too tightly to expand properly. It may lead to low blood pressure, shock, or symptoms of rapidly developing heart failure. This situation requires urgent treatment by draining the fluid from the pericardial sac.

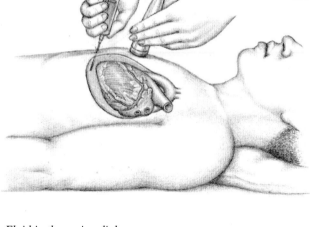

*Fluid in the pericardial sac can accumulate enough to press on the heart and impair its pumping function. The fluid often can be removed by inserting a needle through the skin into the distended pericardial sac, using guidance from an echocardiogram. The fluid can then be drained through the needle.*

### Pericardiocentesis

Pericardiocentesis (centesis means "puncture") involves removing excess fluid from the pericardial sac. To drain the fluid, doctors anesthetize an area of skin over the chest wall or upper abdomen next to the heart and insert a needle directly into the fluid-filled pericardial sac.

Echocardiographic images may be useful to guide the needle's path into the pericardial space. The fluid can be drained either through the needle or through a soft catheter that can replace the needle. If there's concern that fluid may reaccumulate, a catheter can be left in place for several days to continue draining the fluid.

Even in cases of pericardial effusion in which there's no tamponade, it may be advisable to remove at least some of the fluid so that doctors can analyze it and determine the underlying cause.

# Pericarditis

Pericarditis is inflammation of the pericardium, a condition that may produce pain and irritation. Inflammation is one of the causes of excess fluid in the pericardial sac.

## Medications

Pain may be substantially alleviated during the natural healing process by anti-inflammatory medications, such as aspirin, the most common anti-inflammatory agent. Sometimes other anti-inflammatory drugs, such as indomethacin, may be used.

These medications have anti-inflammatory actions similar to those of corticosteroids, although they're not corticosteroids. Thus, they're sometimes called nonsteroidal anti-inflammatory drugs (NSAIDs). Inflammation reduction by any of these medications also decreases the pain.

Rarely, corticosteroids may be required to alleviate pericarditis discomfort. However, a recurring pattern may develop in which pericarditis symptoms ease with the corticosteroid, so its use is stopped, but without the drug the pain recurs.

Treatment with corticosteroids should be avoided because of the significant number of side effects and the increased risk of recurrent pericarditis.

## Surgical treatment

When pericarditis recurs, as it sometimes does, your doctor may advise a surgical procedure to remove the pericardium from the heart's surface. This usually ends your symptoms.

In conditions in which the pericardium becomes thickened and stiff, the resulting pericardial constriction may significantly impede the heart's pumping function. Surgical "stripping" of the pericardium (pericardiectomy: removing the pericardium from the surface of the heart) may be required to reverse this problem. Fortunately, you'll rarely notice any disadvantages to being without your pericardium.

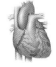

**HEALTHY HEART ♥ TIP**

*Chest X-rays are valuable tools for assessing the health and well-being of your heart. But are they safe?*

*Although you'll receive a small amount of radiation during the procedure, there is virtually no risk to you. In fact, the potential benefits to your health far outweigh any danger. If you're still worried, keep this in mind: Medical X-rays of all kinds account for just over 10 percent of the total radiation exposure for the entire U.S. population. You'll come into contact with about as much radiation as you would on a transcontinental airplane ride.*

# Chapter

# 20 Heart medications

The "Guide to heart medications" (see page 357) contains information about drugs doctors use to treat many aspects of heart disease. For each medication there are specific reasons why it may be especially right (or wrong) for your health problem.

No guide can tell you which, if any, medication is best for you—this can be determined only by your doctor after appropriate evaluation. But the guide does provide useful background information about medications you may be taking, as well as potential alternatives.

## Names of medications

Each medication has several names. The generic name refers to all medications with the same chemical structure, regardless of who manufactures them. Some medications are made by more than one manufacturer; each pharmaceutical company uses a different proprietary (or brand) name.

In general, medications with the same generic name are equal in effectiveness. However, they're usually combined with other substances to make a dosage form such as a tablet, capsule, or liquid (1 milligram of a medicine, for example, is too small to handle conveniently, so it is combined with an inactive substance).

Differences in the inactive substances may affect the way the same generic formula acts. As a result, the dosage form must be the same for the generic form to be considered equivalent to a branded medication. Your doctor may permit a generically equivalent medication. If so, you can discuss your options with your pharmacist. Not all medications are available generically, because they may still be under patent protection.

## Medication dosages

For a medication to be useful, an adequate amount must get into the bloodstream, traveling to the organs and tissues where it produces its effect. Once the medication is ingested, the body (usually the kidneys or liver) begins to eliminate it. If no more medication were taken, eventually there would no longer be any left in the body.

If a sustained effect is desired, an appropriate amount must be taken periodically to maintain an effective level in the body. The size and timing of the dose depends on how much you need to produce the beneficial effect, how well it enters the bloodstream (for example, how much is absorbed from the intestines), and how rapidly the body eliminates it.

Some medications also come in a form that extends their duration, so that doses don't need to be taken as frequently. The names of these "long-acting" or "sustained-release" medications usually have an abbreviation after the brand name, such as LA, SR, XL, or CD.

The specific dose that's best for you must be determined by your doctor. This information isn't included in the guide, because there's no "right" dose for everyone.

## Indications for medications

The reason for giving a medication is the "indication" for its use. Nearly every medication prescribed has been approved for one or more indications by the Food and Drug Administration (FDA) after tests showed it was effective and safe.

Some medications successfully treat indications that haven't been formally authorized by the FDA. A medication endorsed for treating high blood pressure may also effectively control angina and can be used for that purpose, even if it isn't officially approved for that indication.

## Medication combinations

Sometimes you'll need more than one medication to treat a problem. Doctors use some medication combinations frequently enough that pharmaceutical companies have combined them into a single tablet or capsule, giving the combination its own brand name.

## Side effects

Medications may have undesirable effects in some people. Sometimes it's because of an allergy to the medication. Some medications produce unpleasant or even dangerous effects in one person, but not in another. If given in high enough doses (overdose), every medication will produce toxic effects. Then again, what may be an effective dose in one person may be too high for another.

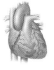

## HEALTHY HEART ♥ TIP

*Exercise is one of the best things you can do for your heart. But if you're out of shape or have heart disease, check with your doctor first. Then remember to:*

- *Exercise regularly. Your cardiovascular risks rise when you alternate intensity and inactivity.*

- *Avoid jarring. Keep your physical exertion continuous with activities like walking or swimming.*

- *Forget competition. You want to exercise, not heighten intensity through competitive sports.*

- *Let your meals settle. Digestion directs blood away from your heart, so wait several hours before exercising.*

- *Can we talk? If you can't talk easily while exercising, you may be overexerting yourself.*

- *Watch the weather. Reduce your speed and distance when it's hot and humid.*

- *Warm up, cool down. Both reduce stress on your heart.*

- *Avoid heavy traffic. Carbon monoxide reduces oxygen supply to your heart.*

- *Listen to your body. If you experience dizziness, nausea, weakness, chest pain or shortness of breath, stop exercising and see your doctor.*

# Precautions and contraindications

For some people, the risk from using a medication will be higher than any benefit; for them, the medication is "contraindicated." Some people are more susceptible than others to adverse effects from certain medications.

The following precautions apply to many or all medications:

- Many medications are potentially risky during pregnancy.

- You can pass some medications on to infants through breast milk.

- The effect of medications must be periodically monitored by appropriate examinations or tests.

- You should take medication as recommended by your doctor and pharmacists (for example, with or without food, at specific times of day).

- When taken together, various medications can interact that can increase, decrease, or change their individual effects. Discuss this possibility with your doctor and pharmacist.

- Do not chew or crush long-acting (slow-release) forms of medications.

- The elderly have a markedly increased risk for adverse reactions and side effects.

- Always complete the course as prescribed.

- Never take antibiotics without first contacting your physician. Your health may be endangered. Also, inappropriate use of antibiotics encourages the development of drug-resistant organisms.

- Ask your doctor if the medication prescribed is available in a convenient, once-a-day preparation.

- Any new symptoms appearing after you start taking a medication may be a side effect. Call your doctor.

# Guide to heart medications

The easy-to-understand tables that follow can be a valuable source of practical information on medications your physician may prescribe for you. You'll find facts on the type and action of a variety of drugs commonly used to manage heart conditions and diseases. Generic names are listed, but you might prefer to look first for the brand name of your medication. Then you can quickly review uses, how the medication is taken, side effects and precautions. The goal is to make you an informed partner in your health care.

## Contents

Medications for angina pectoris

TABLE 1 **MEDICATIONS FOR ANGINA PECTORIS: NITRATES**

(Continued on page 359)

| Medication and action | Generic name | Examples of brand names | Uses | How taken | Specific side effects | Specific precautions |
|---|---|---|---|---|---|---|
| **Nitrates**<br>The nitrates all have the following actions:<br>1. Dilate veins of the body<br>2. Dilate arteries of the body<br>3. Dilate coronary arteries<br>The effects of these actions are:<br>1. Redistribution of some of the volume of blood from the chambers of your heart to the veins of the body. This decreases the amount of stretching of the heart muscle. The less stretch or stress, the less oxygen the heart uses. This is the main way that nitrates lower the heart's demand for oxygen, which is helpful in view of the reduced supply<br>2. Lowering of the resistance the heart encounters in pumping blood into the arteries. This decreases the work load of the heart so that its need for oxygen is reduced<br>3. Increase in the amount of blood that can flow through partially blocked coronary arteries. This enhances the oxygen supply to the heart muscle | Nitroglycerin | *Nitrostat* (tablets) | Shorten angina attack | Let tablet dissolve under tongue at onset of angina, while sitting. If needed, repeat dose twice, 5 minutes between doses | See general side effects listed below<br>Tingling under the tongue is normal | Loses potency 3-6 months after container is opened<br>Remove cotton plug and leave out<br>Keep container tightly closed<br>If angina persists for 15 minutes, go to doctor or emergency room |
| | | | Prevent anticipated angina attack | One tablet under tongue at onset of activity predicted to cause angina | | |
| | | *Nitrolingual* (spray) | Shorten angina attack | 1 or 2 sprays on or under tongue at onset of angina, while sitting. If needed, repeat dose twice, 5 minutes between doses | See general side effects listed below | Do not shake container<br>Do not inhale<br>If angina persists for 15 minutes, go to doctor or emergency room |
| | | | Prevent anticipated angina attack | 1 or 2 sprays on or under tongue at onset of activity expected to cause angina | | |
| | | *Nitrogard* (buccal [extended release] tablets) | Prevent angina attacks | Place tablet between upper lip and gum, or between cheek and gum. Allow to dissolve over 3-5 hours | See general side effects listed below | Do not chew or swallow |
| | | *Nitrol* (ointment)<br>*Nitro-Bid* (ointment) | Prevent angina attacks | Spread (do not rub in) the prescribed amount of ointment in thin layer on hairless area of skin at prescribed schedule. Use applicator paper that is provided | See general side effects listed below<br>Skin irritation | Clean off previous ointment before reapplying<br>Rotate application sites to avoid irritation |

| Medication and action | Generic name | Examples of brand names | Uses | How taken | Specific side effects | Specific precautions |
|---|---|---|---|---|---|---|
| **Nitrates** (cont.) | | *Nitro-Bid* (capsules) | Prevent angina attacks | Swallow tablet at prescribed dose and schedule | See general side effects listed below | Do not stop taking abruptly (to avoid rebound) |
| | | *Minitran* *Nitrodisc* *Nitro-Dur* *Transderm-Nitro* *Deponit* (transdermal patches) *Nitro-Bid IV* *Nitrol IV* *Nitrostat IV* *Tridil* | Prevent angina attacks | Apply skin patch for prescribed duration on hairless skin | See general side effects listed below Skin irritation | Rotate application sites to avoid irritation Avoid skin with nicks or cuts Remove patch for 6-8 hours before replacing (to avoid tolerance) |
| | Nitroglycerin (intravenous) | | Manage heart attack | Given by vein | See general side effects listed below | |
| | Isosorbide dinitrate | *Isordil* (tablets) *Sorbitrate* (tablets) *Dilatrate* (tablets) | Prevent angina attacks Reduce work load of heart | Swallow tablet or capsule at prescribed schedule with full glass of water on empty stomach | See general side effects listed below | Do not stop taking abruptly (to avoid rebound) |
| | Isosorbide mononitrate | *Imdur* *Ismo* *Monoket* | | | | |
| | Pentaerythritol tetranitrate | *Peritrate* (tablets) | Prevent angina attacks | Swallow tablet at prescribed schedule with full glass of water on empty stomach | See general side effects listed below | Do not stop taking abruptly (to avoid rebound) |
| | Erythritol tetranitrate | *Cardilate* (tablets) | Prevent angina attacks | Swallow tablet at prescribed schedule with full glass of water on empty stomach | See general side effects listed below | Do not stop taking abruptly (to avoid rebound) |

General side effects: Headache, dizziness, light-headedness, fast pulse, nausea.

General precautions: After chewing chewable tablets, hold in your mouth for 2 minutes before swallowing.

Alcohol may worsen some side effects (dizziness, light-headedness).

Some side effects (headache) generally lessen after several days of taking the medication.

A rebound effect (sudden worsening of angina or a heart attack) may occur if nitrate use is suddenly stopped. A tapered withdrawal is recommended.

The effect of nitrates diminishes if a constant amount is in the bloodstream all the time ("tolerance"). Skin patches should be removed for a period of time each day.

**Beta-blockers** (see Table 2).   **Calcium channel blockers** (see Table 3).

This list is not comprehensive and does not represent an endorsement of any product listed.

# TABLE 2 MEDICATIONS FOR ANGINA PECTORIS: BETA-BLOCKERS

| Medication and action | Generic name | Examples of brand names | Uses | How taken | Specific side effects | Specific precautions |
|---|---|---|---|---|---|---|
| **Beta-blockers**<br><br>The beta-blockers all have the following actions:<br>1. Slow the heartbeat<br>2. Decrease blood pressure<br>3. Reduce the contraction strength of the heart muscle<br><br>The effects of these actions are:<br>1. Reduction of your heart's need for oxygen by reducing the number of times it beats per minute both at rest and during exertion. This is the main way that beta-blockers lower your heart's demand for oxygen, which is helpful in view of the reduced supply<br>2. Lowering of the pressure your heart must pump against to push blood into the arteries. The lower the pressure, the less oxygen is required | Propranolol<br>Metoprolol<br>Nadolol<br>Atenolol<br>Acebutolol<br>Betaxolol<br>Labetalol<br><br>Penbutolol<br>Pindolol<br>Timolol<br>Carteolol (tablets, capsules)<br>Bisoprolol<br>Sotalol | *Inderal*<br>*Lopressor*<br>*Corgard*<br>*Tenormin*<br>*Sectral*<br>*Kerlone*<br>*Normodyne*<br>*Trandate*<br><br>*Levatol*<br>*Visken*<br>*Blocadren*<br>*Cartrol*<br><br>*Zebeta*<br>*Betapace* | Prevent angina attacks<br>Lower blood pressure<br>Slow or convert fast heart rhythms<br>Lower risk of second heart attack<br><br>Protect aorta | Swallow tablet at prescribed dose and schedule | Abnormal slowing of the heartbeat<br>Fatigue or weakness<br>Lower sexual ability<br>Light-headedness<br>Restless sleep<br>Depression | Asthma, bronchitis, emphysema: may provoke wheezing and breathlessness<br>Claudication: may worsen circulation<br>Heart failure: may worsen heart pumping strength and provoke shortness of breath and edema<br>Diabetes: may lower blood glucose (sugar) or make hypoglycemic episodes (insulin reactions) harder to detect and respond to |
| 3. Lowering of the squeezing strength of your heart's contraction. This lowers the oxygen use by the heart muscle<br>4. Lowering of blood pressure in people with hypertension<br>5. Helping normalize some types of fast or irregular heart rhythms | Intravenous:<br>Propranolol<br>Metoprolol<br>Atenolol<br>Esmolol | *Inderal*<br>*Lopressor*<br>*Tenormin*<br>*Brevibloc* | Rapid control of high blood pressure<br>Rapid control of fast heartbeats<br>To continue beta-blocker in hospitalized patient who cannot take medication by mouth<br>For early treatment of heart attack, to lower chances of further damage | Administered by vein | | Same as above |

**Nitrates** (see Table 1). **Calcium channel blockers** (see Table 3). This list is not comprehensive and does not represent an endorsement of any product listed.

TABLE 3 **MEDICATIONS FOR ANGINA PECTORIS: CALCIUM CHANNEL BLOCKERS** (Continued on page 362)

| Medication and action | Generic name | Examples of brand names | Uses | How taken | Specific side effects | Specific precautions |
|---|---|---|---|---|---|---|
| **Calcium channel blockers**<br><br>The calcium blockers all inhibit the ability of calcium atoms to enter heart muscle and blood vessel muscle cells. This results in the following effects (although each calcium blocker differs from the others in how much it produces each effect):<br>1. Reduction in the heart rate, thus reducing its demand for oxygen<br>2. Lowering of the squeezing strength of the heart's contraction. This lowers the oxygen use by the heart muscle<br>3. Decreasing of blood pressure and the resistance to blood flow through the arteries. This makes the heart's task of pumping blood easier and reduces its need for oxygen<br>4. Dilation of coronary arteries so that blood flow is enhanced. This increases the amount of oxygen delivered to heart muscle<br>5. Helping normalize some types of fast or irregular heart rhythms | Verapamil | *Calan*<br>*Isoptin*<br>*Verelan* | Prevent angina attacks<br>Lower blood pressure<br>Slow or normalize certain fast heart rhythms | Swallow tablet at prescribed dose and schedule | Excessive slowing of heartbeat<br>Excessive lowering of blood pressure<br>Congestive heart failure if heart contraction already weak<br>Constipation | Caution in people with:<br>Abnormally slow heartbeat<br>Weakened heart contraction<br>Low blood pressure<br>Interactions with other medications |
| | Verapamil (intravenous) | *Calan*<br>*Isoptin* | Urgent control of certain rapid heart rhythms | Given by vein | Same as above | Same as above |
| | Nifedipine | *Procardia*<br>*Adalat* | Prevent angina attacks<br>Lower blood pressure | Swallow tablet at prescribed dose and schedule | Excessive lowering of blood pressure<br>Headache<br>Leg edema<br>Flushing sensation | Caution if blood pressure is low<br>Interactions with other medications |
| | Nicardipine | *Cardene* | Prevent angina attacks<br>Lower blood pressure | Swallow tablet at prescribed dose and schedule | Excessive lowering of blood pressure<br>Headache<br>Leg edema<br>Flushing sensation | Caution if blood pressure is low<br>Interactions with other medications |
| | Diltiazem | *Cardizem*<br>*Dilacor* | Prevent angina attacks<br>Lower blood pressure | Swallow tablet at prescribed dose and schedule | Excessive lowering of blood pressure<br>Excessive slowing of heartbeat<br>Rash | Caution if blood pressure is low<br>Interactions with other medications |
| | Isradipine<br>Mibefradil | *DynaCirc*<br>*Posicor* | Prevent angina attacks<br>Lower blood pressure | Swallow capsule at prescribed dose and schedule | Excessive lowering of blood pressure<br>Headache<br>Leg edema<br>Flushing sensation | Caution if blood pressure is low<br>Interactions with other medications |

## TABLE 3 MEDICATIONS FOR ANGINA PECTORIS: CALCIUM CHANNEL BLOCKERS (Continued from page 361)

| Medication and action | Generic name | Examples of brand names | Uses | How taken | Specific side effects | Specific precautions |
|---|---|---|---|---|---|---|
| **Calcium channel blockers** (cont.) | Felodipine | *Plendil* | Prevent angina attacks<br>Lower blood pressure | Swallow tablet at prescribed dose and schedule | Excessive lowering of blood pressure<br>Headache<br>Flushing sensation<br>Fast heartbeat<br>Leg edema | Caution if blood pressure is low<br>Interactions with other medications |
| | Bepridil | *Vascor* | Prevent angina attacks | Swallow tablet at prescribed dose and schedule | Excessive lowering of blood pressure<br>Headache | Caution if blood pressure is low |
| | Amlodipine | *Norvasc* | Lower blood pressure | | | |
| | Nisoldipine | *Sular* | Lower blood pressure | | Nervousness, tremor<br>Nausea<br>Rhythm problems | |

**Nitrates** (see Table 1). **Beta-blockers** (see Table 2).   This list is not comprehensive and does not represent an endorsement of any product listed.

## TABLE 4 MEDICATIONS FOR HEART ATTACK

| Medication and action | Generic name | Examples of brand names | Uses | How taken | Specific side effects | Specific precautions |
|---|---|---|---|---|---|---|
| **Thrombolytics**<br><br>Thrombolytic agents are medications that promote the dissolving of clots<br><br>They are used to restore blood flow through vessels that are obstructed by a blood clot (thrombus) | Urokinase | *Abbokinase* | Dissolve clots in arteries to the lung (pulmonary embolism)<br>Dissolve clots in coronary arteries during heart attack | Given by vein | Bleeding, including internal bleeding, bleeding into brain, bleeding from sites of injury or incisions | Avoid if recent injury or operation, bleeding tendency, severe high blood pressure |
| | Tissue plasminogen activators | | | | | |
| | Alteplase<br>Reteplase | *Activase*<br>*Retavase* | Same as above | Given by vein | Same as above | Same as above |
| | Streptokinase | *Kabikinase*<br>*Streptase* | Same as above | Given by vein | Same as above, and rare allergic reactions | Same as above, and avoid if streptokinase or anistreplase previously received |
| | Anistreplase | *Eminase* | Same as above | Given by vein | Same as above, and rare allergic reactions | Same as above, and avoid if streptokinase or anistreplase previously received |

**Nitrates** (see Table 1). **Beta-blockers** (see Table 2). This list is not comprehensive and does not represent an endorsement of any product listed.

TABLE 5   **LIPID-LOWERING MEDICATIONS**                           **(Continued on page 364)**

| Medication and action | Generic name | Examples of brand names | Uses | How taken | Specific side effects | Specific precautions |
|---|---|---|---|---|---|---|
| **Bile acid sequestrants**<br><br>These medications chemically bind to bile acids in the intestine. Bile acids are made by the body from cholesterol. They normally pass from the liver into the intestine, but a portion returns into the bloodstream through the intestinal wall. These medications do not permit them to return, so more cholesterol is used to make more bile acids, which in turn are also excreted. Eventually, the body's pool of cholesterol decreases<br><br>Gemfibrozil<br><br>This medication reduces triglyceride and VLDL cholesterol, and raises HDL cholesterol. The way it does this is not well understood<br><br>HMG-CoA reductase inhibitor<br><br>This medication enhances your body's ability to rid itself of cholesterol | Cholestyramine | *Questran* (powder)<br>*Prevalite* (powder) | Lower cholesterol | Mix powder with beverage (4-6 oz)—it will not actually dissolve — and drink all the liquid. Mix with other liquid foods if desired (soup, cereal, fruit)<br>Eat it like a candy bar—chew thoroughly | Constipation<br>Abdominal pain and upset<br><br>Constipation<br>Abdominal pain and upset | Avoid taking at same time as other medications<br>Take other medications 1 hour before or 6 hours after taking this medication<br>Double-check possibility of interactions with other medications |
| | Colestipol | *Colestid* (granules) | Lower cholesterol | Mix powder with beverage (4-6 oz) —it will not actually dissolve—and drink all the liquid. Mix with other liquid foods if desired (soup, cereal, fruit) | Constipation<br>Abdominal pain and upset | Other cardiovascular medications that may be affected: digitalis, anticoagulants, propranolol, thiazide, diuretics<br>Do not take as dry powder |
| | Gemfibrozil | *Lopid* | Lower triglycerides<br>Raise HDL cholesterol | Swallow tablet at prescribed dose and schedule | Stomach upset<br>Nausea, diarrhea<br>Rash<br>Muscle pain, weakness<br>Liver function problems<br>Dizziness<br>Blurred vision | Do not take lovastatin while taking this medication. The risk of muscle inflammation increases |
| | Lovastatin<br>Pravastatin<br>Simvastatin<br><br>Atorvastatin<br>Cerivastatin<br>Fluvastatin | *Mevacor*<br>*Pravachol*<br>*Zocor*<br><br>*Lipitor*<br>*Baycol*<br>*Lescol* | Lower LDL cholesterol<br>Lower triglycerides<br>Raise HDL cholesterol (slightly) | Swallow tablet at prescribed dose and schedule | Blurred vision<br>Muscle pain, weakness<br>Stomach upset<br>Liver function problems<br>Insomnia<br>Headache | Do not take gemfibrozil or nicotinic acid (niacin) while taking this medication unless prescribed by a physician. The risk of muscle inflammation increases<br>Other medications that may interact include cyclosporine, other immunosuppressants, warfarin, clofibrate<br>Blood tests for liver function should be performed every 4-6 weeks for the first year<br>Annual eye examination may be advisable |

TABLE 5 **LIPID-LOWERING MEDICATIONS**　　　　　　　　(Continued from page 363)

| Medication and action | Generic name | Examples of brand names | Uses | How taken | Specific side effects | Specific precautions |
|---|---|---|---|---|---|---|
| **Bile acid sequestrants** (cont.)<br><br>Niacin (nicotinic acid)<br>This medication reduces your body's ability to manufacture VLDL cholesterol<br><br>Fenofibrate | Niacin | *Nia-Bid*<br>*Niacels*<br>*Nicobid*<br>*Nicolar*<br>*Slo-Niacin*<br>*Nicotinex* (elixir) | Lower LDL cholesterol<br>Lower triglycerides<br>Raise HDL cholesterol | Swallow tablet (or elixir) at pre-scribed dose and schedule<br>Do not break or crush long-acting forms | Flushing, warm feeling<br>Headache<br>Stomach upset<br>Liver function problems<br>Itching | Side effects can be minimized by starting at low doses, taking with food, and building up to recommended dose |
| | Fenofibrate | *Tricor* | Lower triglycerides | Swallow capsule at prescribed dose and schedule | Stomach upset<br>Rash | Persistent flushing can be reduced by taking 1 aspirin one-half hour before dose<br>Blood tests for liver function should be performed occasionally |
| Clofibrate<br>This medication reduces triglycerides and, to a lesser extent, cholesterol (when triglycerides are also high), but the way it works is not understood | Clofibrate | *Atromid-S* | Lower triglycerides<br>Lower cholesterol | Swallow capsule at prescribed dose and schedule | Gallstones<br>Kidney problems<br>Stomach upset<br>Muscle pain, weakness<br>Pancreatitis<br>Liver function problems | Periodic blood tests for liver function, muscle inflammation (creatine kinase), and blood count are advisable |
| Dextrothyroxine<br>This medication increases your body's ability to break down and remove cholesterol, but the mechanism is unclear | Dextrothyroxine | *Choloxin* | Lower cholesterol | Swallow tablet at prescribed dose and schedule | Heart attack<br>Angina<br>Hyperactive thyroid | Can interact with other medica-tions, especially digitalis and anti-coagulants<br>Avoid if heart dis-ease is already present |

Dietary measures should be attempted first except in severe cases.

Continue to follow dietary recommendations while taking medications.

For all medications, lipid values should be checked within 3 months to determine the degree of success and to decide whether a change in dose or medication is needed.

This list is not comprehensive and does not represent an endorsement of any product listed.

TABLE 6 **MEDICATIONS FOR HIGH BLOOD PRESSURE**

| Medication and action | Generic name | Examples of brand names | Uses | How taken | Specific side effects | Specific precautions |
|---|---|---|---|---|---|---|
| **Centrally acting agents**<br><br>These medications affect control centers in the brain that decrease blood pressure | Methyldopa<br>Guanfacine<br>Guanabenz<br>Clonidine | *Aldomet*<br>*Tenex*<br>*Wytensin*<br>*Catapres* | Decrease blood pressure | Swallow tablet at prescribed dose and schedule | Fluid rentention (edema)<br>Fever<br>Insomnia<br>Lower blood pressure<br>Dizziness<br>Liver function or blood cell count abnormalities<br>Dry mouth | May need to stand slowly from lying position to avoid sudden blood pressure drop and faintness<br>Do not stop taking abruptly (sudden excess rebound in high blood pressure) |
| | Clonidine (skin patch) | *Catapres-TTS* | | Apply skin patch at prescribed schedule | Drowsiness<br>Itching (skin patch) | Double-check possibility of interactions with other medications |
| **Direct-acting vasodilators**<br><br>These medications cause the muscle in the walls of blood vessels to relax | Hydralazine | *Apresoline* | Decrease blood pressure<br>Reduce work load of heart | Swallow tablet at prescribed dose and schedule | Low blood pressure<br>Dizziness<br>Lupus syndrome (blisters, chest pain, joint pain, weakness)<br>Diarrhea<br>Headache | May need to stand slowly from lying position to avoid sudden blood pressure drop and faintness |
| | Minoxidil | *Loniten* | Decrease blood pressure | Swallow tablet at prescribed dose and schedule | Fast heartbeat<br>Flushing<br>Fluid retention (edema)<br>Excessive hair growth | Check resting heart rate periodically<br>Check weight (to assess fluid gain) |
| **Peripherally acting agents**<br><br>These medications exert their effects on the nerves of the body that are involved in blood pressure regulation | Guanadrel<br>Guanethidine<br>Mecamylamine<br>Prazosin<br>Rauwolfia alkaloids<br><br>Terazosin<br>Doxazosin | *Hylorel*<br>*Ismelin*<br>*Inversine*<br>*Minipress*<br>*Harmonyl*<br>*Raudixin*<br>*Rauzide*<br>*Serpasil*<br>*Hytrin*<br>*Cardura* | Decrease blood pressure | Swallow tablet or capsule at prescribed dose and schedule | Fluid retention (edema)<br>Low blood pressure<br>Dizziness<br>Drowsiness<br>Difficulty ejaculating<br>Mental depression<br>Stomach and bowel disturbances | Double-check possibility of interactions with medications<br>May need to stand slowly from lying position to avoid sudden blood pressure drop and faintness |

**Beta-blockers** (see Table 2). **Calcium blockers** (see Table 3). **Diuretics** (see Table 7). **Angiotensin converting enzyme inhibitors** (see Table 7). This list is not comprehensive and does not represent an endorsement of any product listed.

TABLE 7 **MEDICATIONS FOR HEART FAILURE** (Continued on page 367)

| Medication and action | Generic name | Examples of brand names | Uses | How taken | Specific side effects | Specific precautions |
|---|---|---|---|---|---|---|
| **Angiotensin converting enzyme inhibitors** (ACE inhibitors) These medications dilate arteries and decrease resistance to the flow of blood being pumped from the heart. The result is lower blood pressure and easier pumping for the heart | Captopril Moexipril Enalapril Lisinopril Quinapril Benazepril Fosinopril Ramipril Trandolapril | *Capoten* *Univasc* *Vasotec* *Zestril, Prinivil* *Accupril* *Lotensin* *Monopril* *Altace* *Mavik* | Decreased blood pressure Reduce work load of heart | Swallow tablet at prescribed dose and schedule | Low blood pressure Rash Elevated potassium Persistent dry cough Abnormal sense of taste Protein in urine Stomach upset | Avoid taking simultaneously with potassium-sparing diuretics (below) Use with caution in diabetes or with kidney problems |
| **Diuretics** These medications promote the removal of water by the kidneys. This decreases blood pressure and decreases edema | Chlorthalidone Chlorothiazide Hydrochloro-thiazide Methyclothiazide Metolazone | *Hygroton* *Thalitone* *Diuril* *Esidrix* *HydroDIURIL* *Oretic* *Aquatensen* *Enduron* *Diulo, Zaroxolyn* | Milder diuretics for: Decreasing blood pressure Gentle fluid reduction | Swallow tablet at prescribed dose and schedule | Low potassium High calcium Low sodium Elevated blood glucose (sugar) Risk of gout Stomach upset Pancreatitis | Check potassium, sodium, calcium, glucose periodically |
| | Amiloride Spironolactone Triamterene Bendroflumethi-azide Benzthiazide Indapamide Quinethazone Polythiazide Trichlormethi-azide Hydroflumcthi-azide | *Midamor* *Aldactone* *Dyrenium* | As above, but without loss of potassium in the urine ("potas-sium-sparing") | Swallow tablet at prescribed dose and schedule | Male breast enlargement (with spirono-lactone) Elevated potassium Stomach upset | Check potassium, sodium, calcium, glucose periodically Avoid simultane-ous use of ACE inhibitors (may increase potas-sium markedly) |

**Combination medications**

| | | | | | | |
|---|---|---|---|---|---|---|
| | Hydrochloro-thiazide +Amiloride +Spironolactone +Triamterene | *Moduretic* *Aldactazide* *Dyazide,* *Maxzide* | As above, but with reduced loss of potas-sium in the urine | Swallow tablet at prescribed dose and schedule | Male breast enlargement (with spirono-lactone) Variable potassium Stomach upset | Check potassium, sodium, calcium, glucose periodically Avoid simultane-ous use of ACE inhibitors (may increase potas-sium markedly) |

TABLE 7 **MEDICATIONS FOR HEART FAILURE** (Continued from page 366)

| Medication and action | Generic name | Examples of brand names | Uses | How taken | Specific side effects | Specific precautions |
|---|---|---|---|---|---|---|
| **Diuretics** (cont.) | Bumetanide<br>Ethacrynic acid<br>Furosemide (tablet or intravenous)<br><br>Torsemide | *Bumex*<br>*Edecrin*<br>*Lasix*<br><br><br>*Demadex* | Potent diuretics for vigorous reduction of excess fluid | Swallow tablet at prescribed dose and schedule<br>Administer by vein | Excess fluid output<br>Low blood pressure<br>Low potassium<br>Low calcium<br>Low sodium<br>Elevated blood glucose (sugar)<br>Risk of gout<br>Stomach upset<br>Decreased hearing<br>Muscle cramps | Double-check possibility of interactions with other medications<br>Check potassium, sodium, calcium, glucose periodically |
| **Inotropic agents**<br>These medications increase the squeezing strength of the heart muscle. The effect is to increase the amount of blood the heart is able to pump through the circulation. | Digitalis<br>Digoxin<br><br>Digitoxin<br>Digoxin (intravenous) | <br>*Lanoxin*<br>*Lanoxicaps*<br><br>*Crystodigin*<br>*Lanoxin* | Increase pumping strength of heart<br>Help control certain rhythm disorders | Swallow tablet at prescribed dose and schedule<br>Administer by vein | Stomach upset<br>Loss of appetite<br>Visual disturbance<br>Slow or irregular heartbeat | Avoid low potassium level – promotes side effects<br>Check for drug interactions, particularly drugs that can cause digitalis level to become too high, especially verapamil, quinidine |
| | Dopamine (intravenous)<br>Dobutamine (intravenous)<br>Amrinone (intravenous) | *Intropin*<br><br>*Dobutrex*<br><br>*Inocor* | Increase pumping strength of heart | Administer by vein | Rhythm disturbances<br>Nausea<br>Headache<br>Chest pain<br>Cold hands and feet | |

**Nitrates** (see Table 1). **Direct-acting vasodilators** (see Table 6).
This list is not comprehensive and does not represent an endorsement of any product listed.

TABLE 8 **MEDICATIONS FOR RHYTHM DISORDERS** (Continued on page 369)

| Medication and action | Generic name | Examples of brand names | Uses | How taken | Specific side effects | Specific precautions |
|---|---|---|---|---|---|---|
| **Antiarrhythmic agents**<br><br>Medications for fast or irregular heartbeats – alter the way in which electrical currents flow through the conduction system and heart muscle. The change in the electrical characteristics of the heart may reduce the ability of a heart rhythm abnormality to begin or continue | Quinidine | *Cardioquin*<br>*Cin-Quin*<br>*Duraquin*<br>*Quinaglute*<br>*Quinalan*<br>*Quinidex*<br>*Quinora* | Help control various rhythm disorders | Swallow pill at prescribed dose and schedule, or administer by vein | Diarrhea<br>Dizziness<br>Stomach upset<br>Ringing in ears<br>Passing out | Avoid if known sensitivity to quinine<br>Digoxin dose will need to be adjusted because quinidine causes digoxin levels in blood to rise |
| | Procainamide (tablet, capsule, intravenous) | *Procan SR*<br>*Pronestyl*<br>*Pronestyl-SR* | | Oral | Lupus syndrome (blisters, chest pain, joint pain, weakness) | Avoid if known sensitivity to procaine |
| | Disopyramide | *Norpace*<br>*Norpace CR* | | Oral | Blurry vision<br>Urinary obstruction (men)<br>Dry mouth<br>Congestive heart failure | Elderly patients may be more prone to side effects<br>Caution if milk sensitivity – tablets contain lactose (milk sugar) |
| | Lidocaine (intravenous) | *Xylocaine* | | Injection | Confusion<br>Seizures | |
| | Phenytoin | *Dilantin* | | Oral/injection | Overgrowth of gums<br>Drowsiness | |
| | Mexiletine | *Mexitil* | | | Stomach upset<br>Trembling, unsteadiness | |
| | Tocainide | *Tonocard* | | | Stomach upset<br>Trembling, unsteadiness<br>Blood cell abnormalities | |
| | Flecainide | *Tambocor* | | | Congestive heart failure<br>Dizziness, visual disturbance | Avoid after recent heart attack<br>Avoid in heart failure |
| | Moricizine | *Ethmozine* | | | Stomach upset<br>Dizziness, headache | |
| | Propafenone | *Rythmol* | | | Bitter taste<br>Stomach upset<br>Weakness<br>Dizziness | |
| | Bretylium (intravenous) | *Bretylol* | | | Low blood pressure | |

| Medication and action | Generic name | Examples of brand names | Uses | How taken | Specific side effects | Specific precautions |
|---|---|---|---|---|---|---|
| **Antiarrhythmic agents** (cont.)<br><br>Medications for slow heartbeats—act by affecting the nervous system's control of heart rate | Amiodarone | *Cordarone* | Help control various rhythm disorders | | Bluish skin discoloration<br>Overactive or underactive thyroid<br>Lung scarring (fibrosis)<br>Nerve damage<br>Spots in corneas of eyes<br>Liver abnormalities<br>Stomach upset | Digoxin dose will need to be adjusted because amiodarone causes digoxin levels in blood to rise<br>Periodically have blood tests and chest X-ray |
| | Adenosine (intravenous)<br><br>Ibutilide | *Adenocard*<br><br>*Corvert* | For rapid treatment of fast heartbeats originating from the upper parts of the heart (atria and atrioventricular node) | Rapidly injected into a vein<br><br>Rapidly injected into a vein | Chest heaviness<br>Flushing<br>Nausea<br>Headache<br>Shortness of breath/asthma<br>Slow heartbeat<br>Dizziness<br>(All side effects are very brief) | Very short-acting medication<br>Effects enhanced by dipyridamole (see Table 9)<br>Effects reduced by caffeine and certain asthma medications (theophyllines) |
| | Atropine (intravenous) | | For temporary acceleration of certain slow heartbeats | Administered by vein | Rapid heartbeat<br>Mouth dryness<br>Blurred vision<br>Difficulty urinating | Avoid in glaucoma, urinary obstruction |
| | Isoproterenol (intravenous) | *Isuprel* | For temporary acceleration of certain slow heartbeats | Administered by vein | Rapid heartbeat<br>Blood pressure swings | Avoid in angina |

**Beta-blockers** (see Table 2).   **Calcium channel blockers** (see Table 3).

Many antiarrhythmic medications can potentially cause worse rhythm disorders; careful monitoring is necessary.

This list is not comprehensive and does not represent an endorsement of any product listed.

TABLE 9   **MEDICATIONS FOR VASCULAR PROBLEMS**

(Continued on page 371)

| Medication and action | Generic name | Examples of brand names | Uses | How taken | Specific side effects | Specific precautions |
|---|---|---|---|---|---|---|
| **Anticoagulants** These medications reduce the ability of the blood to clot. They act by reducing proteins involved in blood clotting (coagulation) or changing the way they function | Warfarin Dicumarol | *Coumadin Panwarfin* | Prevent blood clotting in high-risk situations such as: Mechanical heart valves Dilated cardiomyopathy Atrial fibrillation Previous blood clot problems | Swallow tablet at prescribed dose and schedule | Bleeding, such as: Internal bleeding into gastrointestinal tract Excess bleeding after cuts Increased nose or gum bleeds Bleeding into joints or muscle Blood in urine Easy bruising Bluish discoloration of toes | Use with caution in liver disease Numerous medications can affect activity of anticoagulants – check with doctor |
| | Heparin Ardeparin Dalteparin Danaparoid Enoxaparin Madroparin Tinzaparin | *Normiflo Fragmin Orgaran Lovenox* | Prevent blood clotting in high-risk situations, such as: All of above In certain hospitalized, injured, or bed-bound patients In heart attack or unstable angina After thrombolytic therapy Pulmonary embolism Compared with warfarin, begins acting faster when medication is started, and effect ends faster when medication is stopped. Often used in place of warfarin, or while beginning warfarin, in hospitalized patients | Administer by vein or by injection under the skin Injection | Bleeding, such as: Internal bleeding into gastrointestinal tract Excess bleeding after cuts Increased nose or gum bleeds Bleeding into joints or muscle Blood in urine Easy bruising Abnormal reduction of blood platelets | Anticoagulant effect must be checked regularly with prothrombin time blood test so that dose can be adjusted if necessary |

TABLE 9   **MEDICATIONS FOR VASCULAR PROBLEMS**                                 (Continued from page 370)

| Medication and action | Generic name | Examples of brand names | Uses | How taken | Specific side effects | Specific precautions |
|---|---|---|---|---|---|---|
| **Antiplatelet medications**<br><br>These medications inhibit the normal function of platelets (blood cells involved in clotting) | Aspirin | | Reduce risk of blood clots, which might contribute to heart attack, stroke, unstable angina | Swallow tablet at prescribed dose and schedule<br>One aspirin (325 mg) or one baby aspirin (81 mg) daily is generally enough for antiplatelet effects | Stomach irritation<br>Increased chance of bleeding or bruising | Generally avoid using with an anticoagulant |
| | Dipyridamole | *Persantine* | Reduce risk of blood clots, which might contribute to heart attack, stroke, unstable angina | Swallow tablet at prescribed dose and schedule<br>Usually not used alone; usually recommended with aspirin or anticoagulant | Upset stomach<br>Increased chest pain<br>Dizziness | |
| | Clopidogrel | *Plavix* | Augment blood flow in blood vessels of the limbs with atherosclerotic blockages | Swallow tablet at prescribed dose and schedule | Irregular heartbeat<br>Stomach upset | Caution if known sensitivity to caffeine or theophylline medications |
| **Hemorrheologic agents**<br><br>This type of medication is intended to affect the way blood flows by decreasing its viscosity ("thickness") and by making red blood cells more flexible. The effect is to make the blood flow through blocked and narrowed vessels more easily | Anagrelide | *Agrylin* | | Swallow capsule at prescribed dose and schedule | Headache<br>Diarrhea | |
| | Ticlopidine | *Ticlid* | | Swallow tablet at prescribed dose and schedule | Diarrhea<br>Rash | |
| | Pentoxifylline<br>Cilostazol | *Trental*<br>*Pletal* | | Swallow tablet at prescribed dose and schedule | | |

This list is not comprehensive and does not represent an endorsement of any product listed.

# Chapter

# 21 Assessing your options

How you deal with heart disease will involve an examination of your own beliefs about health and your quality of life, as well as thorough discussions with your doctors, family, and spiritual advisers. You must ultimately decide your own fate, even though a whole host of options lies before you.

## Weighing the pros and cons

Most medical decisions, whether choosing a test, interpreting the result, or selecting a treatment, involve weighing the pros and cons. You can look at "risk" and "benefit" factors or at "costs" and "benefits," a perspective that's become increasingly important as society grows more concerned about health care.

Modern medicine regularly faces these complex decisions, from escalating health care costs to malpractice lawsuits to ethical dilemmas, such as how to best care for terminally ill people.

But they're also involved in the day-to-day practice of medicine. Their patients want to know: "What are the odds a complication will occur from this procedure?" "How serious might the complication be?" "Will I benefit enough to make the risk worth it?"

Answers to these questions require knowing the following:

- The types of complications that could occur
- The chances of each complication occurring
- The procedure's goals
- The chances of successfully achieving these goals

All of these components should be addressed in discussions with your doctor.

## One example

Consider, for example, the factors that would affect your risks and benefits in a coronary artery catheterization:

- Chances the test will give useful information: *Do the symptoms, examination, and tests point to a problem that requires catheterization to solve?*
- Your stability as a patient: *Is the catheterization being done on a scheduled basis or in the midst of a heart attack?*

- Existence of other problems: *Do you show evidence of peripheral vascular disease or kidney disease? The former may increase difficulty in inserting and advancing a catheter, whereas patients with chronic renal disease will be more sensitive to the effects of radiographic contrast agents on kidney function.*

- Your general medical status: *Are you robust or frail?*

- The severity of the problem being investigated (this may not be known ahead of time): *Is there severe blockage of all the coronary arteries, or minimal blockage in one?*

- The medical team's skill and experience: *Does the team do hundreds of catheterizations each year, or dozens?*

- The availability of support services: *If complications develop, are there ways to deal with them effectively (that is, coronary artery bypass), if necessary?*

Remember, coronary catheterization doesn't generate all your risks. You may miss out on an effective treatment if the coronary catheterization isn't done. The risk of dying during a coronary catheterization is very small—less than 1 chance in 1,000. The risk of dying due to a blockage of the left main coronary artery is about 1 chance in 10 every year, unless you undergo a coronary bypass operation.

Unfortunately, if a person with left main coronary blockage doesn't have a coronary catheterization, the blockage won't be discovered and an operation won't be done. That obviously makes not doing the catheterization the highest risk, and illustrates why it's important to review the possible risks and benefits of all courses of action before undergoing a procedure.

When you undergo any procedure, you take the risks "up front." On the other hand, not doing it may be more risky in the long term.

When determining the value of a medical test or procedure (again, in terms of expense, inconvenience, discomfort, and risk) you should also consider people who care for you (such as friends and family) and society's values. Many major hospitals have chaplains trained to help people reflect on and clarify their values.

Should a patient try everything possible, even expensive and uncomfortable procedures, to extend life in the elderly and terminally ill, or is there more value in seeking comfort and dignity by "supportive" care? There is no single correct answer. Only candid discussions with family and doctor will achieve the appropriate medical care under the circumstances.

Diseases of the heart are often matters of life and death. Evaluating and treating heart disease, therefore, frequently become fateful decisions. Although most doctors and patients direct their attention to saving and enhancing life, there may come a time when it's best to limit these efforts.

This may mean giving instructions for no resuscitation or only limited resuscitation in case of a cardiac arrest. Most doctors with very ill hospitalized patients will seek the

## Deciding on coronary catheterization

**Reasons to do coronary catheterization (benefits)**

- Determine whether coronary blockage is present
- Determine the severity of coronary blockage
- Determine the location of the coronary blockage
- Determine whether bypass operation or balloon angioplasty can be done

**Reasons to avoid coronary catheterization (risks and costs)**

- Small chance of serious complication
- Other tests may give adequate information
- Minor discomfort
- Expense

patient's and family's guidance on these issues; if not, you or your family should bring up the subject. Ideally, families should discuss these serious matters before they occur. Having a "living will" (also called an "advance directive") is one option that can provide guidelines beforehand, and it should be considered by everyone regardless of age.

Whenever you're admitted to a hospital, the Patient Self-determination Act says that you must be asked if you have an advance directive. Think about it before the need arises. A serious component will be to specify who should make decisions for you if you're incapacitated.

## Should you participate in medical research?

Medical knowledge continually evolves and expands. New medications, medical devices, operations, and procedures come from years of testing and refining.

When developing any new heart disease treatment, researchers want the new remedy to provide benefits without undue risk. And they want to be sure it's an improvement on what already exists. How do they do this?

The U.S. Food and Drug Administration (FDA) regulates all developing medications and medical devices. The FDA requires several investigative phases before certifying a new treatment as safe and effective. The ultimate test is whether it produces the desired effect in people who have the disease for which treatment is being sought.

To do this, researchers design studies that must give solid information so that the FDA (as well as doctors and their patients) can be confident the treatment is safe and effective. They must also know what to expect in terms of possible side effects.

Not all trials deal with experimental drugs or devices. Some studies employ treatments that have already been proven but are nonetheless useful because they compare one form of therapy with another to see whether one is better.

For example, several medications with different mechanisms have been prescribed for years to patients with congestive heart failure. As understanding of drugs and their effect on patients with heart failure increases, it's become important to determine how certain combinations compare to others.

Another example of these types of studies compares coronary angioplasty to coronary artery bypass surgery in patients with obstructive coronary artery disease and angina. Both these techniques have been used for at least two decades and yet debate continues over which is more effective than the other in certain situations.

### Participating in a trial

Someone must be among the first to take new medications or use new medical devices, once preliminary tests show reason to believe they might be effective. People willing to be these early recipients participate in a clinical study.

Why would anyone participate in a clinical study? After all, you can't be sure the experimental treatment is effective (that's why it's being studied). Furthermore, researchers design many studies so that some participants may not even get the experimental treatment. Instead, they might actually receive a placebo (inactive substance).

There may be several reasons why you'd choose to be a "study subject." For one, some people get tremendous satisfaction from helping advance medical science. These people believe, "If it can help someone else in the future, I'd like to get involved."

Moreover, some illnesses currently have no effective treatments; a study may offer hope that new medication will be effective and directly help the patient.

Likewise, some patients simply may not benefit from already available medications, and they want to see if a new variety of medication or treatment may possibly help them. Other study participants may feel financial motivation; most clinical studies provide the study medication, many tests, and examinations at no charge (consequently, the patient can receive closely monitored medical care at minimal cost).

Scientists conducting the research monitor the clinical studies, as does a special committee called an institutional review board (IRB) that's composed of scientists from many fields and community representatives. This committee exists by law, and no experiment involving humans can be done without its approval. The IRB is an advocate for human research subjects.

## Defining the study

Doctors, patients, new product manufacturers, and the FDA must all cooperate in assessing the effects of any new treatment. They do this in part by gathering several types of information to determine whether a new treatment is effective.

First, the types of study participants must be carefully defined, specifying "inclusion" and "exclusion" criteria. For example, participants in a study of a congestive heart failure medication might be eligible only if their ejection fraction is less than 35 percent. This criterion assures that only people with diminished pumping function are included.

Even if you have the disease being studied, you might be excluded if you have another major illness. This criterion assures that other diseases won't interfere with the medication's evaluation. For example, researchers would learn little about a congestive heart failure medication's effect in a study participant whose symptoms come mainly from cancer or who may not survive to the study's end.

Second, each study must have methods to measure or determine whether the treatment alters the illness. A new treatment for congestive heart failure would need to assess the medication's effect on the heart's pumping function, on the ability of participants to exert themselves, or on the patients' life span.

Finally, researchers must conduct some type of comparison to determine whether the illness progresses differently with medication than without. Such comparisons can take several forms: One compares groups who receive the treatment with those who don't. Here, random individuals either receive or don't receive the treatment; neither the doctor nor manufacturer can determine who gets the treatment.

Another form of comparison study contrasts how patients fare while they receive treatment with how they do when they're not. In this type of study, participants "cross over" from treatment to nontreatment (or vice versa) after a time. The order of the treatment-nontreatment sequence generally is randomly determined, again to avoid introducing any unintentional bias into the results.

Most comparison forms of study use a "placebo-controlled" format. In this type, patients who don't receive the actual medication (because they were randomized to "control") instead receive an inactive "medication" that looks just like the real thing but contains only sugar or some other inactive ingredient.

Commonly, studies are "double-blind," which means that neither doctor nor patient knows who receives the active medication or the placebo (at least until the study's finished, and then the code identifying the medication is revealed).

In a "randomized, double-blind, placebo-controlled" study, investigators who don't have access to the code analyze the results. The code is revealed only after they finalize the results. (Many studies have a "data monitoring and safety committee" that knows the results as they become available from the investigators. If this monitoring committee sees that one group is doing far worse than the other, they may stop the study early to prevent further risk for members of the group experiencing poor results.) Some studies are "single-blind" (only patients don't know what they receive).

Placebo-control and "blinding" further assure that any effects observed in the actively treated patients really come from the medication and not the biases of the researchers or the subjects. There's a well-recognized tendency for some people who think they're receiving treatment to improve (the "placebo effect"), both subjectively in terms of symptoms and also, surprisingly, in ways you'd think they have no control over. In a sense, placebo-controlled studies provide a "true" assessment of a medication's actual effects.

Doctors and patients are sometimes reluctant to participate in studies in which the patient (who, after all, has a problem that needs treatment) might receive a placebo. If you received the placebo, wouldn't you be deprived of a new and effective form of treatment?

In fact, no one knows, which is the whole point of the study. Reread the section in Chapter 17 (page 343), "Should all palpitations be treated?"and decide whether the treated or "untreated" group was at an advantage. Furthermore, in most studies, conventional treatment continues, even in the control group, so patients aren't deprived of the best known treatment available.

## Use caution

If you have the opportunity to participate in a study, read the consent form carefully. Know what's expected of you and what you can anticipate from participating in the study.

Key elements of the consent form include the study's description and why it's being done, the sequence of events and what tests will occur, alternative noninvestigational treatments that are available, risks of participating in the study, whether there are associated costs, what will be done if complications occur, and whom to contact about questions you may have.

You must sign the consent form to participate, but it's not a contract. The consent form should specify that you can withdraw from the study with no penalty whatsoever.

Once a study is completed, the FDA reviews the data so it can determine whether the treatment should be approved, studied further, or rejected. Often the data are also published in a medical journal. Articles in reputable medical journals are carefully reviewed for accuracy and sound reasoning by other doctors and scientists ("peer review"). This provides further assurance that the information is reliable.

## New research

One of the most exciting areas of research is gene therapy in stimulating the growth of new blood vessels to and from the heart. These new vessels would help restore blood flow to the hearts of people whose arteries were obstructed by cholesterol-rich plaques.

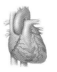

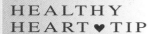

HEALTHY
HEART ♥ TIP

It's hoped that gene therapy could become an addition to other therapies for heart disease which now include low saturated fat diets, exercise, smoking cessation and, in some patients, cholesterol-lowering drugs and procedures such as bypass surgery and angioplasty.

Several studies have dealt with growth factors (FGF-1 and VEGF), which have the ability to cause new blood vessels to grow in the heart. It's possible that these growth factors can be directly injected into the heart muscle or, in the future, by delivery from a stent that has been implanted into the blocked coronary artery.

Some researchers have attached the growth factor protein to a virus that causes the common cold, and this speeds the protein's entry into the heart tissue cells. This is a very exciting area of research, but it's important to emphasize that this is still a glimpse into a very experimental future.

Some "new" medications or treatments gain publicity without ever being subjected to carefully designed studies or peer-reviewed publication. One example is chelation therapy (using agents that bind to calcium and, according to proponents, open blood vessels obstructed by atherosclerosis). Almost invariably, these treatments must be regarded skeptically since they are at best unproven. The claims regarding the treatment are almost exclusively made by those who stand to profit directly from its use.

Those claiming that a treatment provides any benefit, even small, should prove it by careful testing and critical review.

*There are many risk factors associated with heart disease, but perhaps the most perplexing is your own family history. People whose parents and grandparents experienced early heart attacks or death are more genetically predisposed to heart disease themselves.*

*That doesn't mean you're powerless when it comes to your future. Besides family history, you can do much to improve your chances for a long and healthy life. Choose a diet low in saturated fat and cholesterol, don't smoke, exercise regularly, have your blood fats checked and discuss with your doctor whether you need a cholesterol-lowering medication.*

# Chapter

# 22 Women and heart disease

Being male is one of the risk factors for heart disease. So it's not surprising that many women worry about heart disease developing in their husbands, fathers, and other men in their lives. But heart disease is also the number one killer of women. In fact, more than 500,000 women annually die from some form of heart and blood vessel disease (twice the number of deaths from all forms of cancer).

Heart attack alone kills 240,000 women each year, which represents nearly half the total heart attack deaths in the United States. Despite the legitimate concern about breast cancer in women, for example, this disease kills about 42,800 women, or only one-sixth the number of women who annually die of heart attack. Heart disease simply doesn't care about their sex.

The dangerous myth that heart disease affects only men can cause women to close their eyes to reducing risk factors for heart disease. Furthermore, women may ignore symptoms that should send them for urgent medical evaluation. Women who have heart attacks are twice as likely to die as men are within the first few weeks, but women (or their doctors) may tend to misinterpret or discount symptoms suggesting heart attack.

## Have women been undertreated?

Women themselves often downplay or underestimate the severity of heart disease symptoms or attribute them to something else. Evidence shows that when women do enter the medical system, they may be managed less aggressively than men.

Yet it's true that doctors are less likely to find coronary artery obstruction in women with chest pain than in men complaining of similar symptoms. But once they've diagnosed coronary artery disease, women have a prognosis that's similar to men's.

### Diagnosis

Women undergo fewer diagnostic procedures, perhaps because some exams are less accurate in women. For example, some types of exercise tests may indicate more "false-positive" results in women, and doctors may not want to use a test unless it has a high degree of accuracy. However, some diagnostic analyses are quite precise in women, so this reluctance may be unwarranted. In addition, coronary angiography is safe and accurate for women.

## Treatment

There seem to be differences in how some types of heart disease treatments are employed on men and women. For example, figures show that four times as many men as women undergo coronary artery bypass operation. Some of this variance may be more ageism than sex bias. Since women tend to be older when they have heart attacks, they may be viewed as "too old" to endure certain procedures.

## Treatment results

Women also tend to have worse outcomes than men after procedures such as coronary artery bypass operation or balloon angioplasty. Again, women are usually older and sicker when the procedures are done. In addition, women often have smaller coronary arteries, making the procedures more difficult to perform.

But women also seem to have poor post-heart-attack survival rates, even when they're treated with the most effective clot-dissolving medications, exactly like men. Yet the perception remains that heart disease doesn't affect women. Why don't women take this deadly disease more seriously?

For one thing, women aren't affected by heart disease as early as men. Heart disease usually shows up in women almost 10 years later than in men. However, after age 50, it's the leading cause of death in women; by age 65, women's risk almost equals that of men. One in three women over 65 has some form of heart disease.

In addition, most heart disease studies have used men as subjects. For example, the Physicians' Health Study tested only male physicians to find out if aspirin could help decrease heart attack risk in men. The Multiple Risk Factor Intervention Trial, which provided information about risk factors, also studied only men. No one knows whether findings that apply to men pertain equally to women.

The Framingham Study, a large ongoing examination of Framingham, Massachusetts, residents, includes 2,873 women in its study population, and it's provided valuable information concerning the prevalence of and risk factors for heart disease in both men and women. However, many unanswered questions exist, and more research is essential.

So far, nearly all effective therapies for treating heart attack and angina pectoris have also been beneficial in women. However, many studies have shown that women and the elderly are less likely to receive therapies such as aspirin, beta-blockers and coronary revascularization. Fortunately, the National Institutes of Health—the government agency that funds many important studies—has encouraged additional research involving women.

Until results show whether and how prevention, diagnosis, and treatment of heart disease differ for men and women, women should use the information available today to assess their individual risks with their doctors. Guided by this information, you and your doctor can determine the best way to reduce your chances of heart disease.

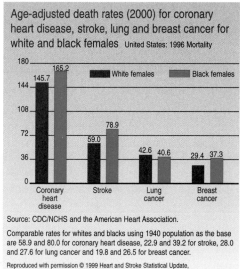

Age-adjusted death rates (2000) for coronary heart disease, stroke, lung and breast cancer for white and black females  United States: 1996 Mortality

Source: CDC/NCHS and the American Heart Association.

Comparable rates for whites and blacks using 1940 population as the base are 58.9 and 80.0 for coronary heart disease, 22.9 and 39.2 for stroke, 28.0 and 27.6 for lung cancer and 19.8 and 26.5 for breast cancer.

Reproduced with permission © 1999 Heart and Stroke Statistical Update, 1998 Copyright American Heart Association.

# Factors that eliminate women's "sex protection"

Although heart disease develops later in women than men, women aren't immune to the ways smoking, diabetes, high blood pressure, obesity, high blood cholesterol level, lack of exercise, and stress influence heart disease. Of course, some risk factors are worse than others. In fact, smoking and diabetes may remove women's "sex protection" altogether.

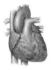

## HEALTHY HEART ♥ TIP

*Pop a daily multivitamin and improve your health. Eat the real thing and benefit even more.*

*One of the advantages of getting vitamins through your food comes from soluble fiber, which regulates your body's production and elimination of cholesterol. Include foods with high levels of soluble fiber, such as apples, lentils, dried beans, peas, barley, citrus fruits, and oats, in your diet every day.*

## Smoking

For women, smoking is the greatest risk factor for heart attack. Women who smoke have 2 to 6 times the risk of heart attack as women who don't smoke. If you smoke and have a heart attack, you will probably die from it.

Women smokers are also 2 to 4 times as likely to die suddenly of heart disease. Smoking seems to promote a more dangerous distribution of body fat. Combining smoking with birth control pills dramatically increases your heart attack risk. Smokers also generally have lower levels of protective HDL cholesterol than nonsmokers.

These are frightening statistics, especially when you consider that teenage girls are the only population group increasing its cigarette use. On the positive side, a woman who quits smoking reduces her risk until it's almost as low as a nonsmoker's within 2 or 3 years.

## Diabetes

Diabetes mellitus occurs when too much sugar (called glucose) remains in the blood stream rather than being transferred into cells throughout the body. Both type I and type II diabetes are associated with a higher risk of cardiovascular disease.

Women with diabetes have cardiovascular disease rates that are 2 to 5 times higher than women without diabetes. These women also experience a higher incidence of "silent or clinically unrecognized" heart attacks than men. This may be because more women than men have diabetes, which is a risk factor for silent myocardial infarction.

Moreover, silent heart attacks occur more frequently in the elderly, an age group in which women claim a majority. For men, diabetes isn't such a strong predictor of heart-related complications.

# Special issues concerning women

Research has started to reveal how factors such as age, menopause, estrogen replacement therapy, and birth control pills affect your risk of heart disease. Some studies suggest that certain risk factors such as blood cholesterol levels may have different implications for women than for men.

## Age and menopause

One major difference between men and women is the age at which their heart disease risk starts to climb. Women's chances for heart disease remain relatively low compared with men's until menopause, when the risk of heart attack increases gradually until it nearly equals men's risk by age 65.

The reasons for this mounting risk are complex and not entirely understood. The female hormone estrogen may exert a protective effect because estrogen tends to raise HDL ("good") cholesterol level and lower LDL ("bad") cholesterol. Even if a woman's total cholesterol level is relatively high, she probably has a higher level of the protective HDL than a man with a similar total cholesterol level. However, after menopause, estrogen production drops drastically and its potentially beneficial effects disappear.

## Estrogen replacement therapy

If estrogen provides some heart disease protection for younger women, why not reverse the sharp decrease in estrogen after menopause? After all, most women can expect to spend at least one-third of their lives after menstruation ceases.

Declining estrogen levels at menopause adversely affect cardiac risk factors (including increased LDL cholesterol and decreased HDL cholesterol) in a number of ways. These changes are at least partially responsible for the observed acceleration of cardiovascular events after menopause.

Estrogen replacement therapy was first used in the 1960s to relieve distressing symptoms such as hot flashes and vaginal dryness that accompany menopause in some women. Studies showed that supplemental estrogen also seems to protect women against heart disease, but high doses increased the risk of endometrial cancer (in the lining of the uterus). Adding the hormone progestin seems to cancel that risk, and it may even protect against endometrial cancer. Unfortunately, it may also partly cancel estrogen's protective advantage against heart disease.

The benefits of estrogen alone or combined with progestational agents may be due to a number of direct and indirect effects on the blood vessels, the serum cholesterol, and other lipid factors, in addition to favorable influences on blood clotting. All of these may provide a plausible explanation for the biologic actions of estrogen but at present, some of these data remain theoretical.

An important 1998 study called HERS was the first randomized, double-blind, placebo-controlled trial of estrogens in 2,763 postmenopausal women who were younger than 80 years with definite coronary artery disease. These patients received either a continuous, combined estrogen and medroxyprogesterone or a placebo. After 4.1 years, the results were disappointing because the combination hormone didn't reduce cardiovascular events, as researchers had expected on the basis of previous, smaller studies.

The unanticipated results of the HERS trial further complicated this already tough issue. The results of this trial may not apply to other patient populations, such as women with no coronary heart disease or those with a prior hysterectomy, and it may achieve different results with other formulations for hormone replacement,

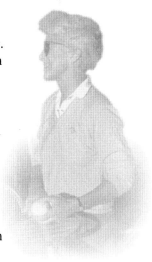

such as estrogen alone or the cyclic use of estrogen and progestin. But for now, this trial suggests that hormone replacement shouldn't be recommended to women with coronary heart disease only to protect the heart.

There are many other reasons why hormone replacement therapy may be prescribed for women. Some researchers say that heart disease risk can be reduced by more than 30 percent in postmenopausal women who take replacement estrogen. This benefit seems to be partly due to increased HDL levels. Estrogen delivered by skin patches (transdermally), however, bypasses the liver and may not improve HDL levels as much.

One study of women between 40 and 59 years in Rochester, Minnesota, suggested that using estrogen could reduce heart disease. However, estrogen couldn't counterbalance the bad effects from smoking.

There is information suggesting that estrogen replacement therapy may reduce heart disease in women, but the evidence is not conclusive. Ongoing studies that pay attention to age, general health and risk factors may clarify this question in years ahead.

The American Heart Association suggests estrogen replacement therapy may not be necessary for women with no menopausal symptoms. Women with a personal or family history of uterine or breast cancer may want to avoid it. However, if you have had your ovaries removed, or have experienced menopause before age 35, estrogen replacement therapy should be considered for its benefit on bone density, general health and, possibly, your heart.

In view of the possible risks of using estrogen replacement therapy, you should discuss your individual situation with your doctor, taking into account your family history and risk factors for heart disease, cancer, and fracture due to osteoporosis.

## Birth control pills

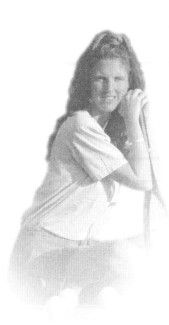

In contrast to the possible benefit of postmenopausal estrogen replacement therapy, using estrogen in birth control pills during the reproductive years may actually increase cardiovascular risk. Earlier studies in women using high-dose oral contraceptives boosted heart attack risk as much as 3 or 4 times over women not taking them—although at that age, the overall risk of heart attack remains very small. Studies using the current formulations of birth control pills, however, haven't shown any significant rise in heart attack risk.

Birth control pills may slightly elevate blood cholesterol level, blood pressure, and blood sugar level in some women. After starting oral contraceptive therapy, you should have your blood pressure monitored; if you experience a large increase in blood pressure, resolve it promptly by discontinuing the oral contraceptives.

Birth control pills also may lead to blood clots, although the risk of deep-vein thrombosis (blood clots in the lower limbs) rises only slightly. The absolute risk of a pulmonary embolism (blood clot to the lungs) or deep-vein thrombosis is very low in premenopausal women, and must be weighed against pregnancy-associated risks. You're 3 times more likely to experience a thromboembolic event if you're pregnant than if you're taking oral contraceptives.

Estrogen levels in birth control pills have declined, which probably reduces risk substantially. Thus, the Food and Drug Administration has recommended that birth control pills can be used safely by women, even women older than 40, if they are otherwise healthy and don't smoke. Simultaneous risk factors tend to multiply, however, which means that concurrent use of birth control pills and smoking boosts the risk of heart attack as much as 39 times, compared with the risk in those who don't smoke or take oral contraceptives.

Overall, oral contraceptives are safe and effective, and have low adverse effects in young, nonsmoking women.

## Blood lipids

Total blood cholesterol is a risk factor for coronary artery disease in women as well as in men. Women whose total cholesterol rises above 265 mg/dL have more than twice the risk for developing coronary artery disease as women with a level below 205 mg/dL. Although the association between coronary artery disease and total cholesterol is significant, women are even more susceptible to the risks of having a low HDL ("good") cholesterol level.

Women's cardiovascular health also seems to be more influenced by triglyceride level than men's. Women with triglycerides higher than 190 mg/dL have a greater risk, whereas men don't appear to increase their chances until triglycerides reach 400 mg/dL.

Women with heart disease should be treated as aggressively as men to lower their LDL cholesterol to below 100 mg/dL. While fewer studies have been performed regarding the benefits of lowering cholesterol in women without coronary disease, studies that have been reported suggest that women will benefit to the same extent as men.

## Body size and type

Women tend to be smaller than men and, in turn, their hearts and coronary arteries are smaller. Some experts believe that smaller coronary arteries can become blocked by atherosclerosis more easily than larger arteries. In fact, some studies suggest that men and women of similar size have similar risks.

Smaller size makes procedures such as balloon angioplasty more difficult in women. They suffer more complications and have a lower success rate with these procedures, although newer, appropriately sized equipment diminishes this problem.

Although women tend to have a higher percentage of body fat than men, the fat usually is distributed differently. Many men are shaped like apples, with fat around the waist, while many women resemble pears, with fat around the hips. However, a woman may be apple-shaped, and this pattern of fat distribution often accompanies a higher risk of coronary artery disease.

Men and women alike should take steps to reduce their risk factors for coronary artery disease. In fact, developing a heart-healthy lifestyle should begin at a young age. Both sexes can play a role in preventing heart disease in future generations.

# Pregnancy and heart disease

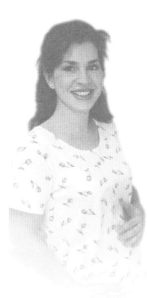

Heart disease in pregnant women requires careful medical management, but consequences have changed substantially. Women with any type of heart disease once were told they shouldn't become pregnant. During the past 50 years, however, doctors have gained a better understanding of changes that occur in a woman's body during pregnancy—especially to her cardiovascular system. Now, many women with heart disease can deliver healthy babies.

Pregnancy puts an extra burden on your heart. Your blood volume increases up to 50 percent by the 32nd week of pregnancy. You therefore have 6 to 8 liters (slightly more than 6 to 8 quarts) more body fluid than before you were pregnant. Your heart has to pump all that extra fluid to your body and your growing baby. To handle this increased load, your heart beats faster and also pumps out more blood with each contraction.

Different kinds of heart disease have different effects on your heart's ability to handle the stresses of pregnancy, labor, and delivery. Therefore, if you have heart disease, you should talk to your doctor before you become pregnant so that you both can evaluate your individual situation.

Most women with heart disease can have a successful pregnancy, especially under the care of both an obstetrician and a cardiologist. But some heart problems (such as cyanotic congenital heart disease, pulmonary hypertension, and severe aortic stenosis) pose a high risk to both mother and fetus. Women with these problems are still advised to avoid pregnancy, unless the problem can be corrected first.

In prenatal counseling, your doctor may discuss possible physical risks for you and your baby during pregnancy, as well as the potential for passing on any congenital heart problems to your child. The rate of congenital heart disease is about 4 to 5 percent in children of women with significant congenital heart disease, but only 1 percent in the general population. In some conditions, the chances of passing along a defect rise as high as 50 percent.

Although necessary for the mother, medication for various heart conditions may pose a potential risk for your baby. Discuss your medication options thoroughly with your doctor before you get pregnant.

Once you're pregnant, your doctor will monitor your fetus's development and the pregnancy's effect on your heart. Your doctor may tell you to cut back on your activities and take frequent breaks for 20 to 30 minutes in bed to give your heart a chance to rest. You should rest on your left side so your uterus doesn't compress your inferior vena cava, the main vein in the lower part of your body that returns blood to the heart.

Other adjustments may include restricting salt in your diet and avoiding hot baths or long hot showers, which may dilate the blood vessels in your arms and legs. Dilated blood vessels are your body's response to hot temperatures, but they divert blood flow from the fetus. It's critical to have early prenatal care and ready access to a high-risk pregnancy center if you experience any problems.

# Rehabilitation

I f you've had a heart attack or a heart operation, you probably have many questions. You most likely want to do everything possible to enhance your recovery. Cardiac rehabilitation helps people who've had a heart attack or heart operation to lead active, productive lives—mentally, physically, and socially.

## Getting with the program

A heart attack or other heart condition doesn't have to leave you weak, anxious, or withdrawn. Each year more than 100,000 people participate in cardiac rehabilitation programs. Going through the rehabilitation process can help restore your strength and vigor and give you the confidence to resume an active life. Many people come out of cardiac rehabilitation feeling healthier and happier than they did before their cardiac event.

Most people with heart disease can benefit from some or all aspects of rehabilitation. This includes those who've had heart attacks, heart operation (including heart transplantation), and percutaneous transluminal coronary angioplasty (PTCA, balloon dilatation), as well as people with angina pectoris, silent ischemia, cardiomyopathy, or valvular heart disease.

Because individual circumstances vary, rehabilitation programs must be tailored to each individual. What's appropriate for one person may not be right for another. For example, you may have experienced a mild heart attack that's left you more psychologically than physically disabled. Or maybe you've had an extensive bypass operation that requires a longer physical recovery. Your doctor's recommendations are crucial in making decisions about your rehabilitation goals.

Recovery from a heart attack or other cardiac event may require several rehabilitation strategies. A diverse group of professionals will help you, bringing together the expertise you need to answer questions about your heart condition and overall health, medications, diet, exercise, and sexual activity, especially during the early stages of your rehabilitation. Program components include supervised exercise, education, and counseling about controlling your risk factors for heart disease.

## Members of the cardiac rehabilitation team

| | |
|---|---|
| Personal doctor | Manages your general medical care |
| Cardiologist | Provides specialized management of your cardiovascular problem: diagnosis, medical prescriptions, treatment procedures, coordination of heart-related care |
| Surgeon | Performs operation (if necessary), provides specialized care after surgical procedures |
| Nursing staff | Provides your daily care in hospital, assists with daily activities, administers medications, instructs, monitors |
| Cardiac rehabilitation coordinator | Organizes various rehabilitation efforts, leads team discussions about your specific goals and outcomes |
| Physiatrist | Oversees physical rehabilitation, provides therapy prescriptions and medical prescriptions during hospitalization |
| Physical therapist | Instructs and assists you in activities to regain and maintain physical and cardiovascular fitness during hospitalization |
| Occupational therapist | Instructs and assists you in adjusting to daily life and compensating for any limitations you may have |
| Psychiatrist | Provides specialized management of significant emotional diff~culties that may arise, discussion, prescriptions for appropriate medications if needed |
| Psychologist | Provides ongoing counseling and evaluation of emotional or psychological problems when necessary |
| Exercise physiologist | Analyzes your body's exercise capabilities or limitations, makes recommendations for improving or adapting function of heart and body during outpatient rehabilitation |
| Outpatient cardiac rehabilitation nurse | Oversees ongoing rehabilitation efforts after hospitalization, monitors progress, confers with cardiologist and exercise physiologist |
| Exercise specialist | Teaches specific exercises and conducts exercise sessions with patients individually or in groups |
| Registered dietitian | Analyzes nutritional needs, develops and instructs you in food selection and preparation to meet goals of reducing cholesterol level and losing weigh |
| Chaplain | Provides support for your spiritual needs in hospital |
| Pharmacist | Reviews concerns about medications, such as interactions and side effects |
| Social worker | Assists and oversees special needs such as arranging for nursing facilities or financial assistance options if needed |
| Smoking cessation counselor | Makes recommendations and provides support for stopping smoking if needed |

A rehabilitation team helps you:

- Adjust physically and emotionally to your situation
- Understand your condition
- Learn ways to reduce your symptoms or limitations
- Improve your capacity for physical exercise
- Optimize a heart-healthy lifestyle to reduce cardiovascular risk factors and the chance of further problems

Rehabilitation begins as soon as you're medically stable after the cardiac event. Individual and group discussion and counseling sessions help you adapt psychologically to your illness. The sessions also provide information on diet, risk factors, medications and physical activity, and address any concerns you may have.

Rehabilitation efforts focus on creating an action plan that meets your individual needs. This book cannot provide recommendations that meet all of your specific objectives, but it's useful for describing how a general plan might work.

## The rehabilitation plan

Programs generally involve a minimum of 6 months of rehabilitation, divided into 4 phases: hospitalization, early recovery, late recovery, and maintenance.

### Phase 1: Hospitalization

This phase usually continues throughout hospitalization after your heart attack, operation, or other illness. Consequently, it doesn't last long.

During your hospitalization, you begin nonstrenuous activities such as sitting up in bed and simple range-of-motion exercises. Initially, the range-of-motion exercises are passive, which means the therapist will move your limbs for you, but you quickly progress to active exercises. With these activities, you want to maintain muscle tone and joint flexibility, even though you're restricted in overall activity.

You then progress to walking and limited stair climbing. Without such efforts, you can lose up to 15 percent of muscle strength in as little as 1 week in the hospital.

### Gaining momentum

The physical activity program in the hospital follows a step-by-step progression. You usually advance 1 step, or activity level, each day. The following schedule follows a 6-day plan, but your doctor may adjust the timing depending on your condition.

**Day 1 morning**

Remain in bed, except to use the bedside commode (avoid straining)

You may brush your teeth or dentures; the nurse will assist you as necessary

You may wash your face and hands, but the nurse will help you with your sponge bath

You may feed yourself, with your elbows supported on the tray table; the nurse will set up your tray

A physical therapist will exercise your arms and legs for you

You will need adequate rest; therefore, it will be important for you to observe the rest period

**Day 1 afternoon**

You may sit in the chair 15 to 30 minutes, depending on your tolerance

Your educational program begins

**Day 2 morning**

You may sit in the chair up to 60 minutes

You may divide your time in the chair as you choose

You may begin to exercise with the assistance of a physical therapist

**Day 2 afternoon**

You may sit in the chair up to 90 minutes

**Day 3 morning**

You may sit in the chair up to 2 hours; this period will include class time

You may walk in your room with professional assistance

You may have bathroom privileges and take a wheelchair shower

You may attend classes and discussion groups

**Day 3 afternoon**

You may walk around the nurses' station with professional supervision

You may sit in the chair as much as you like and can tolerate

**Day 4**

You may be up in your room and walk around the nurses' station as much as you like

You are encouraged to dress in street clothes

You may take a standing shower with a nurse's assistance

**Day 5**

You may continue walking around the nurses' station as much as you like

You may climb stairs with professional assistance

**Day 6**

Your home-going instructions will be finalized

Recent guidelines have been modified to accommodate shorter stays in the hospital, which naturally compresses the rehabilitation program. Activities for a 3- to 4-day hospitalization period, as opposed to a 6-day or longer stay, would be at the discretion of your nurse caring or physician team. Patients scheduled for a shorter hospitalization can usually leave the Coronary Care Unit (CCU) in less than 24 hours.

## Phase 2: Early recovery

The next 2- to 12-week phase of your rehabilitation begins when you go home from the hospital. During this time, you gradually assume self-care, increase your general activity level under supervision, and, instead of the physical therapist moving your arms and legs, you use your own strength to keep your limbs and joints limber. Your doctor may suggest home exercises that include walking, stationary cycling, and gentle calisthenics during the first few days.

After you leave the hospital, you may be advised to participate in medically supervised exercise at your local hospital or cardiac rehabilitation center. These programs generally encourage aerobic exercise and some muscle strengthening at your individually tolerated level, usually determined with an exercise test.

This phase of rehabilitation also continues to emphasize health and nutrition education and psychological counseling and support.

### Gradually increasing physical activity

If you've had a heart attack, a typical plan for your post-hospital activity progression may proceed as follows:

**Week 1**

Any light activity that can be done while sitting

Walking slowly for about 10 minutes on a level surface once or twice a day or using a stationary cycle with minimal resistance

Light housework such as dishes, cooking, dusting, or sweeping with a broom

Personal hygiene such as shaving, showering, and dressing

**Week 2**

Social activity such as playing cards at home, visiting neighbors, or riding in the car

Walking at a relaxed pace for about 20 minutes on a level surface once or twice a day or riding a stationary cycle with slight resistance

Housework such as making beds, ironing, minor appliance repair, bench work, or supervising yard work

Resume sexual activity

**Week 3**

Driving with a backup motorist present

Housework such as vacuuming

Increase social activity such as movies, attendance at place of worship, and concerts

Walking at a moderate pace for about 30 minutes once or twice a day or continuing stationary cycling

Lifting a few (10 to 15) pounds

**HEALTHY HEART ♥ TIP**

*If your doctor told you to monitor your blood pressure at home, you'll need a measuring device with a sphygmomanometer and a stethoscope. The three types of measuring devices—mercury, aneroid and electronic or digital readout—have advantages and disadvantages.*

*A mercury sphygmomanometer is easy to read and doesn't require readjustment, but it can be bulky, and spilling the mercury would be hazardous. Aneroid equipment is inexpensive and portable, but it's fairly delicate and complicated. Electronic or digital readout equipment is easy to use and carry, but it's fragile and may require repair and readjustment.*

*Remember that home blood pressure measurement is not a substitute for periodic evaluation by your doctor. But the maintenance of a log of home blood pressure recordings may be very useful in helping your physician decide whether your blood pressure is controlled or not.*

**Week 4**

Driving alone

Light gardening

Pitch-and-putt golfing

Social group activities such as club meetings, parties, and dancing

Grocery shopping (no heavy lifting)

Walking or stationary cycling for 30 minutes, once or twice a day

Perhaps a return to work part time

During the next 2 to 4 weeks, you should do aerobic exercise (in addition to your usual daily activities) for up to 40 minutes at a moderate intensity. Doctors usually recommend exercising 5 to 7 times per week, with 3 or fewer of the sessions at the rehabilitation center. Recommendations will vary for each individual.

Ideally, you should exercise in a medically supervised environment for several weeks after leaving the hospital. In reality, however, many people don't have access to these programs and must exercise on their own. Nonetheless, get your doctor's opinion before beginning an exercise program after a cardiac event. Your rehabilitation team will tell you what symptoms to watch for, the type of exercise permitted, kinds of equipment you might need, the importance of warm-up and cool-down exercises, and proper techniques for pacing yourself during exercise.

This phase is also a good time to consider joining a community support group, such as a local "coronary club," to help you learn how to better manage your heart disease.

Near the end of this phase, your doctor evaluates your overall progress to determine your readiness to return to work and other activities. Follow-up visits to the rehabilitation center at several points, such as at 3, 6, and 9 months after you complete phase 2, helps ensure you continue with your good efforts.

Regarding driving and work restrictions, two general guidelines may help: wait 1 to 2 weeks before driving and 2 to 4 weeks before returning to work. Obviously these recommendations should be modified if work involves heavy lifting, high stress, or long work days. These schedules can be further adjusted to include activities such as home maintenance and retirement activities.

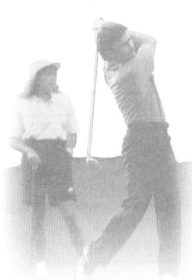

## Phase 3: Late recovery

You probably will have settled into your own comfortable exercise routine at home or at local exercise facilities about 6 to 12 weeks after your hospitalization. By this time you should also be making good progress with controlling your other cardiovascular risk factors such as smoking, high blood pressure, high blood cholesterol, obesity, or stress.

Diet is an important aspect of a rehabilitation program. A registered dietitian (R.D.) can suggest ways to reduce fat, cholesterol, and salt, if necessary, in your diet. Alcohol and caffeine may or may not be allowed, depending on your condition. Following the dietary recommendations also will help you lose weight, if that's one of your rehabilitation program's goals.

## Phase 4: Maintenance

This phase lasts indefinitely, and in some ways it's the most important part of your rehabilitation. At this point, you should regain your independence and work toward a lifelong commitment to the changes you started earlier in your recovery.

Periodic visits with your rehabilitation team can help reinforce your "heart-healthy" lifestyle. Some maintenance aspects include psychological adjustments, resuming normal sexual activity, and obtaining appropriate social support.

## Psychological adjustments

It's natural to react to a heart attack with panic and anxiety. You face the stress of the illness itself, unfamiliar surroundings, pain, discomfort, and the threat of death.

Even after your condition has stabilized and you've left the hospital, restrictions and alterations in previously routine activities can be stressful. Burdens may fall, at least temporarily, on your spouse or other family members. You may have to reverse certain responsibilities within a relationship.

After a cardiac event, you may have to take new medications and alter your lifestyle drastically, including diet changes that may affect other family members. And, of course, the thought of death or a recurrence or worsening of your condition lingers in the background.

## Emotional responses to cardiac events

Emotional responses to a heart attack often follow a common pattern. Your spouse and family often experience these same emotions on a delayed time schedule.

Denial that a heart attack has occurred, or that it may be serious, happens frequently at the first sign of a heart attack. In fact, denial may have been present long before the actual attack, as you may have continued smoking and eating a high-fat diet despite advice from many sources and in the face of fatigue, shortness of breath, and chest discomfort.

When you can no longer deny the problem, distress and fear usually follow. Anger prevails—sometimes taking the form of "why me?"—and is often directed at medical personnel, your spouse, and yourself.

Within days of the event, you may experience depression, probably related to the perceived loss of physical ability. Depression may be mild and brief or severe and long-lasting, depending on the disease's severity, your psychological makeup, and the type and amount of therapy provided. Some people become depressed only after they return home, while others seem to experience no feelings of depression at all.

## Looking for the silver lining

Believe it or not, most people eventually view a cardiac event as a positive experience in their lives. They commonly report physical improvements such as weight loss and enhanced fitness. They quit smoking and eat a more healthful diet. In addition, they identify social and psychological benefits, such as stronger relationships with their spouse and families, healthier self-image, better ability to deal with work pressures, and an awakened enthusiasm for the simple pleasures in life.

In some cases, people even see a message or spiritual meaning in the cardiac event, and this gives them a sense of spiritual enlightenment or helps to resolve long-standing conflicts or doubts.

People who effectively resolve crises such as a heart attack, and go on to experience personal growth, adopt one or more of these strategies:

- Remember that someone always has it worse than you do.

- Accept some responsibility for the event, then change that behavior to reduce the risk of future events.

- Look for the event's message or meaning and identify the changes or experiences that have been positive.

With new medications and medical procedures, in addition to changing your lifestyle and learning new ways to deal with stress, you can maintain or even improve the quality of your life after a heart attack or other cardiac event.

Depression may be characterized by complaints of fatigue, dizziness, nonspecific discomfort, sleep disturbance, weeping, and an inability to enjoy things, among a host of more subtle complaints. Depression is often under recognized, but individuals who experience prolonged melancholy may respond well to psychological counseling and antidepressant medication.

You may go through a bargaining stage where you try to get reassurance from your doctor to erase the event: "If I watch my diet closely, can I get the cholesterol out of my arteries and repair the damage to my heart?" Or from God: "Let me live through this and I'll start praying daily."

Most people go through a period of excessive concern in which they fear that every little muscle twitch and upset stomach signals another heart attack. Unfortunately, even if you fully comply with doctors' recommendations, total recovery and freedom from any future problems can't be guaranteed. Adapting to this stage requires a realistic perspective.

Many cardiac rehabilitation programs recognize the emotional stress of heart disease and begin to help patients and their families address these issues as soon as possible.

Outpatient programs, in addition to providing exercise classes, often include special group sessions where you can discuss stress related to the event itself and also the more general stress issues you encounter as you return to work and normal activities.

Psychological screening may help identify people who remain angry or depressed beyond a reasonable period. Many say that learning to better handle stress was the most important change they made after a cardiac event.

## Sexual activity after a heart attack

It's common for people to reduce the frequency of sexual activity for many months after a heart attack or other cardiac event. Sexual dysfunction also prevails. Although you may worry about the physical demands of sex after a cardiac event, research indicates this concern is unfounded.

Most people can return to sexual activity by the second week after a heart attack or heart operation. The demands sexual intercourse places on your heart approximate those of taking a brisk walk, scrubbing a floor, or climbing 1 or 2 flights of stairs. In a way, sexual activity parallels any other physical exertion: Your heart rate, breathing rate, and blood pressure increase, so you should proceed sensibly, with caution but without fear.

Just as with your other activities, proceed gradually with sex. As your confidence in the health of your heart grows, you'll resume your usual sexual patterns. It's important to talk to your partner to alleviate fears and concerns. Be reassured that it's normal for your needs to have changed temporarily.

Some medications, such as beta-blockers, can reduce sexual function, although this effect more often comes from depression or anxiety rather than the medication. Discuss reduced sexual desire with your doctor or the appropriate member of your rehabilitation team.

If you're taking long-acting nitrates for coronary artery disease, don't attempt to improve sexual performance with Viagra. This medication can cause a marked drop in blood pressure and is potentially dangerous.

You should also be very cautious about using Viagra if you have severe or difficult-to-control hypertension or congestive heart failure, especially if you're on diuretics. Although Viagra is an important medicine in treating patients with cardiovascular disease who have erectile dysfunction, it's particularly important to consult with your doctor before taking the drug.

Talk to your doctor about any other fears and concerns, too. If you experience chest pain, extreme shortness of breath, or irregular heartbeat during sexual activity, stop. Don't try to do too much too fast.

## Social support

When it comes to hastening psychological recovery after a cardiac event, you can't overemphasize the importance of social support from friends and family. Although professional counseling can work wonders, time heals most wounds, and people usually have a tendency to forget the most unpleasant parts of their ordeal. Those around you can help with this perspective.

## Ways to enhance your psychological recovery after a heart attack

### Understand your condition

A heart attack occurs when a lack of blood and oxygen permanently damages a part of your heart muscle. However, having one heart attack doesn't mean you will have another. Look at the heart attack as a warning that you should seriously consider changing your lifestyle to reduce your risk of future problems.

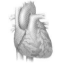

**HEALTHY HEART ♥ TIP**

*Your kids are couch potatoes, and you don't know what to do. Take heart: You can find plenty of ways to get them up and moving—and increase their chances of growing into heart-healthy adults.*

- *Lead by example, then invite your children to share in the exercise.*

- *Plan family outings and vacations that involve outdoor activities such as hiking, bicycling or swimming.*

- *Give them household chores that require physical exertion, such as mowing lawns, raking leaves, scrubbing floors and taking out the garbage.*

- *Observe what activities appeal to them, then find out about lessons and clubs.*

- *Stay involved in their physical education classes at school.*

## Stay active

Don't fall for the common myths that say people with heart disease shouldn't drive, exert themselves, or have sexual intercourse.

Follow your doctor's prescription for your individual level of activity. Exercise should be high on your list of things to do. Activity affirms that you're still alive and not an invalid.

You should rank these items at the top of your priority list: Don't smoke, don't eat too much, don't hurry, and don't worry.

## Get involved

Your local coronary club can be an excellent resource. Regularly exchanging information and experiences with other people who are also learning to live with heart disease can help you regain your confidence and sense of well-being.

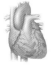

## HEALTHY HEART ♥ TIP

*It's easy to find out if you're exercising too hard. Just count your heart rate while engaging in vigorous activity. In general, your maximum heart rate should be approximately 220 minus your age. Here's what to aim for:*

### Target Heart Rate

| Age (Years) | Average rate (BPM)* | Maximum rate (BPM)* |
|---|---|---|
| 20 | 100-150 | 200 |
| 25 | 98-146 | 195 |
| 30 | 95-142 | 190 |
| 35 | 93-138 | 185 |
| 40 | 90-135 | 180 |
| 45 | 88-131 | 175 |
| 50 | 85-127 | 170 |
| 55 | 83-123 | 165 |
| 60 | 80-120 | 160 |
| 65 | 78-116 | 155 |
| 70 | 75-113 | 150 |

*BPM: beats per minute

## Can coronary artery disease go away?

The possibility that a medication can "dissolve" atherosclerotic blockages in arteries understandably generates great interest and hope. Likewise, people want to believe that removal or treatment of heart disease risk factors could reduce atherosclerotic blockages that are already present.

Medical studies do indicate ways to force atherosclerosis to "regress," or diminish its severity. Not unexpectedly, most of these methods involve improving the lipid profile by lowering cholesterol (especially LDL cholesterol) and triglycerides and by raising HDL cholesterol. Researchers have found evidence that improving cholesterol and triglyceride levels with medication, diet, or even (in rare cases) special blood-filtering equipment (somewhat like a kidney dialysis machine) can reverse atherosclerosis.

However, the observed reductions in artery narrowing after aggressive interventions have been small, and don't occur in everyone. For example, one study showed evidence of reduced narrowing in the coronary arteries of men with angina or previous heart attacks when they followed diet guidelines and used cholesterol-lowering medication.

But this effect occurred in only about one-third of the men, and the degree of improvement was small (the average coronary artery narrowing decreased by only a 1/10th of a millimeter after 3 years). Remarkably, the treated men did have considerably less coronary artery disease progression and fewer new symptoms of heart problems.

Other studies have made similar observations: Some (but not all) people at high risk for cardiovascular problems show evidence of less worsening of coronary blockages and, in some cases, slight improvement in blockages if they successfully amend their lipid profile with medications. Furthermore, this upgrading in the lipid profile results in fewer heart attacks or heart-related deaths and less need for coronary artery bypass or angioplasty.

Although evidence indicates that regression occurs in few people, the benefit of treating lipids may "stabilize" atherosclerotic plaques, which makes them less prone to rupture and consequently reduces cardiac events such as heart attacks and sudden death.

It's therefore essential to focus on controlling cholesterol and eliminating other risk factors even if the direct benefits on regression are small. Prevention remains the best strategy, even if it only slows the process that blocks the coronary arteries.

# Index

oxygen
   in blood, 6, 234-235, 262-263
   delivered during CPR, 288

**P**

pacemakers, A14, 332-336
   after heart attack, 317-318
   cautions, 335-336
   external, 295
   one-wire, 333
   rate-responsive, 334
   two-wire (dual-chamber), 333-334
palliative operations, 61
pallor, 40
palpitations, 38-39, 332. *See also*
   irregular heartbeats
   when not to treat, 343-344
papillary muscles, 11
paralysis, 41
paroxysmal nocturnal dyspnea, 32
paroxysmal supraventricular
   tachycardia, 113-114
patent ductus arteriosus, 62-63
pentoxifylline, 345, 371
percutaneous transluminal coronary
   angioplasty (PTCA), 318-320
perfusion scans, 249-250
pericardial constriction, A16, 134-135
pericardial effusion, A16, 133-134, 352
   diagnosis, 257
pericardiectomy, 353
pericardiocentesis, echo-guided, 259,
   352
pericarditis, A16, 133, 353
   after heart attack, 96
pericardium, A4, A5, A9, A16, 23, 257
peripheral vascular disease, 145
personality "type," 166
"phen fen," 177
phlebitis, 127-128
   and chronic venous insufficiency, 129
photoangioplasty, 322
physical examination, 226-231
phytochemicals, 188, 194
plaques (in arteries), 87, 313
platelets, 313
Plavix, 345
polyarteritis nodosa, 124
polyunsaturated fat, 166, 173
popliteal pulse, 228
positive inotropic medications, 297,
   367
positive thinking, 215
positron emission tomography (PET)
   scans, 279
potassium loss and diuretics, 300

pregnancy and heart disease, 384
presyncope (light-headedness), 37
prevention, 168-219
   effectiveness, 142
   exercise, 207-212
   functional foods, 188
   healthy diet, 172-182, 189-205
   managing stress, 212-217
   quitting smoking, 168-172
   vitamins and supplements, 184-187
primary angioplasty, 315
Prinzmetal's angina, 89, 90
prostheses (artificial devices)
   heart, 305
   left ventricular assist, 305
   valves, A8, 310
prothrombin time, 235-236, 299
psyllium, 188
pulmonary angiography, 263
pulmonary artery, A1, A2, A3, 18
pulmonary circulation, A3, 6
pulmonary edema, 34
   diagnosis, 246
pulmonary embolism, 128-129, 250,
   350
   diagnosis, 250, 263
pulmonary hypertension, 44, 131-132,
   350-351
   diagnosis, 257
pulmonary regurgitation, 84-85
pulmonary thromboendarterectomy,
   351
pulmonary valve, A1, A6, 11-12
pulmonary valve stenosis, 83-84
   balloon valvuloplasty, 308-309
pulmonary veins, A1, A2, A3
pulse
   anatomy of, 5
   brachial, 229
   carotid, 228
   counting during exercise, 210
   femoral, 228
   maximal, 19, 395
   normal, 8, 18, 99
   popliteal, 229
   radial, 228
   resting, 18, 19
   venous, 229
pulse volume recording, 273

**R**

radial arteries, 323
radial pulse, 228
radiofrequency catheter ablation, A13,
   111, 269, 342-343

radionuclide ventriculography, 248-249,
   252-253
rapid breathing, 33
Raynaud's phenomenon, 40, 125
   diagnosis, 274
reddish skin color (erythema), 40
rehabilitation, 385-395
   early recovery phase, 389-390
   hospitalization phase, 387-388
   late recovery phase, 390-391
   maintenance, 391
   social support, 393, 394
rejection of transplanted organs, 304
research studies, participating in,
   374-377
research trends, 218-219
restaurant meals, 204
resuscitation orders, 373-374
rheumatic fever, 72-73
   and endocarditis risk, 71
rhythm disorders. *See* arrhythmias
risk factors, 138-167
   age, 140-141, 379
   body mass index, 161
   diabetes, 163-164
   excess weight, 160-163
   heredity, 140
   high blood pressure, 147-153
   high cholesterol, 153-159
   interactions among, 139
   primary prevention, 142
   reducing risks, 168-219
   secondary prevention, 142
   sedentary lifestyle, 164-165
   sex, 141, 379, 381-382
   smoking, 144-147
   stress and personality, 166-167
rotational burr atherectomy, A11, 321

**S**

salt. *See* sodium intake
salt substitutes, 179
saphenous vein, 322
saturated fat, 166, 173
scleroderma, 57
sclerotherapy, 130
second opinions, 279
semilunar valves, 11-12
sestamibi (perfusion) scans, 249-250
sexual activity after heart attack,
   392-393
sheath, catheterization, 265, 319
shock, 41
   cardiogenic, after heart attack, 96
shock treatment. *See* cardioversion

*You want the latest health information. But who can you trust?*

A question of health?
Mayo Clinic books
are the answer.™

*Available wherever books are sold, or order online at www.mayohealth.org (Click on "Products")*

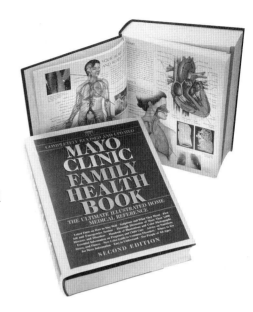

## Mayo Clinic Family Health Book—Second Edition

The health information you need at your fingertips! Over 1 million copies sold. It's the ultimate illustrated home medical reference, with detailed, current information on hundreds of medical conditions.

ISBN 0-688-14478-0, $42.50, 1,438 pages, hardcover, product #268140

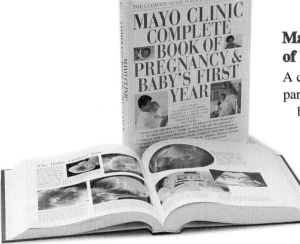

## Mayo Clinic Complete Book of Pregnancy & Baby's First Year

A comprehensive guide for expectant or experienced parents and grandparents, from pregnancy through the baby's first year of life. Offers reliable, easy-to-read information and advice.

ISBN 0-688-11761-9, $33.00, 750 pages, hardcover, product #268178

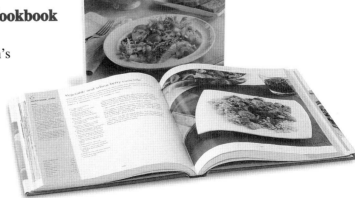

## The Mayo Clinic|Williams-Sonoma Cookbook

Eating well has never been easier—or tastier. Mayo Clinic has joined forces with the nation's leading cookware retailer, Williams-Sonoma, to offer the ultimate guide to preparing healthful appetizers, side dishes, entrees, and desserts.

ISBN 0-7370-0008-2, $29.95, 272 pages, hardcover, product #268300

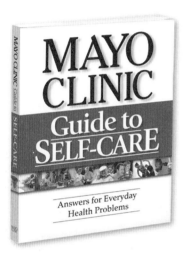
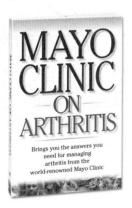
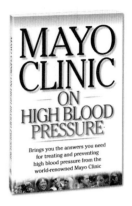
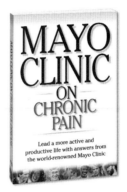
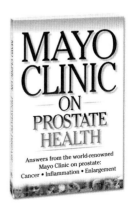